To Erica,

At the 2018 GRC.

So wonderful to talk

with you,

Dave Russ

ENGINEERING POLYMER SYSTEMS FOR IMPROVED DRUG DELIVERY

ENGINEERING POLYMER SYSTEMS FOR IMPROVED DRUG DELIVERY

Edited by

Rebecca A. Bader
David A. Putnam

WILEY

Library of Congress Cataloging-in-Publication Data:
Engineering polymer systems for improved drug delivery / edited by Rebecca A. Bader, David A. Putnam.
    pages cm
  Includes bibliographical references and index.
  ISBN 978-1-118-09847-9 (cloth)
  1. Polymeric drug delivery systems. 2. Polymeric drugs. 3. Polymers in medicine. 4. Drug delivery systems. I. Bader, Rebecca A., 1977- editor of compilation. II. Putnam, David A., 1966- editor of compilation.
  RS201.P65E54 2013
  615.1—dc23
                                                                                              2013016292

Printed in the United States of America.

10 9 8 7 6 5 4 3 2 1

CONTENTS

FOREWORD

The body is made up of tens of trillions of human cells and an even greater number of microorganisms, each of which impact health in ways that scientists, physicians, and engineers are still trying to fully comprehend. Overall, the amount of information encoded in each of these cells and their surroundings is staggering, leading to the organization of approximately 7 octillion atoms (a 7 followed by 27 zeros) into a well-oiled, living, breathing, and reproducing machine. Importantly, the myriad of cells in the body do not act in isolation, but rather in concert with one another, sometimes with subsecond precision and timing, forming a countless network of signals and interactions that is nothing short of awe-inspiring.

In contrast, the current state of medicine is somewhat less impressive. Even the most modern medicine is still administered in a way so as to expose a drug to all cells in the body indiscriminately, even though that drug's goal is to elicit a specific response from a specific cell type. In the few instances where this is not the case, any observed cell-specific localization could be completely accidental. Consequently, the total costs to the US Healthcare system associated with side effects from these kinds of drugs (including costs associated with deleterious effects from patients not properly taking these drugs) currently exceeds the amount of money spent on treating both cancer and heart disease combined. It may be surprising to hear that a solution to these problems was described four decades ago with the first demonstration of polymers for the controlled and localized release of biologic molecules. Using polymers that are extremely safe (some of which can completely disappear in the body following action), it was envisioned that it was not only possible to limit a drug's effects to a specific location or specific cell population, but also quite possible to achieve effects over extremely long durations of time, making the common, daily dosing of drugs obsolete. Yet, only a handful of these advanced drug delivery systems have ever been translated to clinical practice given a slower than anticipated learning curve in the understanding of the nature of polymeric delivery systems and the engineering of their behavior.

Most recently, however, there have been exciting advances in understanding and practice in the field of polymeric drug delivery systems so as to increase the effectiveness of new drugs while minimizing (or even completely eliminating) their toxicity and side effects. These advances are built on the foundations laid by the founders and luminaries in the field by the next generation of leaders, many of whom were personally trained by these founders and luminaries.

It is for this reason that I could not have been more excited to hear that Dr. Rebecca Bader and Dr. David Putnam (who are both outstanding teachers and well-respected scholars in the field) have taken on the task of bringing together an impressive team of these next generation leaders to contribute to the book that you are reading right now and to provide an overview of the state of the art in the field of polymeric drug delivery. Also, as expected, Dr. Bader and Dr. Putnam provide excellent historical and topical context in this work as well as a well-grounded understanding of the important current problems in the field. The following chapters (arranged by mode of administration) cover an extremely broad array of advances ranging from micro and nano particulate systems to implantable matrices, to rate controlling membranes, to advanced, stimuli responsive and affinity-based systems. Importantly, each of these chapters has been carefully composed by individuals who have each contributed to the modern understanding of the respective polymeric drug delivery systems. I am excited to have this extremely valuable resource on my bookshelf.

It is also important to mention that given the expected impacts that the information contained in this book will have on the field, I am sure that this volume could not have come at a better time. It is my opinion that we will soon pass a critical point in time where our understanding will lead to drug delivery systems that enable the scores of promising drugs that would have otherwise been discarded. It is also my strong belief that we are extremely close to this critical point. If that is true, the person reading this text right now may very well be one of the ones who will use this information to create the next generation of medical treatments that will improve the quality of life and the cost of healthcare for our children and our grandchildren. Now is indeed a very exciting time in the field, one that has the potential to redefine medicine forever.

STEVEN LITTLE

CHAIRMAN, DEPARTMENT OF CHEMICAL ENGINEERING UNIVERSITY OF PITTSBURGH

PREFACE

Pharmaceutical treatment of disease has evolved from "the botanical era," when herbal remedies were the mainstay, to the present "age of biologics," marked by the use of nucleic acid- and protein-based drugs to alter disease pathology. Although these exciting, new therapeutics offer the possibility of curing diseases that were previously thought to be incurable, a myriad of problems have arisen that have prevented translation to widespread clinical use. Of primary concern is the unwanted delivery of these compounds to normal, healthy tissue, rather than the disease site, which can result in unexpected and/or severe adverse side effects (see Fig. 1). For example, in 2006, TGN1412, a monoclonal antibody that activates T cells, caused multiple organ failure in all six human volunteers recruited for the Phase I clinical trial, despite proven preclinical safety and efficacy. The antibody was intended to target only regulatory T cells to suppress, rather than induce, inflammation, thereby providing an effective treatment for those who suffer from autoimmune diseases such as rheumatoid arthritis. However, TGN1412 instead is thought to have indiscriminately activated T cells throughout the body, leading to an abnormal immune response as well as destruction of healthy tissue [1].

In this example, the question remains as to whether this drug could have been formulated in such a way so as to have enhanced specificity and efficacy, thereby preventing the horrific outcome that was observed. The goal of *Engineering Polymer Systems for Improved Drug Delivery* is to provide an overview of how polymers can be used to control not only what the drug does to the body but also what the body does to the drug. In so doing, polymers provide the key to maximizing the potential of old and new therapeutics alike, including those that would previously be eliminated from consideration as nonviable drug candidates. The cooperation of pharmaceutical scientists and polymer engineers may mark the beginning of an era in which diseases can be treated with increased certainty of a positive outcome.

This book, intended for undergraduate or graduate student instruction, begins with the basics of drug delivery (Chapters 1 and 2), continues through injectable (Chapters 3–6), implantable (Chapters 7 and 8), and oral polymer-based drug delivery systems (Chapters 9–11), and concludes with advanced polymeric drug delivery techniques (Chapters 12 and 13). Each chapter is written so as to give a broad overview of a topic and is concluded with key points, worked problem(s), and homework problems. By taking this approach, we are hopeful that we will inspire the next generation of scientists to make meaningful contributions to the field of drug delivery.

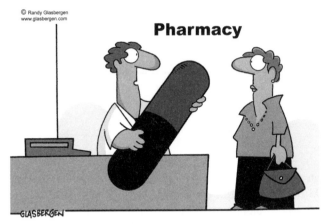

© Randy Glasbergen
www.glasbergen.com

Pharmacy

GLASBERGEN

**"Each capsule contains your medication,
plus a treatment for each of its side effects."**

Figure 1. The advent of new therapeutic treatments has been accompanied by an increase an adverse side effects. Our hope is that polymeric drug delivery can help eliminate some of these side effects.

We would like to thank all the authors for their valuable contributions. Special thanks are due to Patricia Wardwell for her help in organizing the chapters, obtaining permissions, and for providing assistance in general.

REBECCA A. BADER AND DAVID A. PUTNAM

REFERENCE

1. Attarwala H. TGN1412: from Discovery to Disaster. J Young Pharm 2010;2(3):332–6.

CONTRIBUTORS

Rebecca A. Bader Syracuse Biomaterials Institute, Syracuse University, Syracuse, NY, USA

Giuseppe Battaglia Department of Chemistry, University College London, London, UK

Danielle S.W. Benoit Department of Biomedical Engineering, University of Rochester, Rochester, NY, USA

James Blanchette Department of Biomedical Engineering, University of South Carolina, Columbia, SC, USA

Angela Carlson Department of Radiology, Case Western Reserve University, Cleveland, OH, USA

Colleen E. Clark Department of Chemical Engineering, Villanova University, Philadelphia, PA, USA

Noelle K. Comolli Department of Chemical Engineering, Villanova University, Philadelphia, PA, USA

Zhanwu Cui Department of Biomedical Engineering, University of Rochester, Rochester, NY, USA

James C. DiNunzio Pharmaceutics Division, College of Pharmacy, The University of Texas at Austin, Austin, TX, USA; Hoffmann-La Roche, Inc., Nutley, NJ, USA

Thomas D. Dziubla Department of Chemical and Materials Engineering, University of Kentucky, Lexington, KY, USA

Agata A. Exner Department of Radiology, Case Western Reserve University, Cleveland, OH, USA

Cristina Fante School of Pharmacy, University of Reading, Reading, UK

Andrew S. Fu Department of Biomedical Engineering, Case Western Reserve University, Cleveland, OH, USA

Francesca Greco School of Pharmacy, University of Reading, Reading, UK

Adrian S. Joseph Department of Biomedical Science, The University of Sheffield, Sheffield, UK

Justin M. Keen Pharmaceutics Division, College of Pharmacy, The University of Texas at Austin, Austin, TX, USA

David Mastropietro Department of Pharmaceutical Sciences, College of Pharmacy, Nova Southeastern University, Fort Lauderdale, FL, USA

James W. McGinity Pharmaceutics Division, College of Pharmacy, The University of Texas at Austin, Austin, TX, USA

Srinath Muppalaneni Department of Pharmaceutical Sciences, College of Pharmacy, Nova Southeastern University, Fort Lauderdale, FL, USA

Hossein Omidian Department of Pharmaceutical Sciences, College of Pharmacy, Nova Southeastern University, Fort Lauderdale, FL, USA

Nisa Patikarnmonthon Department of Biomedical Science, The University of Sheffield, Sheffield, UK

David A. Putnam Department of Biomedical Engineering, Cornell University, Ithaca, NY, USA

Horst A. von Recum Department of Biomedical Engineering, Case Western Reserve University, Cleveland, OH, USA

James D. Robertson Department of Biomedical Science, The University of Sheffield, Sheffield, UK

Gregory Russell-Jones Mentor Pharmaceutical Consulting Pty Ltd, Middle Cove, Australia

Matthew Skiles Department of Biomedical Engineering, University of South Carolina, Columbia, SC, USA

Luis Solorio Department of Radiology, Case Western Reserve University, Cleveland, OH, USA

Amy Van Hove Department of Biomedical Engineering, University of Rochester, Rochester, NY, USA

Andrew L. Vasilakes Department of Chemical and Materials Engineering, University of Kentucky, Lexington, KY, USA

Patricia R. Wardwell Syracuse Biomaterials Institute, Syracuse University, Syracuse, NY, USA

Paritosh P. Wattamwar Teva Pharmaceutical Industries Ltd., West Chester, PA, USA

Haoyan Zhou Department of Radiology, Case Western Reserve University, Cleveland, OH, USA

PART I

INTRODUCTION

1

FUNDAMENTALS OF DRUG DELIVERY

Rebecca A. Bader

Syracuse Biomaterials Institute, Syracuse University, Syracuse, NY, USA

1.1 INTRODUCTION: HISTORY AND FUTURE OF DRUG DELIVERY

As depicted in Fig. 1.1, as drug discovery has evolved, the need for innovate methods to effectively deliver therapeutics has risen. In the early 1900s, there began a shift away from the traditional herbal remedies characteristic of the "age of botanicals" toward a more modern approach based on developments in synthetic chemistry [1, 2]. Through the 1940s, drug discovery needs were directed by the needs of the military, that is, antibiotics were developed and produced to treat injured soldiers [3]. As more pharmaceuticals were rapidly identified by biologists and chemists alike, people became more cognizant of the impact therapeutics could have on everyday life. During the late 1940s to the early 1950s, drugs were, for the first time, formulated into microcapsules to simplify administration and to facilitate a sustained, controlled therapeutic effect [4]. For example, Spansules®, microcapsules containing drug pellets surrounded by coatings of variable thickness to prolong release, were developed by Smith Kline and French Laboratories and rapidly approved for use [5]. Many of these early microencapsulation techniques, particularly the Wurster process, whereby drug cores are spray coated with a polymer shell, are still in use today [6, 7].

Engineering Polymer Systems for Improved Drug Delivery, First Edition.
Edited by Rebecca A. Bader and David A. Putnam.
© 2014 John Wiley & Sons, Inc. Published 2014 by John Wiley & Sons, Inc.

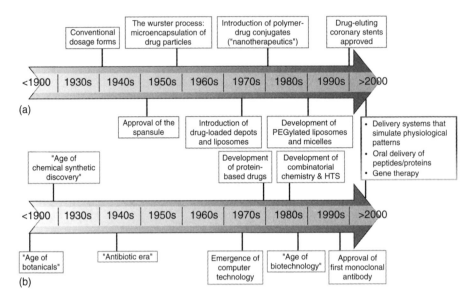

Figure 1.1. Drug delivery (a) and drug discovery (b) have followed similar trajectories with the need for drug delivery rising with the identification of new therapeutic compounds.

Although a number of advanced methods for controlled and/or targeted drug delivery were proposed in the 1960s, building on the conventional drug delivery method of microencapsulation, these techniques were not fully implemented until the 1970s [8, 9]. During this decade, biotechnology and molecular biology began to play a significant role in the drug discovery process, culminating in an increased understanding of the etiology of numerous diseases and the development of protein-based therapeutics. Likewise, computer screening, predictive software, combinatorial chemistry, and high throughput screening significantly accelerated the rate at which lead compounds for new therapeutic compounds could be identified [1, 4]. As is discussed further in Chapter 2, drug carrier systems, such as implants, coatings, micelles, liposomes, and polymer conjugates, were proposed to address the growing need to deliver the newly identified therapeutic compounds with maximum efficacy and minimal risk of negative side effects [8, 9] (Fig. 1.2).

In sum, over time, as technology has advanced for drug discovery, there has been a paradigm shift in drug delivery from simplifying the administration of old drugs to creating systems that can make new drugs work. This is particularly true as we continue to identify and develop therapeutics based on proteins and nucleic acids that are difficult to administer in a patient-friendly manner and/or with the necessary site-specificity to reverse adverse consequences. However, as drug delivery technology has advanced for new drugs, many of the old drugs have likewise benefited through increased predictability of pharmacokinetic/pharmacodynamic profiles, decreased side effects, and enhanced efficacy. This text is intended to explain how these advanced drug delivery techniques, particularly those related to the application of polymers, have

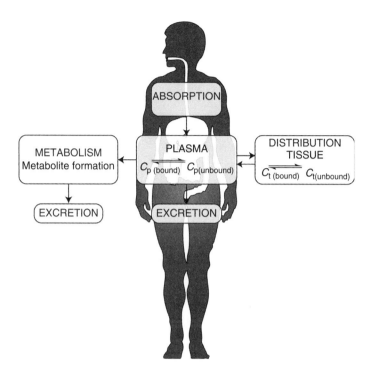

Figure 1.2. The temporal and spatial distribution of drugs is impacted by absorption, distribution, metabolism, and excretion (ADME).

improved the efficacy of old and new drugs alike. Chapter 1 serves as the foundation for all subsequent chapters, defining the necessary terminology related to drug delivery and pharmaceutics.

1.2 TERMINOLOGY

1.2.1 Pharmacology

Pharmacology, the science of drugs, is composed of two primary branches, pharmacodynamics and pharmacokinetic. In broad terms, pharmacokinetics refers to what the body does to the drug whereas pharmacodynamics describes what the drug does to the body. In the subsequent sections, a brief overview of these two branches of study are given in order to highlight some of the basic pharmacological terminology frequently encountered in both drug discovery and delivery

1.2.1.1 Pharmacokinetics. Pharmacokinetics tracks the time course of drugs and drug delivery systems through the body. The processes that impact the temporal and spatial distribution of drugs are absorption, distribution, metabolism, excretion (ADME). Following administration, the drugs are absorbed by the bloodstream,

TABLE 1.1. Pharmacokinetic Parameters

Process	Parameter	Definition
Absorption	Absorption rate constant (k_a)	First-order rate constant for absorption
	Bioavailability (F)	The extent of drug absorption
Distribution	Plasma drug concentration (C_p)	The concentration of drug in the plasma
	Volume of distribution (V_d)	The mass amount of drug given (dose) divided by the plasma concentration (C_p). V_d is an apparent volume with no direct physiological relevance
	Unbound fraction	The fraction of drug not bound to protein, that is, pharmaceutically active
Elimination (metabolism and excretion)	Metabolism rate constant (k_m)	First-order rate constant for elimination by metabolism
	Excretion rate constant (k_{ex})	First-order rate constants for elimination by excretion
	Elimination rate constant (k_e)	$k_e = k_{ex} + k_m$
	Extrarenal (metabolic) clearance	The volume of plasma cleared of drug per unit time by metabolism
	Renal clearance	The volume of plasma cleared of drug per unit time by metabolism
	Total clearance	Total clearance = renal clearance + extrarenal Clearance
	Half-life ($t_{1/2}$)	The time necessary for the plasma drug concentration to be reduced 50%

distributed to tissues and organs throughout the body, and eventually eliminated by metabolism or excretion. Although a summary of these processes with associated parameters is provided in Table 1.1, each of these terms are described in further detail in Section 1.3 [10, 11].

1.2.1.2 Pharmacodynamics. Because pharmacodynamics broadly refers to what the drug does to the body, pharmacodynamics measurements involve looking at toxicity, as well as therapeutic efficacy. These measurements frequently involve examining dose–response curves to determine the optimal range over which drugs can be administered with maximum therapeutic impact and minimal negative side effects. Pharmacodynamics also involves examining the mechanism by which drugs act, that is, drug–receptor interactions. Typically, these studies are used to identify the amount of drug necessary to reduce interactions of endogenous agonists with the receptor [12]. These concepts related to pharmacodynamics will be explored in greater detail in Section 1.4.

1.2.2 Routes of Administration

The route by which drugs are administered can have a profound impact on the pharmacokinetic properties given in Table 1.1. One of the goals of drug delivery is to facilitate administration by routes that normally have an adverse impact on the associated therapeutic pharmacokinetic properties. For example, as is discussed further in Chapter 2, effective oral administration of numerous drugs is not feasible because of poor uptake through the mucosal epithelial barrier of the intestine and a low resultant bioavailability. Furthermore, orally administered drugs are subject to what is referred to as the first pass effect, whereby the bioavailability is reduced by metabolism within the liver and/or gut wall. Carrier systems have been designed to (i) increase intercellular transport by disrupting the epithelial barrier, (ii) facilitate intracellular transport through targeting of the absorptive epithelial cells, and/or (iii) reduce the destruction of drugs by liver enzymes [13–16].

The most explored routes of drug administration are summarized in Table 1.2. Although 90% of drugs are administered orally due to convenience and high patient compliance, oral drug delivery is associated with low and/or variable bioavailability as a result of the harsh environment of the gastrointestinal tract and the impermeable nature of the mucosal epithelial barrier. In contrast, parenteral forms of administration (intravenous, subcutaneous, and intramuscular) yield rapid effects and high bioavailability (100% for intravenous); however, patient compliance is extremely low as a result of the discomfort because of the injection. Transdermal delivery is

TABLE 1.2. Routes of Administration for Drug Delivery

Route of Administration	Advantages	Limitations
Parenteral	Immediate effects Reproducible High bioavailability	Low patient compliance Often requires a clinician
Oral	Convenient High patient compliance	Highly variable Harsh environmental conditions Low absorption of many drugs
Transdermal	Continuous delivery	Limited to lipophilic drugs
Pulmonary	High absorptive surface area Rapid absorption of small molecule drugs	The morphology of the lung tissue makes systemic delivery difficult Limited absorption of macromolecules
Nasal	Rapid absorption of lipophilic drugs High bioavailability of lipophilic drugs	Limited absorption of polar molecules

a favorable route of administration because of high patient acceptability and ready access to the site of absorption; however, this method has historically been limited to small, lipophilic drugs that can passively diffuse through the skin barrier [17, 18]. New techniques are currently being developed to extend transdermal delivery to polar and/or macromolecular compounds. For example, ultrasound and iontophoresis provide a driving force for the passage of small, charged drugs, while electroporation and microneedles disrupt the outermost layer of the skin for delivery of macromolecules, particularly peptides and proteins [19]. Nasal and pulmonary drug deliveries are also attractive routes of administration because of the high potential surface area available for drug absorption; however, as with transdermal delivery, the nature of the epithelial barriers in both regions limits this to lipophilic compounds [17, 18].

1.2.3 Drug Delivery

1.2.3.1 Controlled Release. Controlled drug delivery systems, also referred to as prolonged and sustained release systems, aim to minimize dosing frequency by maintaining the local and/or systemic concentrations of drugs for extended periods of time. Although difficult to achieve, ideal release of drugs from controlled release delivery systems follow zero-order release kinetics, whereby the rate of drug release does not change with time until no drug remains. As a result, constant drug levels within the body can be maintained. A variable release rate with drugs provided to the body at a nonconstant, time-dependent rate is more common. If first-order kinetics are followed, the release rate decreases exponentially with time until the majority of the drug has been released, at which time zero-order release kinetics are approached (Fig. 1.4) [9, 20–23].

1.2.3.2 Active Versus Passive Targeting. Inflammatory tissue and solid tumors both possess an increased vascular permeability that can be exploited for improved drug delivery. The diseased tissue can be passively targeted by developing systems (such as liposomes, micelles, and nanoparticles) with a hydrodynamic radius large enough to prevent renal filtration, but small enough to pass through the leaky vasculature. In cancer, the change in vasculature is accompanied by a reduction in lymphatic drainage, thereby increasing the passive targeting capacity of carrier systems through "enhanced permeation and retention" [24–26]. The site-specificity of drug delivery systems can be further improved through the addition of a ligand, such as an antibody, polysaccharide, or peptide, that will actively target receptors overexpressed in the diseased region [27–30]. The concepts of active and passive targeting will arise throughout this book.

1.3 BASIC PHARMACOKINETICS

1.3.1 Compartment Models

Compartment models are used as a simple method to describe the time course of a drug through a physiological system on administration. One and two compartment models are depicted in Fig. 1.3. The simplest pharmacokinetic model is the one compartment open model for drugs administered by intravenous (IV) bolus with first-order elimination, that is, the rate at which the amount of drug in the body changes is proportional to the amount of drug remaining in the body. To apply a one compartment open model, the assumption must be made that the drugs are instantaneously, homogenously distributed between tissues on administration, thereby allowing the body to be described as a unit from which drugs are cleared. While the one compartment model for IV bolus administration will be presented herein, more complicated models, such as those required when drugs are not instantaneously distributed, are beyond the scope of this text. Readers are encouraged to look at several excellent textbooks on basic pharmacokinetics for additional information [10, 11, 31]

As mentioned in brief above, elimination after IV bolus administration can be described using a first-order kinetic equation when applying a one compartment model. This equation can be derived by assessing the rate of change for either drug concentration (Eq. 1.1) or drug amount (Eq. 1.2)

$$\frac{dC_p}{dt} = -k_e C_p \qquad (1.1)$$

$$\frac{dM}{dt} = -k_e M \qquad (1.2)$$

where C_p is the plasma concentration of drug, M is the mass amount of drug, and k_e is a first-order elimination rate constant. Although an identical analysis can be applied to the rate of change of drug amount, all subsequent pharmacokinetic parameters will be derived using the rate of change of drug concentration (Eq. 1.1). Thus, integration of Eq. 1.1 gives:

$$C_{p,t} = C_{p,0} e^{-k_e t} \qquad (1.3)$$

Equation 1.3 in conjunction with the area under the curve (AUC) described in Section 1.3.2, serves as a spring board from which other pharmacokinetic parameters are derived. Note that C_p is not equal to the concentration of drug in other tissues;

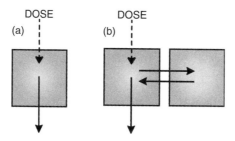

Figure 1.3. (a) One and (b) two compartment models can be used to describe the time course of drugs in the body after administration.

however, changes in drug concentration within the plasma are directly proportional to those in other tissues as a consequence of describing the body as a homogenous, single compartment.

1.3.2   Bioavailability and Area Under the Curve (AUC)

Bioavailability refers to the rate and extent to which a drug has reached the systemic circulation for delivery to the site of action. Thus, the most common indicator of bioavailability is C_p. From a plot of C_p versus time, the AUC provides a quantitative measure of how much drug stays in the body and for how long [10, 31].

For an IV bolus with first-order elimination kinetics, an exact solution for the AUC can be obtained by analytical integration [10, 31]. For example, consider the C_p versus time plot shown in Fig. 1.4. As derived in Section 1.3.1, C_p at a given time can be determined from Eq. 1.3. Using calculus, the AUC is equal to the integral from $t = 0$ to an infinite time point. Therefore, taking the integral of Eq. 1.3 gives

$$\text{AUC} = \int_0^\infty C_{p,t}\, dt \tag{1.4}$$

$$\text{AUC} = \int_0^\infty C_{p,0}\, e^{-k_e t}\, dt = C_{p,0}\left[\frac{e^{-k_e t}}{-k_e}\right]_0^\infty \tag{1.5}$$

$$\text{AUC} = C_{p,0}\left[\frac{e^{-k_e \infty} - e^{-k_e 0}}{-k_e}\right] \tag{1.6}$$

$$\text{AUC} = \frac{C_{p,0}}{k_e} \tag{1.7}$$

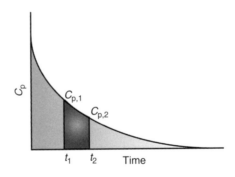

Figure 1.4. After IV bolus administration, elimination can be described using a first-order kinetic equation if a one compartment model is assumed.

Alternatively, $C_{p,0}$ if and/or k_e are unknown, the AUC can be found using the trapezoidal rule. Using Fig. 1.4, the AUC for the highlighted segment can be found with

$$\text{AUC}_{1-2} = \frac{C_{p,1} + C_{p,2}}{2}(t_2 - t_1) \tag{1.8}$$

Extrapolating the first segment to determine $C_{p,0}$, assuming the last points follow an exponential decay that defines k_e, adding all possible segments together yields.

$$\text{AUC} = \text{AUC}_{0-1} + \text{AUC}_{1-\text{last}} + \text{AUC}_{\text{last}-\infty} \tag{1.9}$$

$$\text{AUC} = \frac{C_{p,0} + C_{p,1}}{2}t_1 + \frac{C_{p,1} + C_{p,2}}{2}(t_2 - t_1) + \cdots + \frac{C_{p,\text{last}}}{k_e} \tag{1.10}$$

1.3.3 Elimination Rate Constant and Half-Life

The elimination rate constant, k_e, introduced above can be found by converting Eq. 1.3 to natural logarithmic form to give

$$\text{Ln}(C_{p,t}) = \text{Ln}(C_{p,0}) - k_e t \tag{1.11}$$

Thus, k_e is the slope of a plot of $\text{Ln}(C_p)$ versus time:

$$k_e = \frac{\text{Ln}(C_{p,1}) - \text{Ln}(C_{p,2})}{t_2 - t_1} \tag{1.12}$$

Note that the elimination rate constant includes both excretion and metabolism. From k_e, the half-life, that is, the time necessary to decrease C_p to one half of $C_{p,0}$, can be determined. Considering Eq. 1.12 and solving for the time when $C_{p,2} = C_{p,1}/2$ gives

$$t_{1/2} = \frac{\text{Ln}2}{k_e} = \frac{0.693}{k_e} \tag{1.13}$$

Equation 1.13 shows that the half-life is independent of drug concentration. Thus, regardless of $C_{p,0}$, the half-life can be used to describe when most of the drug has been eliminated from the body. For example, after five half-lives, $C_p = C_{p,0}/32$ and 96.875% of the initial amount of drug in the body has been lost [10, 31].

1.3.4 Volume of Distribution

Despite the importance of this parameter in pharmacokinetics, the volume of distribution, V_d, does not have any direct physiological relevance and does not correlate with a true volume. V_d can be defined as the ratio of dose, D, to the plasma concentration at $t = 0$

$$V_d = \frac{D}{C_{p,0}} \tag{1.14}$$

Likewise, V_d can be obtained by taking the ratio of the mass amount to the concentration of drug at any given time point. If V_d is high, the drug is highly distributed to tissues/organs throughout the body, rather than being confined primarily to the plasma; while if V_d is low, the drug is not well distributed to tissue/organs and resides, for the most part, in the plasma [10, 31].

1.3.5 Clearance

Drug clearance (CL) is a proportionality constant relating the elimination rate, dM/dt, to the plasma concentration C_p [10, 31].

$$CL = \frac{dM}{dt} \cdot \frac{1}{C_p} \tag{1.15}$$

Substituting in Eq. 1.2 and noting that volume of distribution is equal to the amount of drug divided by the concentration of drug gives

$$CL = k_e V_d \tag{1.16}$$

Half-life is related to k_e through Eq. 1.13. Thus,

$$CL = \frac{0.693 V_d}{t_{1/2}} \tag{1.17}$$

1.4 BASIC PHARMACODYNAMICS

1.4.1 Therapeutic Index and Therapeutic Window

The goal in the development of new therapeutic agents, as well as drug delivery systems, is to maximize efficacy while minimizing the potential for adverse drug events. Thus, dose–response curves, will examine both therapeutic response and toxicity, as shown in Fig. 1.5. The ratio of the median toxic dose (TD_{50}), that is, the dose that causes toxicity in 50% of the population, to the median effective dose (EC_{50}), that is, the dose required to elicit a response in 50% of the population, is referred to as the therapeutic index (TI). A drug with a high TI can be used over a wide range of doses, referred to as the therapeutic window, without adverse side effects. In contrast, a low TI suggests a narrow therapeutic window [12, 32].

1.4.2 Ligand-Receptor Binding

Although some drugs act through chemical reactions or physical associations with molecules within the body, a number of other drugs are used to elicit, change, or prevent a cellular response via ligand-receptor binding interactions. For this mechanism of action, the drug serves as an exogenous ligand that either (i) prevents interactions

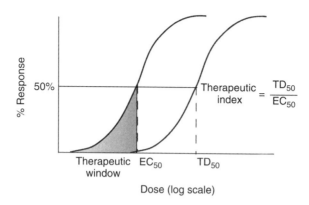

Figure 1.5. Typical dose–response curves looks at both efficacy and toxicity. The therapeutic window is the dosing range that can be used to safely treat a disease.

of the receptor with an endogenous ligand (e.g., a cytokine or hormone), that is, the drug acts as an antagonist, or (ii) elicits a physiological response equal to or greater than what would result from the binding of an endogenous ligand, that is, the drug acts as an agonist. Ligand (drug)–receptor interactions are governed by affinity, as indicated by the ratio of the association to dissociation rate constants. The inverse of the affinity, that is, the dissociation divided by association rate constant, is referred to as the dissociation constant (K_D), the most frequently reported indicator of the strength of drug–receptor interactions [33, 34]. The concept of ligand–receptor binding is critical in understanding how to design a carrier system such that the therapeutic efficacy of the drug can be maintained and/or active targeting can be implemented. Section 1.5.2.2 takes a more quantitative approach toward helping readers understand the importance of drug/drug delivery system–receptor interactions.

1.5 MASS TRANSFER

Learning the basics of mass transfer is critical to understanding how drugs travel through/out of polymeric matrices of carrier systems and through the surrounding tissue. Numerous examples using the principles of mass transfer are given throughout this text. Mass transfer describes the tendency of a component in a mixture to move from a region of high concentration (i.e., the source) to an area of low concentration (i.e., the sink). This transport can occur as a result of molecular mass transfer, or diffusion, whereby movement occurs through a still medium, or convective mass transfer, whereby transfer is promoted by fluid flow. The interested reader is referred to conventional texts on mass transfer and transport phenomena [35–37].

1.5.1 General Flux Equation and Fick's First Law

The total mass transported can be expressed as the sum of the mass transported by diffusion and the mass transported by bulk motion of the fluid. Considering a mixture of two species with one dimensional transport along the z axis, the molar flux of species 1, N_1, is given by

$$N_1 = J_1 + c_1 v^*$$ (1.18)

where J_1 is the flux due to pure diffusion, c_1 is the molar concentration, and v^* is the molar average velocity. v^* can be determined as the sum of the velocity contributions from the components in the mixture.

$$v^* = \frac{1}{c} \sum_i c_i v_i = \sum_i x_i v_i$$ (1.19)

where x_i is the mole fraction of species i in the mixture. $c_i v_i$ is equivalent to the molar flux of species i relative to stationary coordinates.

$$N_i = c_i v_i \left(\frac{\text{mol}}{\text{m}^2\text{s}} \right)$$ (1.20)

Thus, in a binary mixture

$$v^* = \frac{1}{c} \sum_i c_i v_i = \frac{1}{c}(c_1 v_1 + c_2 v_2) = \frac{1}{c}(N_1 + N_2)$$ (1.21)

Referring back to Eq. 1.18, $c_1 v^*$ is the flux generated by processes other than diffusion, such as convection/fluid flow. The flux, owing to diffusion, J_1, can also be expressed in the form of Fick's First Law in one dimension

$$J_1 = -D_1 \frac{dc_1}{dz}$$ (1.22)

where D_1 is a proportionality constant referred to as the diffusion coefficient. Combining Eqs. 1.18, 1.21, and 1.22 yields the General Flux Equation [35, 36]:

$$N_1 = -D_1 \frac{dc_1}{dz} + \frac{c_1}{c}(N_1 + N_2)$$ (1.23)

Of note, for dilute solutions, as would be found for a drug moving though a polymer matix or tissue, the general flux equation reduces to Fick's first law.

$$N_1 = -D_1 \frac{dc_1}{dz}$$ (1.24)

1.5.2 Mass Conservation and Fick's Second Law

Referring to Fig. 1.6, consider a material balance on species 1 along diffusion path length z and through fixed cross sectional area for flux A.

By conservation of mass in − out + generation = accumulation, expressed mathematically as

$$N_1 A|_z - N_1 A|_{z+\Delta z} + \psi_1 A \Delta Z = \frac{c_1|_{t+\Delta t, \bar{z}} - c_1|_{t, \bar{z}}}{\Delta t} A \Delta Z \qquad (1.25)$$

Division of Eq. 1.25 by A, rearrangement, and division by ΔZ yields

$$-\left[\frac{N_1|_{z+\Delta z} - N_1|_z}{\Delta Z} \right] + \psi_1 = \frac{c_1|_{t+\Delta t, \bar{z}} - c_1|_{t, \bar{z}}}{\Delta t} \qquad (1.26)$$

If the limit of $\Delta Z \to 0$, $\Delta t \to 0$ is taken, the following equation is obtained:

$$-\frac{\partial N_1}{\partial z} + \psi_1 = \frac{\partial c_1}{\partial t} \qquad (1.27)$$

Using Eq. 1.27 with the General Flux Equation (Eq. 1.23), assuming that D_1 is constant, gives

$$D_1 \frac{\partial^2 c_1}{\partial z^2} - \frac{\partial(c_1 v^*)}{\partial z} + \psi_1 = \frac{\partial c_1}{\partial t} \qquad (1.28)$$

If the total system density is also constant, Eq. 1.28 can be further simplified to

$$D_1 \frac{\partial^2 c_1}{\partial z^2} - v^* \frac{\partial c_1}{\partial z} + \psi_1 = \frac{\partial c_1}{\partial t} \qquad (1.29)$$

In a situation with no fluid motion ($v^* = 0$) and no productive term ($\psi_1 = 0$), this equation reduces to Fick's Second Law, which facilitates prediction of concentration changes with time because of diffusion [35, 36].

$$D_1 \frac{\partial^2 c_1}{\partial z^2} = \frac{\partial c_1}{\partial t} \qquad (1.30)$$

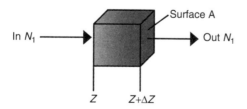

Figure 1.6. A generalized mass balance for a volume element.

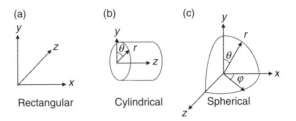

Figure 1.7. One dimensional flux equations can be derived for (a) rectangular, (b) cylindrical, and (c) spherical geometries.

TABLE 1.3. One Dimensional Flux Equations for Different Geometries

Rectangular	$D_1 \dfrac{\partial^2 c_1}{dz^2} = \dfrac{\partial c_1}{\partial t}$
Cylindrical	$D_1 \left[\dfrac{\partial^2 c_1}{dr^2} + \dfrac{1}{r} \dfrac{\partial c_1}{\partial r} \right] = \dfrac{\partial c_1}{\partial t}$
Spherical	$D_1 \left[\dfrac{\partial^2 c_1}{dr^2} + \dfrac{2}{r} \dfrac{\partial c}{\partial r} \right] = \dfrac{\partial c_1}{\partial t}$

Although Fick's Second Law was derived for one dimension flux in a rectangular coordinate system above, these concepts can readily be extended to spherical and cylindrical coordinate systems (Fig. 1.7). The equations for one dimensional flux in different geometries are summarized in Table 1.3. Detailed derivations of solutions to Fick's Second Law, including those given for the problems in Section 1.5.2.1, can be found in Crank's book on the mathematics of diffusion [38].

1.5.2.1 Application of Fick's Second Law in Drug Delivery.

Applications of Fick's Second Law will appear throughout this text; however, two in depth examples will be provided to here to show how Eq. 1.30 can be used to predict the concentration of drug as a function of time and distance away from or through a controlled release system. First, consider a cylindrical hydrogel with a radius of 4 mm and a height of 0.75 mm loaded with keratinocyte growth factor (KGF) at a high concentration ($c_{KGF,0}$) intended for use as a wound healing dressing (Fig. 1.8) [39]. Assuming that diffusion only occurs in one dimension through the surface placed in contact with the wound and taking into account that $h \ll r$, the system can be modeled with Fick's Second Law using a rectangular coordinate system.

$$D_1 \frac{\partial^2 c_1}{dz^2} = \frac{\partial c_1}{\partial t} \qquad (1.31)$$

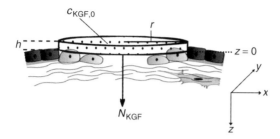

Figure 1.8. KGF release from a cylindrical hydrogel with $h << r$ can be modeled as one dimensional flux in the z direction (i.e., a rectangular coordinate system).

If we assume that (i) a high concentration of drug is maintained at the surface of the cylinder, (ii) KGF is not initially present in the underlying tissue, and (iii) there is no KGF at an infinite distance from the cylinder, the following boundary conditions can be applied to determine the drug concentration as a function of time and distance into the underlying tissue.

$$c_{KGF}(z, 0) = 0 \quad \text{for } 0 < z < \infty, t = 0 \tag{1.32}$$

$$c_{KGF}(0, t)(\text{surface}) = c_{KGF,0} \quad \text{for } z = 0, t > 0 \tag{1.33}$$

$$c_{KGF}(\infty, t) = 0 \quad \text{for } z = \infty, t > 0 \tag{1.34}$$

Solving Eq. 1.31 with the method of combination of variables gives the following solution

$$\frac{c_{KGF}(z, t) - c_{KGF}(z, 0)}{c_{KGF,0} - c_{KGF}(z, 0)} = \text{Erfc}\left(\frac{z}{2\sqrt{D_{KGF}t}}\right) \tag{1.35}$$

Which, given that $c_{KGF}(z, 0) = 0$, can be reduced to

$$\frac{c_{KGF}(z, t)}{c_{KGF,0}} = \text{Erfc}\left(\frac{z}{2\sqrt{D_{KGF}t}}\right) \tag{1.36}$$

Taking D_{KGF} to be 4.86×10^{-9} cm^2 s^{-1}, the concentration of KGF as a function of distance from the hydrogel wound healing dressing is plotted for several time points in Fig. 1.9.

Next, consider the release of 10 mg of Dramamine from a spherical capsule ($r = 0.30$ cm) (Fig. 1.10). Using a spherical coordinate system and assuming that diffusion only occurs in the radial direction, Fick's Second Law can be used to predict the change in drug concentration within the capsule over time.

$$D_1\left[\frac{\partial^2 c_1}{dr^2} + \frac{2}{r}\frac{\partial c}{\partial r}\right] = \frac{\partial c_1}{\partial t} \tag{1.37}$$

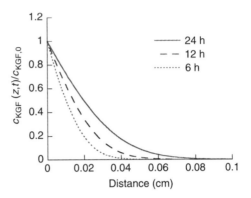

Figure 1.9. Distance of penetration of KGF into the wound site following release from cylindrical hydrogels at three time points (6, 12, and 24 h), as determined from Eq. 1.36.

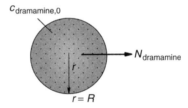

Figure 1.10. Release of Dramamine from a spherical capsule can be model as one dimensional flux in the radial direction.

The following boundary conditions can be applied assuming that (i) the capsule radius remains constant, (ii) the capsule possesses radial symmetry, and (iii) the drug is immediately swept away from the surface of the capsule on release.

$$c_d(r, 0) = c_{d,0} \text{ for } 0 < r < R, t = 0 \tag{1.38}$$

$$\frac{\partial c_d(0, t)}{\partial r} = 0 \text{ for } r = 0, t \geq 0 \tag{1.39}$$

$$c_d(R, t)(\text{surface}) = 0 \text{ for } r = R, t > 0 \tag{1.40}$$

An analytical solution to Eq. 1.37 can be obtained following the separation of variables method.

$$\frac{c_d(r, t) - c_{d,0}}{c_d(R, t) - c_{d,0}} = 1 + \frac{2R}{\pi r} \sum_{n=1}^{\infty} \frac{-1^n}{n} \sin\left(\frac{n\pi r}{R}\right) e^{\frac{-D_d n^2 \pi^2 t}{R^2}} \tag{1.41}$$

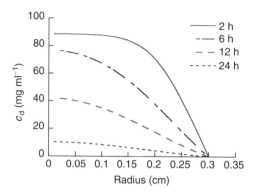

Figure 1.11. Dramamine concentration throughout the spherical capsule was predicted for several time points based on Eq. 1.42.

which, given that $c_{\text{dramamine}}(R, t) = 0$, can be simplified to

$$\frac{c_d(r, t) - c_{d,0}}{-c_{d,0}} = 1 + \frac{2R}{\pi r} \sum_{n=1}^{\infty} \frac{-1^n}{n} \sin\left(\frac{n\pi r}{R}\right) e^{\frac{-D_d n^2 \pi^2 t}{R^2}} \tag{1.42}$$

Figure 1.11 illustrates the change in Dramamine concentration with distance outward from the center of the capsule for several different time points. Alternatively, by using $r = R$ and $m_{d,0} = c_{d,0} \times (4/3)\pi R^3$, where $m_{d,0}$ is the initial mass amount of Dramamine loaded into the capsule, the equation can be revised to predict the time necessary for near complete drug release. Figure 1.12 uses Eq. 1.43 to demonstrate the fractional release of drug $(1 - m_{d(t)}/m_{d,0})$ as a function of time.

$$\frac{m_d(t)}{m_{d,0}} = \frac{6}{\pi^2} \sum_{n=1}^{\infty} \frac{1}{n^2} e^{\frac{-D_d n^2 \pi^2 t}{R^2}} \tag{1.43}$$

1.5.2.2 Fick's Second Law and Ligand Binding. As discussed previously, there are many instances, particularly in regard to biologics; efficacy is dependent on the therapeutic agent not only diffusing to the cells within the active site, but also on binding to the cell surface. For these cases, the assumption cannot be made that the drug disappears immediately on reaching the cell, that is, the drug concentration at the surface is equal to 0. Instead, the drug disappears at a rate that is governed by binding kinetics.

Consider the system illustrated in Fig. 1.13. At the surface, the drug can bind to or dissociate from the receptor. This relationship can be described by

$$C_R + C_L \underset{k_{\text{off}}}{\overset{k_{\text{on}}}{\rightleftharpoons}} C_R C_L \tag{1.44}$$

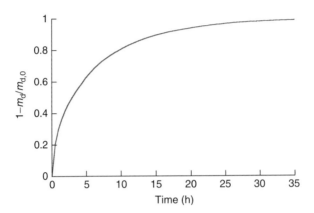

Figure 1.12. Equation 1.43 can be used to predict when most of the Dramamine will be released from the spherical capsule.

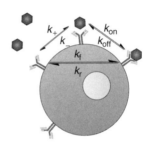

Figure 1.13. For a ligand (i.e., drug) to associate with a cell surface receptor, the drug must first diffuse to the cell surface.

where k_{on} and k_{off} are the rate constants of binding and dissociation, respectively; C_R is the concentration of the receptor; C_L is the concentration of ligand (drug); and $C_R C_L$ is the concentration of ligand bound to receptor. At equilibrium, C_R, C_L, and $C_R C_L$ remain unchanged with time. Thus,

$$\frac{d(C_R C_L)}{dt} = C_R \cdot C_L \cdot k_{on} - C_R C_L \cdot k_{off} = 0 \tag{1.45}$$

$$C_R \cdot C_L \cdot k_{on} = C_R C_L \cdot k_{off} \tag{1.46}$$

Equation 1.46 can be rearranged and expressed with the equilibrium dissociation constant, K_d.

$$\frac{C_R \cdot C_L}{C_R C_L} = \frac{k_{off}}{k_{on}} = K_d \tag{1.47}$$

Likewise, an equilibrium exists between the drug diffusing to and from the receptor, as defined by k_+ and k_-. Taken together, the overall forward and reverse rate constants are given by k_f and k_r, respectively.

By assuming that (i) flux only occurs in the radial direction, (ii) the ligand does not degrade within the physiological solution, (iii) the cell radius remains constant, and (iv) the rate of ligand disappearance is equal to the rate of diffusion at the surface, expressions can be developed to determine k_f and k_r. Because there is a constant source (the ligand in solution) and a constant sink (the cell surface), the system is at steady state. Thus, Fick's second law for a spherical geometry can be written as

$$D_L \left[\frac{d^2 c_L}{dr^2} + \frac{2}{r} \frac{dc_L}{dr} \right] = 0 \tag{1.48}$$

The following boundary conditions can be applied based on the assumptions given above.

$$c_L(r) = c_{L,0} \text{ for } r = \infty \tag{1.49}$$

$$4\pi R^2 \cdot N_L = k_{on} \cdot C_R \cdot C_L \text{ for } r = R \tag{1.50}$$

The second boundary condition equates the rate of ligand disappearance at the surface, as given by $k_{on} \times C_R \times C_L$, to the rate of diffusion at the surface, as given by the surface area $(4\pi R^2)$ times the flux (N_L). Thus, this boundary condition can be rewritten as

$$4\pi R^2 \cdot D_L \frac{dc_L}{dr} = k_{on} \cdot C_R \cdot C_L \text{ for } r = R \tag{1.51}$$

Solving with the specified boundary conditions yields the ligand concentration as a function of radius.

$$C_L(r) = \frac{-k_{on} C_R R C_{L,0}}{4\pi Dr + k_{on} C_R} \cdot \frac{1}{r} + C_{L,0} \tag{1.52}$$

If binding is diffusion-limited, that is, $4\pi Dr \ll k_{on}$, the rate of ligand disappearance at the cell surface $(r = R)$ can be given by

$$\text{Rate of ligand disappearance} = -D(4\pi R^2) \frac{dC_L}{dr} \tag{1.53}$$

Substituting in Eq. 1.52 into Eq. 1.53 gives

$$\text{Rate of ligand disappearance} = 4\pi D \frac{k_{on} C_R R C_{L,0}}{4\pi DR + k_{on} C_R} \tag{1.54}$$

where $4\pi DR$ is equivalent to k_+. By equating the overall rate of ligands diffusing toward and binding to the cell surface receptors, $k_f C_{L,0}$, to Eq. 1.54, the overall rate constant k_f can be expressed in terms of k_+, the rate constant for diffusion-limited binding, to $C_R k_{on}$, the intrinsic binding rate [40, 41].

$$k_f = \frac{k_+ C_R k_{on}}{k_+ + k_{on} C_R} \tag{1.55}$$

As an example, consider that antibody fragments conjugated to PEG can be used for the active, targeted delivery of therapeutics to cancer cells that possess specific cell surface antigens. The hydrodynamic radius and diffusion coefficient of the antibody-PEG fragment in PBS at $37\,^\circ$C have been determined to be 2.5 nm and 8.4×10^{-7} cm^2 s^{-1} respectively. The intrinsic association constant, k_{on}, is 6.1×10^4 M^{-1} s^{-1} [42]. Assuming that binding is diffusion limited, the transport rate constant, k_+, and the overall rate constants for ligand binding, k_f, for a normal cell that has 20,000 surface receptors ($C_R = 20,000$) and a cancerous cell that has 2,000,000 receptors ($C_R = 2,000,000$) can be determined.

$$k_+ = 4\pi DR$$

$$k_+ = 4\pi (8.4 \times 10^{-7} \text{ cm}^2 \text{ s}^{-1})(2.5 \times 10^{-7} \text{ cm})$$

$$k_+ = 2.64 \times 10^{-12} \text{ cm}^3 \text{ s}^{-1} \text{ ligand}^{-1}$$

$$k_+ = \frac{2.64 \times 10^{-12} \text{ cm}^3}{\text{ligand}} \times \frac{6.022 \times 10^{23} \text{ ligands}}{\text{mole}} \times \frac{1 \text{l}}{1000 \text{ cm}^3}$$

$$k_+ = 1.59 \times 10^9 \text{ M}^{-1} \text{ s}^{-1}$$

$$k_f = \frac{k_+ C_R k_{on}}{k_+ + C_R k_{on}}$$

For normal cells:

$$C_R = 20,000$$

$$k_f = 6.90 \times 10^8 \text{ M}^{-1} \text{ s}^{-1}$$

For cancer cells:

$$C_R = 2,000,000$$

$$k_f = 1.57 \times 10^9 \text{ M}^{-1} \text{ s}^{-1}$$

Thus, the overall forward rate constant for cancer cells is greater than that for normal cells, lending credence to the possibility of active targeting by carrier systems modified with a ligand for receptors overexpressed by diseased cells. Note that while the above calculations were made on a per cell basis, careful attention should be given to units when solving for problems related to ligand binding interactions.

1.6 KEY POINTS

- As drug discovery has evolved to encompass compounds that are less physiologically soluble and/or stable, the need for drug delivery has increased.
- Pharmacokinetics refers to what the body does to the drug, while pharmacodynamics refers to what the drug does to the body.
- The route of absorption can have a profound impact on pharmacokinetic properties.
- Compartmental models can be used to describe the absorption, distribution, metabolism, and excretion of drugs by/from the body.
- In many cases, Fick's second law can be used to predict the release of a drug from a polymer-based drug delivery system.

1.7 HOMEWORK PROBLEMS

1. Discuss why 100% bioavailability is difficult to obtain by oral drug delivery.
2. Apo2L/TRAIL (tumor necrosis factor-related apoptosis-inducing ligand) has demonstrated anticancer efficacy. Recently, a recombinant, water soluble form of Apo2L/TRAIL was developed for clinical application. Before clinical studies, several *in vivo* models were used for pharmacokinetic evaluation. For all animals, Apo2L/TRAIL was administered via an IV bolus. The following average data was obtained from chimpanzees administered Apo2L/TRAIL at a dose of 1 mg^{-1} kg [43].

Time, min	C_p, ng ml^{-1}
10	20,000
20	15,000
45	9000
60	6000
90	2000
120	900
180	200

Construct a semi-log plot of serum concentration versus time and determine the best fit exponential equation for the curve. Determine the following pharmacokinetic parameters, assuming a chimpanzee weight of 60 kg:

a. Elimination rate constant, k_e
b. Half-life, $t_{1/2}$
c. Volume of distribution, V_d
d. Clearance, CL

3. The diffusion coefficients for the antibiotic cefoperazone through agar gel, fibrin gel, and cerebral cortex tissue were determined by applying a solution of drug in PBS at a concentration of 5 mg ml^{-1} to the top of the appropriate matrix and measuring the concentration as a function of depth at a predetermined time point. Experiments with brain tissue were performed *in vivo* on rats, while experiments with agar and fibrin gel were performed on matrix prepared in Petri dishes (thickness $= 0.5$ cm, diameter $= 10$ cm). The following data was obtained [44]:

Matrix	D, cm^2 s^{-1}
Agar gel	6.10E−07
Fibrin gel	7.00E−07
Cortex tissue	2.50E−08

a. Construct a model of cefoperazone penetration into agar, fibrin, or cortex tissue by (i) drawing the physical situation, (ii) listing at least three assumptions, (iii) specifying the boundary and initial conditions, and (iv) formulating the correct differential equation for mass transfer.
b. Assuming that the correct differential equation and boundary/initial conditions were identified, the analytic solution is

$$c_{\text{Cefazolin}}(z, t) = c_{\text{Cefazolin},0} \times \text{Erfc}\left(\frac{z}{2\sqrt{Dt}}\right)$$

Construct plots showing (i) the concentration of cefoperazone as a function of depth (0–500 μm) at a time of 30 min and (ii) the concentration of cefoperazone as a function of time (5–30 min) at a depth of 100 μm for agar gel, fibrin gel, and cortex tissue.

4. To control inflammation around implantable glucose sensors, researchers have suggested controlled release of dexamethasone at the site of implantation. In an experimental study with rats, dexamethasone was released from osmotic pumps implanted subcutaneously. Drug delivery from the pump was achieved from the spherical tip (radius $= 0.6$ mm) of a catheter attached to the pump. The osmotic pump maintains a constant concentration in the catheter tip. The following data was obtained for the concentration versus distance profile of dexamethasone at 6 h after implantation. Distance is expressed as the radial distance (r) from the center of the catheter tip, while concentration in the tissue is expressed relative to the concentration at the tip (C_s) [45].

r (distance from the center of the catheter tip, cm)	C/C_s
0.06	1
0.085	0.72
0.110	0.54
0.135	0.32
0.16	0.25
0.21	0.13
0.26	0.11
0.31	0.073
0.36	0.06
0.41	0.05

a. Construct a model to describe the controlled release of dexamethasone from the spherical tip of the catheter. Draw a picture of the physical system, list at least three assumptions, decide on the most appropriate coordinate system, formulate the differential equation for mass transfer, and specify the boundary/initial conditions.

b. The solution for the release of dexamethasone from the spherical tip of the catheter can be given by

$$\frac{C}{C_s} = \frac{a}{r}\text{erfc}\left[\frac{r-a}{2\sqrt{Dt}}\right]$$

where a is the radius of catheter, r is the distance from the center of the catheter, and C/C_s is the concentration in the tissue relative to the concentration at the tip.

Given the information about the radius of the catheter tip and the concentration profile of dexamethasone obtained at a time point of 6 h, plot the above equation and determine the diffusion coefficient for dexamethasone.

c. Evidence suggests that dexamethasone can be eliminated from the site of implantation. To account for this, an elimination rate constant (k_e) can be incorporated into the solution for predicting the concentration as a function of radius.

$$\frac{C}{C_s} = \frac{a}{2r}\left\{\exp\left[-(r-a)\sqrt{\frac{k}{D}}\right]\text{erfc}\left[\frac{r-a}{2\sqrt{Dt}} - \sqrt{kt}\right]\right.$$

$$\left. + \exp\left[(r-a)\sqrt{\frac{k}{D}}\right]\text{erfc}\left[\frac{r-a}{2\sqrt{Dt}} + \sqrt{kt}\right]\right\}$$

Plot this equation using the diffusion coefficient determined in part (b). Comment on whether or not you think elimination plays a significant role in the observed concentration profile.

REFERENCES

1. Kong DX, Li XJ, Zhang HY. *Where is the hope for drug discovery? Let history tell the future.* Drug Discov Today 2009;14(3-4):115–119.

2. Schmidt B et al. A natural history of botanical therapeutics. Metab Clin Exp 2008; 57(7):S3–S9.

3. Persidis A. Antibacterial and antifungal drug discovery. Nat Biotechnol 1999;17(11): 1141–1142.

4. Rosen H, Abribat T. The rise and rise of drug delivery. Nat Rev Drug Discov 2005; 4(5):381–385.

5. Helfand WH, Cowen DL. Evolution of pharmaceutical oral dosage forms. Pharm Hist 1983;25(1):3–18.

6. Wesdyk R et al. Factors affecting differences in film thickness of beads coated in fluidized-bed units. Int J Pharm 1993;93(1–3):101–109.

7. Wesdyk R et al. The effect of size and mass on the film thickness of beads coated in fluidized-bed equipment. Int J Pharm 1990;65(1–2):69–76.

8. Yokoyama M. Drug targeting with nano-sized carrier systems. J Artif Organs 2005; 8(2):77–84.

9. Hoffman AS. The origins and evolution of "controlled" drug delivery systems. J Control Release 2008;132(3):153–163.

10. Makoid MC, Vuchtich PJ, Banakar UV. Basic Pharmacokinetics. Virtual University Press; 1996. http://eglobalmed.com/opt/FB4D/pharmacy.creighton.edu/pha443/pdf/pkin00.pdf

11. Winter ME. Basic Clinical Pharmacokinetics. 5th ed. Philadelphia: Wolters Kluwer/ Lippincott Williams & Wilkins Health xii; 2010. p 548.

12. Tozer TN, Rowland M. Introduction to Pharmacokinetics and Pharmacodynamics: The Quantitative Basis of Drug Therapy. Philadelphia: Lippincott Williams & Wilkins; 2006. p 326.

13. Zhang N et al. Synthesis and evaluation of cyclosporine A-loaded polysialic acid-polycaprolactone micelles for rheumatoid arthritis. Eur J Pharm Sci 2013 submitted.

14. des Rieux A et al. Nanoparticles as potential oral delivery systems of proteins and vaccines: a mechanistic approach. J Control Release 2006;116(1):1–27.

15. Gaucher G et al. Polymeric micelles for oral drug delivery. Eur J Pharm Biopharm 2010;76(2):147–158.

16. Galindo-Rodriguez SA et al. Polymeric nanoparticles for oral delivery of drugs and vaccines: a critical evaluation of in vivo studies. Crit Rev Ther Drug Carrier Syst 2005; 22(5):419–464.

17. Zempsky WT. Alternative routes of drug administration--advantages and disadvantages (subject review). Pediatrics 1998;101(4 Pt 1):730–731.

18. Hilery AM, Lloyd AW, Swarbrick J. Drug Delivery and Targeting: For Pharmacists and Pharmaceutical Scientists. 1st ed. New York: Taylor & Francis Inc; 2001. p 496.

19. Paudel KS et al. Challenges and opportunities in dermal/transdermal delivery. Ther Deliv 2010;1(1):109–131.

20. Nair LS, Laurencin CT. Polymers as biomaterials for tissue engineering and controlled drug delivery. Adv Biochem Eng Biotechnol 2006;102:47–90.

21. Szycher M. Controlled drug delivery: a critical review. J Biomater Appl 1986; 1(2):171–182.

22. Langer RS, Peppas NA. Present and future applications of biomaterials in controlled drug delivery systems. Biomaterials 1981;2(4):201–214.

23. Zaffaroni A. Systems for controlled drug delivery. Med Res Rev 1981;1(4):373–386.

24. Gillies ER, Frechet JM. Dendrimers and dendritic polymers in drug delivery. Drug Discov Today 2005;10(1):35–43.

25. Lee CC et al. A single dose of doxorubicin-functionalized bow-tie dendrimer cures mice bearing C-26 colon carcinomas. Proc Natl Acad Sci U S A 2006;103(45):16649–16654.

26. Padilla De Jesus OL et al. Polyester dendritic systems for drug delivery applications: in vitro and in vivo evaluation. Bioconjug Chem 2002;13(3):453–461.

27. Pasquetto MV et al. Targeted drug delivery using immunoconjugates: principles and applications. J Immunother 2011;34(9):611–628.

28. Bhattacharjee H, Balabathula P, Wood GC. Targeted nanoparticulate drug-delivery systems for treatment of solid tumors: a review. Ther Deliv 2010;1(5):713–734.

29. Venkatraman SS et al. Polymer- and liposome-based nanoparticles in targeted drug delivery. Front Biosci (Schol Ed) 2010;2:801–814.

30. Ulbrich W, Lamprecht A. Targeted drug-delivery approaches by nanoparticulate carriers in the therapy of inflammatory diseases. J R Soc Interface 2010;7(Suppl 1):S55–S66.

31. Dhillon S, Kostrzewski A. Clinical Pharmacokinetics. London; Chicago: Pharmaceutical Press xvii; 2006. p 262.

32. Golan DE, Tashjian AH. Principles of Pharmacology: The Pathophysiologic Basis of Drug Therapy. 3rd ed. Philadelphia: Wolters Kluwer Health/Lippincott Williams & Wilkins xxi; 2012. p 954.

33. Ouellette RG, Joyce JA. Pharmacology for Nurse Anesthesiology. Sudbury, MA: Jones and Bartlett Learning xvi; 2011. p 544.

34. Kenakin TP. Pharmacology in Drug Discovery: Understanding Drug Response. 1st ed. Amsterdam: Academic Press xi; 2012. p 247.

35. Welty JR. Fundamentals of Momentum, Heat, and Mass Transfer. 4th ed. New York: Wiley xii; 2001. p 759.

36. Cussler EL. Diffusion: Mass Transfer in Fluid Systems. 2nd ed. New York: Cambridge University Press xviii; 1997. p 580.

37. Bird RB, Stewart WE, Lightfoot EN. Transport Phenomena. 2nd, Wiley international ed. New York: John Wiley & Sons, Inc. xii; 2002. p 895.

38. Crank J. The Mathematics of Diffusion. 2d ed. Oxford, England: Clarendon Press viii; 1975. p 414.

39. Bader RA, Kao WJ. Modulation of the keratinocyte-fibroblast paracrine relationship with gelatin-based semi-interpenetrating networks containing bioactive factors for wound repair. J Biomater Sci Polym Ed 2009;20(7–8):1005–1030.

40. Erickson J et al. The effect of receptor density on the forward rate constant for binding of ligands to cell surface receptors. Biophys J 1987;52(4):657–662.

41. Berg HC, Purcell EM. Physics of chemoreception. Biophys J 1977;20(2):193–219.
42. Kubetzko S, Sarkar CA, Pluckthun A. Protein PEGylation decreases observed target association rates via a dual blocking mechanism. Mol Pharmacol 2005;68(5):1439–1454.
43. Kelley SK et al. Preclinical studies to predict the disposition of Apo2L/tumor necrosis factor-related apoptosis-inducing ligand in humans: characterization of in vivo efficacy, pharmacokinetics, and safety. J Pharmacol Exp Ther 2001;299(1):31–38.
44. Meulemans A. A model of cefoperazone tissue penetration: diffusion coefficient and protein binding. Antimicrob Agents Chemother 1992;36(2):295–298.
45. Moussy Y, Hersh L, Dungel P. Distribution of [3H]dexamethasone in rat subcutaneous tissue after delivery from osmotic pumps. Biotechnol Prog 2006;22(3):819–824.

2

CHALLENGES OF DRUG DELIVERY

Patricia R. Wardwell and Rebecca A. Bader

Syracuse Biomaterials Institute, Syracuse University, Syracuse, NY, USA

2.1 INTRODUCTION

Recent advances in drug development have led to the discovery and production of a variety of therapeutic molecules with the potential to target and treat many diseases [1]. Their use is somewhat limited, however, by the drug delivery methods available today and by the obstacles put in place by the human body. The body is essentially a complex network of compartments within which the desired sites of action lie. In order to reach these targets, the drug molecules have to cross a variety of boundaries, usually in the form of epithelial or mucosal barriers, as well as face exposure to a harsh environment of degrading enzymes and varying pH levels [2]. In including hydrodynamic radius, charge, hydrophilicity, and permeability can sometimes affect movement [3]. The impact of these obstacles on bioavailability differs among users, and, consequently the therapeutic efficacy is likewise variable [4].

In general, the ability of the drug molecule to reach its target organ and have the desired effect is hindered by obstacles that can be broken into three interrelated categories: (i) *in vivo* drug solubility, (ii) *in vivo* drug stability, and (iii) physical barriers to absorption (Fig. 2.1) [5, 6]. In order to travel to the site of action and have maximum

Engineering Polymer Systems for Improved Drug Delivery, First Edition.
Edited by Rebecca A. Bader and David A. Putnam.
© 2014 John Wiley & Sons, Inc. Published 2014 by John Wiley & Sons, Inc.

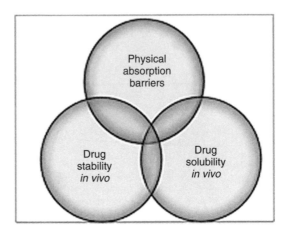

Figure 2.1. Several intertwined factors affecting the design of a drug delivery system.

efficacy, the drug must be soluble and stable within the aqueous environment of the body. Furthermore, soluble and stable therapeutic agents are better able to permeate the physical barriers that hinder absorption. On the basis of the obstacles introduced above, development and enhancement of methods for improving delivery of therapeutic molecules that lack stability and solubility is imperative. Many methods for improved delivery rely on polymer-based compounds in the form of (i) implantable networks for controlled release; (ii) carrier systems including nanoparticles, liposomes, and micelles for therapeutic encapsulation; and (iii) polymer–drug conjugates. Each of these topics will be explored in depth in subsequent chapters.

This chapter will provide an overview of the various physical and chemical challenges encountered in the physiological environment that prevent therapeutics from reaching the site of action. Additionally, the concept of dosing maintenance and the therapeutic window will be explored. Finally, a brief introduction will be given on how polymer-based carrier systems and polymer conjugates can be used to overcome these barriers.

2.2 HISTORY AND CHALLENGES OF DRUG DELIVERY

With the advancement of science, the discovery of potential drug molecules is increasing. However, owing to the complexity of both the human body and the drug molecules themselves, application of new therapeutics in and of themselves is somewhat limited. Thus, as new drug discoveries were made, advances in delivery mechanisms became increasingly necessary [7]. To optimize efficacy and minimize negative effects, a high concentration of the nonmetabolized drug must reach the site of action preferentially over nontarget tissues [8].

As discussed in Chapter 1, the advent of new delivery systems started in the mid-1900s. Until then, most drugs were delivered through conventional methods such as injections (parentaral, intramuscular, subcutaneous), oral delivery (solutions, tablets), or transdermal application in the form of a cream or ointment [9]. Each of these methods, although effective at the time, comes with disadvantages. The injection route is painful, invasive, and often requires administration by a trained clinician; thus patient compliance is low, resulting in reduced therapeutic efficacy [10]. Additionally, as the drug is often injected directly into the blood stream, the effect is somewhat short lived, thereby reducing the potential for sustained effect. Oral delivery methods are associated with high patient compliance, but many drug molecules cannot survive the harsh environment of the gut or be absorbed through the intestinal epithelial barrier [11, 12]. Topical delivery, again, generally improves patient compliance, but this method is limited to local delivery, as many therapeutics cannot diffuse through the protective layers of the epidermis [13]. Drug delivery systems aim to mitigate the limitations of these conventional delivery methods.

In the 1950s, a breakthrough in drug delivery systems was made with the Wurster process (see Chapter 1) [14]. This in turn led to the development of other microencapsulation methods. In the late 1960s, Alejandro Zaffaroni, a pioneer in drug delivery research, designed the first controlled release drug delivery system in the form of a transdermal patch [15]. His research is considered by many to have laid the foundation of all subsequent drug delivery research.

Liposomal systems were also developed in the 1960s for controlled release. A liposome is an artificial vesicle made from two lipid bilayers, resulting in a hydrophilic outer shell and an inner core, with a hydrophobic layer between the two. The dual attitude toward water allows the encapsulation of both hydrophobic and hydrophilic drug molecules within the carrier system. Current liposomal systems incorporate poly(ethylene glycol) (PEG) to reduce undesired uptake by the reticuloendothelial system (RES). Liposomes are beyond the scope of this chapter, but are covered in depth in References 16–20.

Polymer–drug conjugates, also referred to as polymeric prodrugs, with a variety of architectures have been explored as drug delivery systems. Through conjugation, the drug molecule can be held in an inactive form until release at the site of action, thereby reducing nonspecific toxicity and enhancing therapeutic efficacy. Conjugation can likewise increase therapeutic stability and solubility. These concepts will be discussed further in Chapters 4 and 7 on polymer–drug conjugates and dendrimers, respectively. Drug delivery systems, particularly those based on polymers, have allowed scientists to overcome the barriers frequently encountered in vivo.

2.3 PHYSICAL BARRIERS

In order to reach the systemic circulation and/or the site of action, all molecules must cross a series of physiological barriers, particularly epithelial, mucosal, and endothelial membranes. These membranes exist throughout the body, with varying complexity, thickness, and permeability [21]. Membrane properties allow some molecules to cross easily, while others are not able to cross them at all. The barriers to drug delivery, and their associated properties, will be discussed in detail in this section.

2.3.1 Epithelial Membranes

Epithelial membranes line the interior and exterior of numerous organs. As individual organs serve distinct purposes and functions, epithelial membranes differ in cellular morphology and arrangement. The epithelium functions mainly in protection and transport, but also assists in the regulation of secretion, absorption, excretion, filtration, and diffusion of molecules, such as nutrients, waste, and drugs [22, 23]. As shown in Fig. 2.2, epithelial cells can be categorized as squamous, cuboidal, or columnar on the basis of their shape [24]. These cells can be arranged into layers by a process known as stratification. Squamous cells are generally flat and wide, as illustrated in Fig. 2.2a and b. Consequently, these cells are typically found in areas with a high amount of material exchange. The lungs, for example, utilize a simple squamous epithelium

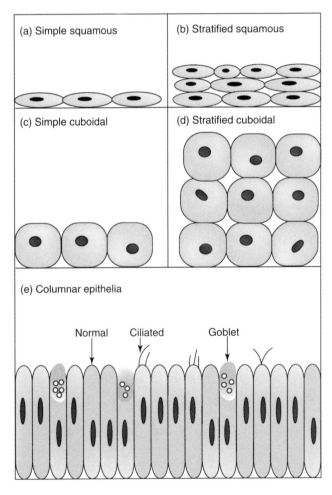

Figure 2.2. Epithelial cell classification by morphology and alignment.

(Fig. 2.2a) to allow rapid exchange of gases, as thinner membranes are easier to cross. Cuboidal cells (Fig. 2.2c and d) are most commonly found in the epidermis and mainly function as structural maintenance cells. Like the simple squamous cells of the lungs, columnar epithelial cells (Fig. 2.2e) are also found in areas that require a large surface area for material exchange; however, this morphology facilitates greater regulation of the exchange. As columnar cells are more elongated than squamous cells, they allow an increased number of lateral cell junctions which regulate the connectivity of the membrane. For example, a simple columnar epithelium is found in the small intestine to allow the absorption of ingested nutrients. Columnar epithelial cells can be specialized with cilia that sweep unwanted particles away from the area, thereby enhancing the protective nature of the membrane. Ciliated columnar cells are found in other areas aside from the small intestine, including the respiratory passages. Additionally, specialized cells known as goblet cells are often scattered among other columnar epithelial cells. As will be discussed further below, goblet cells secrete mucus which protects the body from potential pathogens and provides a medium for transport. As a general rule, as the complexity of an epithelial membrane increases, the permeability of molecules, including drugs, decreases.

Contact between neighboring epithelial cells is provided by several types of cell junctions, which can reduce permeability of the membrane to select molecules. These junctions include tight junctions, adherens junctions, desmosomes, and gap junctions (Fig. 2.3). Tight junctions are paracellular connections, often found toward the apical

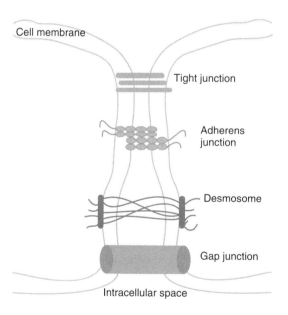

Figure 2.3. Tight junctions, adherens junctions, desmosomes, and gap junctions serving as connections between epithelial cells and acting to reduce the membrane permeability of molecules.

surface, that seal off the pathway between cells, thereby preventing harmful substances and therapeutic molecules from traveling through the membrane [25]. Tight junctions are composed of transmembrane proteins with adhesive properties, including occludins, claudins, and the recently discovered tricellulin [25]. Adherens junctions are typically located below the tight junctions. The primary components of these cells are cadherins, which are adhering proteins requiring the presence of calcium to maintain adhesiveness. These junctions include actin and myosin filaments on the intracellular side of the membrane, resulting in an ability to generate contractile force, which in turn acts to control and maintain the cell's proper shape and tension. The combination of tight and adherens junctions is referred to as the junctional complex [25]. Desmosomes are the next type of junctions found moving away from the apical surface. Desmosomes are also composed of calcium-dependent adhesive molecules; however, they are specifically called desmosomal cadherins. Desmosomes primary job is to connect epithelial cells to each other on the lateral surface, giving the membrane strength and durability. They differ from tight junctions in their level of permeability. As desmosomes' primary function is not to create a seal between two compartments, the level of permeability is much higher. Unlike the other junctions discussed in this section, gap junctions allow transport between cells and do not have a significant role in strengthening cell–cell structural connections. They can be thought of as small, water-filled channels spanning the intracellular space between two adjacent cells. The channels themselves are composed of proteins called connexins, which assemble to form a ring structure and are able to span the intracellular space.

The major limiting factor to absorption of orally administered drugs is the low permeability of the gastrointestinal epithelial membrane [26]. Within the gastrointestinal tract, drug absorption occurs primarily in the lower portions of the small intestine where the tight junctions and, consequently, the epithelium are most permeable [27]. This leakiness of tight junctions is associated with a decreased transepithelial electrical resistance (TEER). The realization of the importance of tight junctions and TEER in transepithelial movement has led to the development of several methods to enhance permeability. For example, several investigators have found methods to target occludins and cladins, the primary proteins involved in tight junctions [28, 29]. While useful for drug delivery applications, the disruption of tight junctions also reduces the protective function of the epithelial membrane; therefore, application of tight-junction modulation must be highly specific and easily reversible.

Rather than targeting intercellular delivery through the tight junctions, other investigators in the realm of drug delivery have focused on enhancing absorption through the primary columnar epithelial cells of the intestine, namely the enterocytes. Enterocytes possess villi and microvilli on the apical surface, which increases the surface area for absorption [30]. Among enterocytes are specialized cells known as M cells, or membranous cells. They typically are found covering what are known as Peyers patches, sections of lymphoid tissue. M cells present antigens that can be targeted to enhance the efficiency of the transcytosis of macromolecules and nonbioactive molecules compared to enterocytes [31]. Enterocytes produce the glycoprotein enzymes necessary for transporting materials across the epithelia. Recently, enterocytes were found to express many of the same drug-metabolizing enzymes originally thought to be found only in the liver [32]. Actions such as co-administration of enzyme competitor molecules to decrease the catalytic activity of enzymes (belonging to the cytochrome P450 family, see Section 2.3.1) on the primary administered drug can be taken to enhance absorption and efficacy. Absorption can be further hindered by other columnar epithelial cells, goblet cells, and ciliated epithelial cells [33]. Goblet cells secrete mucus, which forms the basis of the mucosal membrane, as discussed below. Ciliated cells hinder absorption through the enterocytes by creating drug molecule movement [33].

Transdermal drug delivery is another favored noninvasive route of administration hindered by the relative impermeability of the epithelial membrane. The major limiting factor of transdermal delivery is the outermost layer of skin known as the stratum corneum. This layer is 10–20 μm thick and can be thought of as a brick-and-mortar type of system, where the bricks are the cells, composed mainly of cross-linked keratin, and the mortar is a dense mass of extracellular matrix proteins and lipids. This architecture requires drug transport to take a tortuous path of diffusion through the intercellular lipid mass. Thus, only a limited number of molecules, specifically those that are lipophilic, have a low effective dosing requirement, and possess a molecular weight of less than 500 Da, can travel in this route [34]. Below the stratum corneum is the avascular epidermis, composed primarily of squamous epithelial cells near the stratum corneum and cuboidal epithelial cells approaching the dermis [35]. The epidermis provides another nonvascularized barrier that must be traversed by the drug before reaching the dermis, which is the desired destination of most transdermally administered drugs. This is the inner most layer of the skin epithelium containing blood vessels and nerve endings [34].

2.3.2 Endothelial Membranes

Drugs that enter and exit systemic circulation must cross the endothelial barrier provided by the blood vessels. The anatomy of blood vessels varies with the type; however, each artery, vein, and capillary consists of a thin inner membrane of squamous endothelial cells, which provides the main barrier to drug absorption [36]. In most healthy systemic vessels, this endothelial sheet is continuous with cells, connected by impermeable tight junctions and adherens junctions.

Capillaries, consisting of a single endothelial membrane and a small amount of connective tissue, are the most common type of blood vessel and the site of blood/tissue–material exchange. Therefore, capillaries are of interest in many drug delivery applications. The capillary endothelium can be targeted using ligands specific to receptors expressed by endothelial cells. Angiogenic vessels associated with tumors and inflamed tissue provide several examples of the specific targeting idea. For instance, the endothelium of newly formed vessels often overexpress key proteins and molecules, including the vascular endothelial growth factor (VEGF), adhesion molecules such as the vascular adhesion molecule (VCAM), and e-selectin [37]. Atherosclerosis, a disease characterized by vascular inflammation, stiffening, and plaque buildup, also is characterized by upregulated adhesion molecules (VCAM-1, ICAM-1, selectins). Potential plaque "rupture" provides further prospective targets as proteins such as fibrin are released into the vessel near the plaque [38]. Additionally, endothelial cells contain vesicles specifically designed to transport materials across the cytoplasm [39]. In highly angiogenic states, as often associated with pathologies such as tumor growth and inflammation, the capillary endothelium becomes increasingly discontinuous. This discontinuity, which results from the rapid and somewhat disorganized assembly of vessels, can be used to facilitate enhanced permeation and retention (EPR) of drug molecules, as will be discussed in subsequent sections [39].

2.3.3 Mucosal Membranes

Many epithelial layers, particularly the gastrointestinal tract membrane, are accompanied by another barrier membrane known as the mucosal membrane. The mucosal membrane contains a viscoelastic gel-like substance, namely mucus, comprised of the glycoprotein mucin. The mucosal membrane has several physical and chemical properties that affect the absorption and bioavailability of therapeutics [40]. For example, the diffusion coefficient of various macromolecular compounds, including therapeutics, is typically 30–50% of that of the same compounds in an aqueous environment [41, 42]. Furthermore, mucosal membranes can serve as physical barriers to absorption. The viscoelastic properties of mucus result in entrapment of compounds and agglomeration of particles. This agglomeration effectively increases the size of compounds and, thus, contributes to the reduction in the diffusion coefficients [42].

The decrease in diffusion coefficients of agglomerated drug/mucin particles indicates a general size restriction for diffusion through mucus. This can be described by the Stokes–Einstein equation (Eqs. (2.1 and 2.2)) [40].

$$D = \left(\frac{kT}{6\eta\pi r} \right) \tag{2.1}$$

$$P = \left(\frac{kT}{6\eta\pi rh} \right) \tag{2.2}$$

2.3.4 Routes of Transport

There are several classifications regarding how a molecule moves across biological barriers. Active transport (requiring an energy input) and passive transport (not requiring an energy input) are the two main categories of movement, with passive transport having numerous subcategories. Transport mechanisms can also be divided into paracellular (between cells) and transcellular (through cells) routes. Figure 2.4 provides a pictorial representation of the different transport routes.

The structure of the cell membrane plays an important role in drug transport. Cell membranes are composed of phospholipid bilayers, with hydrophilic head groups on the edges and hydrophobic tails composing the core. This structure imposes the following limitations on the types of drugs that can cross the membrane by transcellular passive diffusion: (i) the drug must be lipid-soluble, (ii) the drug must possess a low molecular weight, and (iii) the drug must be in a position to travel from an area of high concentration to an area of low concentration. Drugs can also cross a membrane

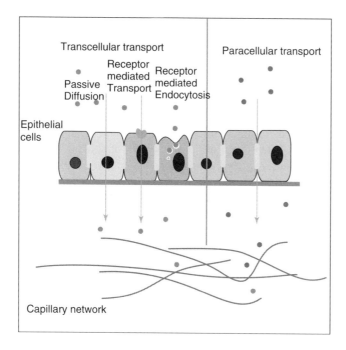

Figure 2.4. General paths a drug molecule can take to cross a membrane. Typically, small, polar molecules (light gray dots) can passively diffuse across an epithelial membrane by passing between the cells. This is particularly prevalent in the lower portions of the small intestine. Lipid-soluble molecules have the ability to diffuse across a membrane but not between cells (gray dots).

by passive diffusion paracellularly. This type of transport requires the drug molecule to be water soluble and of low molecular weight, and traveling along a concentration gradient. In both paracellular and transcellular passive diffusion, the driving force is the concentration gradient. The concentration gradient is the fundamental idea behind all types of diffusion, as shown by the Fick's law discussed in Chapter 1. Depending on the cellular architecture of the barrier, the drug molecule may have to diffuse through or between more than one layer of cells. Under these circumstances, each different layer must be accounted for, resulting in an effective barrier to drug absorption. For a given drug molecule undergoing passive diffusion, the rate of absorption will be linear with respect to the concentration [43].

A variation of passive diffusion is a process known as facilitated diffusion. This process still relies on the concentration gradient as the driving force and requires no energy input; however, membrane-embedded proteins are required for entry to the cell. Facilitated diffusion can be thought of as belonging to two different categories as well: carrier-mediated transport and channel-mediated transport. Carrier-mediated transport requires transport proteins that function by binding to the molecule to be transported, moving across the membrane, and releasing it on the other side. No direct change is made to the transport protein in this process. These proteins are structurally selective for the drugs that they transport and are saturable. Thus, the maximum rate of absorption will be dependent on the concentration of receptor, not on the concentration of the drug [44]. Channel-mediated diffusion requires continuous aqueous pores spanning a lipid bilayer membrane. Charged or polar drugs are able to travel through these channels faster than by passive diffusion through the membrane; therefore, the rate of drug absorption is increased [44].

The transport mechanisms discussed above rely on the concentration gradient for the driving force and therefore do not require any outside input of energy. In contrast, active transport most often refers to the movement of solute against a concentration gradient but does require an energy input. In drug delivery applications, active transport typically refers to transmembrane pumps that use adenosine triphosphate (ATP) to transport drug molecules from areas of low concentration to areas of high concentration. Protein pumps can move molecules either into or out of a cell and are also crucial in maintaining ion balances across membranes. Some examples of transmembrane protein pumps include the sodium potassium pump (Na+/K+), the sodium hydrogen pump in the gastrointestinal tract, and the calcium ion pump [44, 45].

2.3.5   The Blood–Brain Barrier

The blood–brain barrier (BBB) is a general term for the system of membranes acting in a protective manner to keep the central nervous system (CNS) impermeable to molecules from the systemic circulation. The CNS is the most convenient route of delivery for therapeutics capable of treating nervous system disorders, including stroke, many types of cancer, Alzheimer's disease, and the human immunodeficiency virus (HIV) [46]. Unfortunately, the physiology of the BBB makes transport into the CNS from systemic circulation difficult. The BBB is comprised mainly of cerebral microvascular endothelial cells, which give rise to structural differences in brain capillaries compared to other systemic capillaries. As shown in Fig. 2.5, endothelial cells

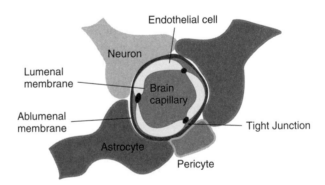

Figure 2.5. Representative cross-sectional view of the blood–brain barrier. The BBB is comprised of the endothelial cells of brain capillaries connected by nearly impermeable tight junctions. Additionally, the astrocytes, pericytes, and neurons lining the capillaries further hinder transport of drugs into the central nervous system (CNS).

lining the brain capillaries contain tight junctions, creating a less permeable barrier between the blood and the CNS [47]. Non-brain capillaries contain endothelial cells as well, but the spaces between them generally contain more, and larger, openings than brain capillaries. As a result, molecules less than 500 Da can passively diffuse through the openings and reach the tissues. In contrast, the tight-junction-regulated brain capillaries do not allow diffusion between cells, leaving only membrane diffusion as a means of transport into the brain [48]. Small (<500 Da) lipophilic drug molecules have the best chance of achieving transport with this process [48]. This requires solutes to diffuse through two membranes; the lumenal and ablumenal membranes of the endothelium. Furthermore, surrounding the ablumenal membrane of the capillary are astrocytes, pericytes, and neurons, which provide additional membrane barriers between the systemic and brain blood flows [49].

A number of transmembrane transport systems are present in the endothelial cells of the BBB. These transporters are generally facilitative, with the main function being to allow the uptake of nutrients [50]. These transport systems can be exploited in applications to improve delivery to the BBB. In addition to facilitative transport systems, transmembrane transport systems exist within the endothelial cell layer that function to keep the molecules out. Known as efflux pumps, these transport systems are also present in the intestinal tract and liver. Many efflux transport pumps employ ATP hydrolysis as energy to power the pump, and thus are termed the ATP binding cassette family proteins, or ABC transporters. This class of proteins is very large and structurally diverse, giving rise to individual ABC pump subfamilies. The subfamilies are denoted with the letters A–G, and are distinguished from each other by the types of drugs they transport. In general, ABC substrates are typically hydrophobic or amphipathic, and the differences that distinguish the substrates of each subfamily are subtle. For example, lipids, bile salts, and peptides are all transported by subfamilies A, B, and G. Additionally, organic anions, as well as conjugates with anionic residues such as glutathione, sulfate, or glucuronyl have receptor specificity for ABCC [51, 52]. In addition to the discussion here, efflux pumps will be covered in further detail in Section 2.3.1.

P-glycoprotein (P-gp) is a well-characterized efflux pump present in the BBB. This protein is associated with the expression of the multidrug resistant gene family (MDR family). A variety of lipophilic drugs have been identified as substrates for P-gp. For example, cyclosporine A (CysA), an immunosuppressive agent, has been shown to be hindered by P-gp when crossing the BBB. However, in the presence of agents shown to suppress the MDR genes, including chlorpromazine and various steroid hormones, uptake of CysA can be significantly improved [53]. P-gp is a transporter present in many other tissues, including the liver, intestines, and kidneys, and will be further discussed in Section 2.4.1.

2.4 METABOLIC AND CHEMICAL CONCERNS

The mechanism of transport of drug in the body depends on several chemical and physical properties, including the molecular weight, hydrodynamic radius, lipid solubility, partition coefficient, and polarity [54]. To affect the target tissue, a drug must enter the cells in an active form. In general, drugs are metabolized, resulting in either a decrease in the usable concentration of drug molecules or an increase in the amount of metabolite concentration which will have an undesirable effect on the target tissue. Knowledge of the physiochemical properties of drug molecules *in vivo* is essential for predicting their therapeutic efficacy. This section will discuss the effects of drug metabolism on drug absorption, including the use of transport proteins and enzymes to hinder or aid absorption.

2.4.1 The First-Pass Effect

First-pass metabolism (first-pass effect) occurs mostly in oral delivery applications when the concentration of the administered therapeutic is reduced by metabolic efforts of the body before systemic circulation is reached. The principal organs involved in first-pass metabolism are the small intestine and the liver [55].

2.4.1.1 Enzymatic Hepatic Metabolism. Despite the several barriers to absorption in the intestine, many drugs are able to cross the epithelium and enter systemic circulation. However, they are not yet ready to travel to the site of action and effect a response. All drugs absorbed through the intestinal epithelium are carried to the liver via the hepatic portal vein. The liver is responsible for breakdown and metabolism of a variety of substances synthesized by an individual, including steroids, sterols, bile acids, and eicosanoids. Though vital for normal function, the liver provides an undeniable barrier to drug delivery. Drug molecules with structural or chemical properties similar to those of the natural liver substrates will be metabolized in the liver via the same metabolic pathways. Some drugs (e.g., the glyceryl trinitrate, used to treat angina, and lidocaine, an analgesic) are rendered useless when delivered orally because of extensive metabolism by the liver [56].

The cytochrome P450 (CYP) enzyme family is the major source of enzyme activity involved in hepatic metabolism. The CYP450 family is a large gene family composed of 57 different members. The majority (70–80%) of phase-1 drug metabolism is carried out by about 15 of these, belonging to classes designated CYP1 and CYP3. Phase-1 metabolism refers to modifications of the basic structure of a drug molecule. CYP enzymes can catalyze modifications, including hydroxylation, O, S, and N dealkylation, oxidation, demethylation, and deamination. The results of these modifications are structurally changed metabolites, which are either eliminated immediately, are used as substrates for phase-2 metabolism, or retain the ability to be therapeutically active. Codeine, for example, typically undergoes an O-demethylation catalyzed by CYP2D6, resulting in a structural change to morphine, a drug with an increased activity level [56]. Although the goal of phase-1 metabolism is generally to detoxify compounds transported in the bloodstream, the opposite effect can sometimes occur, resulting in a secondary metabolite that is more toxic than the original drug molecule. For instance, phase-1 metabolism of the chemotherapeutic Tamoxifin results in a metabolite with genotoxic hepatocarcinogenic properties. In instances such as this, phase-2 metabolism is extremely important in preventing the toxic molecule from not only damaging the liver but also entering systemic circulation once again [57].

Phase-2 metabolism is carried out by a class of enzymes known as transferases. As the name implies, transferases catalyze the transfer of material. In the case of drug metabolism, the transferase catalyzes the transfer of a hydrophilic moiety from a donor molecule to the metabolite molecule, typically reducing the toxicity or allowing neutralization reactions to occur. Like the CYP enzymes, transferases are also typically thought of as gene superfamilies. Some of the major transferase families include glutathione-S transferase (GST), sulfotransferase (SULT), N-acetyltransferase (NAT), and UDP-glucuronosyltransferase (UGT). GST catalyzes reactions with nonpolar compounds, SULT results in sulfation of steroid hormones and bile acids, NAT results in acetylation of amine groups, and UGT leads to glucuronidation of molecules, such as the hepatic product bilirubin, pain reliever acetaminophen (toxic in instances of overdose), pain reliever morphine, and other nonsteroidal anti-inflammatory drugs (NSAIDs) [56]. Toxicity of a phase-1 metabolism byproduct is highly dependent on its rate of production in relation to its rate of reaction with phase-2 metabolizing transferases.

2.4.1.2 Enzymatic Intestinal Metabolism.
In addition to physical barriers preventing absorption, metabolic enzymes, including lipases, proteases, and glycosidases, are present in the gastrointestinal tract to breakdown ingested food and release energy and nutrients [58]. While highly efficient at providing energy and nutrients, these enzymes are also responsible for the degradation of drug products, preventing absorption and/or resulting in a loss of function. Two major proteins responsible for metabolizing drugs in the gastrointestinal tract are CYP3A and the P-gp efflux pump [59]. These complexes are found in several locations, including the intestine and liver. In the intestinal tract, they are often found within the membrane of individual enterocyte cells, which are the primary cells for drug absorption. Methods to circumvent CYP metabolism of drugs in the intestine include co-administration of a CYP inhibitor or inducer. A simple method of inhibition is the co-administration of a secondary drug which competes with the primary drug for access to the active site of a CYP enzyme. Drugs with a high affinity for CYP450 that can be used as secondary drugs for competition include cimetidine (used to treat ulcers), ketoconazole (used to treat fungal infections), and Indinavir, a protease inhibitor used to treat viral infections [56]. Additionally, a metabolite of the primary administered drug may sometimes form an inactive complex with the catalytic site of the CYP enzyme. This method of inhibition is often known as mechanism-based P450 inhibition [60]. CYP inhibitors decrease the effect of the enzyme, allowing increased absorption of drugs, including sirolimus, cyclosporine, and tacrolimus [59].

The most prevalent and important enzyme of the CYP family in intestinal metabolism of drug molecules is CYP3A4. Found in large quantities in the liver, CYP3A4 is also present in the jejunum portion of the small intestine, primarily located on the villi [30]. Studies have shown the enzyme activity and concentration of jejunum CYP3A4 to be equal to those of the microsomes of the liver [61]. CYP3A4 has a broad range of structurally diverse substrates, with an equally broad range of therapeutic function; however, hydrophobicity is a commonality across substrates. Biotransformation reactions of drug molecules by CYP enzymes are typically considered to be phase-1, referring to a basic structural change of the molecule [30].

2.4.2   Efflux Systems

Efflux systems are energy-dependent transport systems whose function is to protect the body by preventing harmful substances from traversing membranes and entering other body compartments [58]. They are present in many different areas of absorption, but play the most significant role in the gastrointestinal tract and the BBB. The most well-known and well-classified efflux pumps are members of the P-gp family, as mentioned previously. P-gp was first characterized as the transport system behind tumor resistance to chemotherapeutics, as it was able to transport the therapeutic agents out of the cell. This efflux pump is transcribed as a result of the multidrug resistant gene MDR-1 [30]. P-gp has a large variety of substrates, similar to CYP3A, many of which are large and amphipathic [59]. Additionally, in the intestine, expression of P-gp increases longitudinally throughout the tract, in contrast to the levels of CYP3A expression. This results in a constant source of molecular absorption prevention throughout the gastrointestinal tract, as P-gp's main effect is to pump drug molecules back into the lumen [11].

 In sum, the mechanism of membrane crossing for solutes traveling into the brain is usually by receptor-mediated transport or slow diffusion. Properties of drug molecules can be tailored to make crossing the BBB more feasible and efficient. If the molecular weight of the molecule in question falls at 500 ± 100 Da, the permeability of that molecule increases linearly with the partition coefficient of the molecule. This relationship can be shown graphically by constructing a plot of the log of permeability versus the log of the partition coefficient divided by the square root of the molecular weight, as described by Tsugi and Tamai and shown in Fig. 2.6 [53]. An alternative to the molecular weight explanation of decreased permeability is the presence of the P-gp efflux system. This system, also present in the gut, serves to restrict transcellular flux of drug molecules, thus decreasing permeability.

2.5   PHYSICAL PROPERTIES OF THERAPEUTICS

Several factors are involved in both the amount of and the extent to which a drug molecule will affect the target tissue. In addition to the physiological and chemical properties discussed previously, the route of administration and delivery method, dose and release profile, as well as physiology changes due to pathology play a role in determining the biological effect of a drug molecule.

2.5.1   Bioavailability

As discussed in Chapter 1, bioavailability is defined as the amount of drug reaching the systemic circulation out of the amount of drug that was administered [62]. Careful

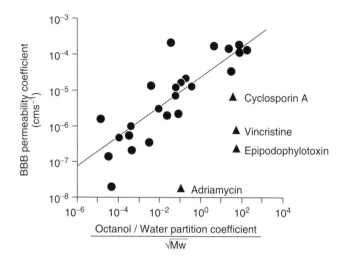

Figure 2.6. Permeability of the BBB shown to increase linearly with the partition coefficient relative to the square root of the molecule weight for drugs with a molecular weight of 500 ± 100 Da. P-gp efflux pump has been shown to account for discrepancies, as the outlier drugs in the graph are known to be P-gp substrates. Reprinted from Reference 53, Copyright (1997), with permission from Elsevier.

dosing and administration is necessary for efficacious treatment. The amount of drug available at the desired site of action must fall within the therapeutic window [4].

Achieving reproducible oral bioavailability is particularly difficult because there are several factors that must be considered on the basis of the path the drug must travel before reaching systemic circulation. In this case, the overall bioavailability (F) is the product of the portion of drug absorbed (F_a), that is, the fraction that passes into the hepatic portal blood unaffected by the enzymes of the gut and intestine, and the fraction of drug that escapes metabolism by the liver (F_h) [30, 62]. This value will vary between drugs as a result of the differential effects of enzymes, including CYP and P-gp, on individual drugs.

In addition to the effect of the body's metabolism, properties of the drug molecule itself have a large impact. Solubility, for example, is one of the leading factors hindering oral absorption and reducing bioavailability, and a great deal of effort is being put into determining methods to increase solubility of therapeutics in aqueous environments [63]. For example, chemical modifications to the drug molecules to generate prodrugs with increased aqueous solubility are being explored, as are methods of solid dispersion. Solid dispersions typically consist of a hydrophilic matrix material with a hydrophobic drug dispersed throughout. The result is an increased dissolution rate and higher bioavailability of hydrophobic drugs. The degree of therapeutic solubility (or dissolution rate) is dependent on the diffusion coefficient of the drug, the concentration of the drug within the dissolution medium, and the solubility of the drug within the dissolution medium. Additionally, physical factors, including the surface area of the formulation available for dissolution and the thickness of the diffusion boundary the drug must travel through, must be accounted for [64].

2.5.2 Release Profiles

The amount of drug released into the bloodstream over time is known as the release profile. Release profiles typically depend on the dosage form of the drug, the method of release, and the properties of the carrier system. These release profiles are often categorized as controlled release, pulsatile release, and burst release, as shown in Fig. 2.7. Controlled release is characterized by a gradual increase in the plasma concentration with time until a maintenance concentration is reached. This is often the desired treatment method, although somewhat more difficult to attain. Pulsatile release similarly begins with an increase in plasma concentration to a desired level, followed by decreases in concentration, which are counteracted with additional dosing, thereby maintaining the concentration within the therapeutic window. Burst release consists of an initial dose generating a steep rise in plasma concentration. When the drug begins to dissipate, however, it is not supplemented with additional doses, resulting in a short time period when the plasma concentration is within the designated therapeutic window [65].

Of particular importance are the carrier system properties that modulate how the drug molecules are released. Diffusion always plays a role in drug release; however, depending on the properties of the source (i.e., the carrier system), the concentration profile will differ. The two primary methods of degradation are bulk and surface erosion (Fig. 2.8). Surface erosion results in a reduction of the overall volume of the carrier system as degradation occurs at the surface of the material. This also results in a turnover of the surface; a new layer of the material is constantly being exposed to the

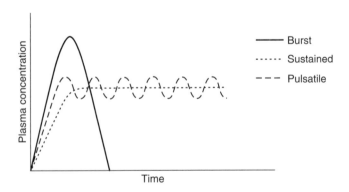

Figure 2.7. Three release profiles commonly observed for drug carrier systems. Sustained/controlled release is characterized by an increase in plasma concentration until a desired maintenance concentration is reached. Pulsatile release is characterized by a cyclic fluctuation in plasma concentration. Burst release is characterized by a large initial increase in plasma concentration, followed by a sharp decline.

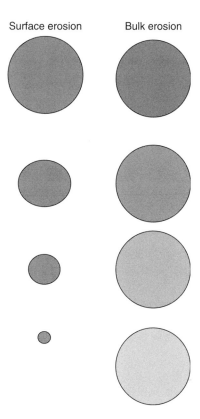

Figure 2.8. Surface and bulk erosion as two methods for degradation of carrier systems. Surface erosion results in a decrease in overall volume, shown here by a reduction in size. Bulk erosion results in a decrease in the amount of material within the matrix.

environment. In contrast, bulk erosion does not result in a volume reduction; rather, the material is lost uniformly throughout the entire volume of the carrier system [66].

Different applications require different release profiles, but, as mentioned previously, a sustained plasma concentration is generally most desirable. For example, release of drugs dispersed within polymer constructs, as will be covered in subsequent sections, is dependent on the rate of degradation of the polymer substrate, as well as on the diffusion rate of the drug. If the degradation rate is slower than the diffusion rate, the release will follow the pattern of bulk erosion. If polymer degradation is faster than the diffusion rate, the release will follow the pattern of surface erosion [67].

2.6 POLYMER CARRIERS AS A SOLUTION TO CHALLENGES

The term "polymer" refers to a long-chain molecule composed of many repeating molecules. Polymer encapsulation of and/or modification to drug molecules increases

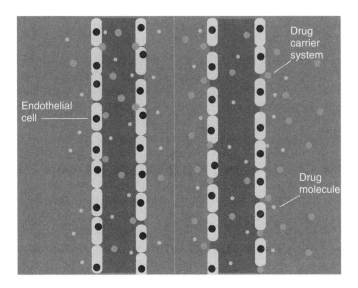

Figure 2.9. Enhanced permeation and retention (EPR) facilitating passive targeting of drug delivery systems. (a) Vessels within healthy tissue have narrow gaps between endothelial cells. (b) Vessels within diseased tissue have larger ("leaky") gaps.

the circulation time of the drugs in the body by increasing their size, thereby decreasing the amount of filtration by the kidneys [1]. Additionally, targeting of drugs to specific sites of pathology can be improved by the increase in size through a phenomenon referred to as enhanced permeation and retention or EPR [2]. For example, cancer tumors and sites of inflammation show increased angiogenesis and a characteristic "leaky" vessel endothelium (Fig. 2.9). The leaky vasculature is caused by rapid and disorganized vessel formation, which results in larger pore spaces between endothelial cells. Polymeric drug delivery systems may be taken into the tissue by transcellular transport, but this is a time-dependent process and generally not efficient. In diseased tissue, however, the larger gaps between vascular endothelial cells allow relatively easy uptake of the drug carriers [2].

In general, polymer carrier systems should have several common characteristics. These characteristics include (i) an ability to be produced easily and on a large scale, (ii) applicability to a wide range of drugs, (iii) physiological stability, (iv) biocompatibility, and (v) acceptability by regulatory committees, such as the U.S. Food and Drug Administration (FDA) [3].

2.6.1 Colloidal Polymer Carrier Systems

Several kinds of polymer carrier systems can be utilized for drug delivery applications to help avoid some of the previously discussed challenges. In general, colloidal polymer carrier systems are small, spherical particles with varying layers and thicknesses [1]. The spherical particle shape of these formulations increases the surface area of

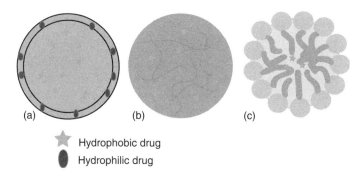

Figure 2.10. Colloidal polymer carrier systems. (a) Liposomes. (b) Nanoparticles. (c) Micelles.

the system, allowing increased absorption. Different particle carrier systems include micelles, liposomes, and nanoparticles [4]. Simplified versions of these carrier systems are depicted in Fig. 2.10 and discussed in depth in subsequent chapters.

Micelles are small, soluble particles that can self-assemble by means of hydrophilic/hydrophobic segregation. In addition to hydrophobic interactions, electrostatic interactions, metal complexation, and hydrogen bonding may contribute to micelle formation [2]. A block copolymer with separate hydrophobic and hydrophilic segments will have the ability to assemble in a hydrated environment such that the hydrophobic segments form a core in the center and the hydrophilic segments form a shell surrounding the particle, thus greatly increasing the aqueous solubility of hydrophobic therapeutics. A popular choice for hydrophilic block copolymer sections is PEG, a widely used polymer in drug delivery applications and the gold standard for "stealth cloaking" of carrier systems. Stealth cloaking is a means of avoiding nonspecific uptake once administered, and functions by creating an aqueous layer around the particle to avoid detection by the immune system [5]. Nonspecific uptake by the RES is a major obstacle to micelles and other small colloidal carrier systems. The RES is part of the body's defense mechanism and includes cells such as macrophages and monocytes. These cells are phagocytic in nature, and function by engulfing potential threatening substances, eventually accumulating in the liver and spleen for degradation and elimination [6]. This poses a problem for drug carrier systems because uptake by these cells will reduce the amount of therapeutic in the systemic circulation [6]. Poly-L-amino acids, such as poly(D,L-lactic acid) (PDLLA), are frequently used as the hydrophobic portion of micellar block copolymers. For example, Genexol PM, a PEG–PDLLA copolymer micelle loaded with the chemotherapeutic paclitaxel, is currently approved in Korea for the treatment of breast cancer and is undergoing clinical trials in the United States for use in pancreatic cancer treatment [7]. Micelle formation is influenced by factors such as the molecular weight of the copolymer, the ratio of copolymer blocks to each other, and the amount of polymer involved. The minimal amount of polymer necessary to form a micelle is referred to as the critical micelle concentration (CMC)

[8]. Above this concentration, all additional polymer molecules will be formed into micelles.

Nanoparticle-based drug delivery systems consist of submicrometer-sized spherical particles, ranging from 10 to 1000 nm, although the desired size is often around 100 nm [9]. Nanoparticles are typically made of a biocompatible, degradable material and contain drugs either dispersed or dissolved within a core matrix. Two classes of nanoparticles have been identified on the basis of the way the drug is incorporated. *Nanocapsules* contain drug molecules confined to the interior of the polymeric shell of the particle, while with *nanospheres* the drug molecules are uniformly dispersed within the polymeric matrix system [10]. Once inside the body, drugs can be released from the particles by means of diffusion, degradation, swelling, or erosion. Efficacy of nanoparticle carrier systems is based on the size, particle stability, the amount of drug that can be incorporated, the type of drug that can be incorporated (i.e., hydrophilic or hydrophobic drug molecules, siRNAs or DNA for gene therapy, or proteins), and the potential for different routes of administration (i.e., oral delivery, inhalation, intravenous). Nanoparticles have been shown to be more effective in intravenous delivery than microparticles, which have an increased potential of becoming trapped in the capillaries, some of which are only 5–6 μm in diameter. In addition, *in vitro* studies with Caco2 intestinal cells demonstrated that 100 nm particles result in a 2.5-fold increase in uptake compared to 1 μm diameter particles and a sixfold increase in uptake compared to 10 μm particles [11]. Furthermore, particles smaller than 200 nm have the ability to escape processing of the liver and kidney for several circulation cycles, increasing their time in the systemic circulation and hence the level of effectiveness [12]. However, a diameter larger than 200 nm will increase the risk for RES uptake, reducing the circulation time and thus the efficacy.

As mentioned in brief previously, materials used to generate the nanoparticle systems must be nontoxic, nonimmunogenic, noninflammatory, and nonthrombogenic (all of which fall under the general category of biocompatibility). Additionally, the nanoparticles must be stable and able to avoid detection and uptake by the RES and to be used as carrier systems for a broad array of drug types, including proteins, nucleic acids, and hydrophilic and hydrophobic drug molecules [6]. Some commonly used materials for the generation of nanoparticle systems include poly(lactide) (PLA), poly(glycolide) (PGA), poly(lactide-*co*-glycolide) (PLGA), poly(cyanoacrylates), and poly(caprolactone) [6, 9]. Currently, there are no approved drug-encapsulated nanoparticles or on-going human clinical trials in the United States, although a great deal of research and development regarding nanoparticle formulations is ongoing.

Liposomes are another form of small, spherical drug carrier systems. They consist of a lipid bilayer (similar to a cell membrane) surrounding an interior space. This morphology allows the entrapment and delivery of both hydrophilic and hydrophobic drug molecules. Hydrophobic molecules can be entrapped within the bilayer, while hydrophilic molecules can be carried within the core. The physiochemical properties of the liposomal constituents, including the membrane fluidity, permeability, charge density, and steric hindrance, have influence on the types of interactions the liposomes will have with blood and tissue constituents [13].

There are several different types of liposomes. Long-circulating liposomes (LCLs) can be formed by incorporating hydrophilic polymers into the lipid bilayer to create an aqueous coat on the surface, which prevents marking by immune system opsonins and thereby reduces uptake by the RES. An example of this modification is called PEGylation, where chains of PEG are attached to the particle surface [14]. As discussed above, "stealth" PEG coating generates an aqueous layer. Additionally, LCLs can be tailored with ligands to target specific cell types. For example, LCLs prepared with a PEG coating and loaded with Doxorubicin, an anticancer chemotherapeutic, were approved by the FDA in 1995. The efficacy of this system has been further improved via linkage to mAb 2C5, a monoclonal antibody that specifically targets a variety of tumors [15].

Active cationic liposomes have a high affinity for cell membranes and deliver materials to cells by fusing with cell membranes and depositing material into the cell [13]. Nucleic acids are the most common therapeutic form delivered with cationic liposomes. As nucleic acids are negatively charged, stability is increased when complexed with cationic liposomes for delivery. Phase-1 clinical trials were completed for liposomes containing pGT-1, a regulatory gene involved in cystic fibrosis, to the respiratory epithelium. These studies have shown promising early results; however, the regulatory gene expression was fairly low and relatively short lived, despite efficient liposomal delivery [16].

2.6.2 Polymer–Drug Conjugates

Another method of increasing the targeting specificity of drug molecules and avoiding detection and subsequent elimination by the RES is to chemically conjugate polymers to drug molecules. Polymer conjugation serves several purposes. Many chemotherapeutic drugs are very cytotoxic, as their efficacy is generally dependent on their ability to cause death of cancerous cells. These same drugs are also often insoluble in aqueous environments, as found in the human body. Covalent attachment of a water-soluble polymer to an insoluble drug molecule increases the amount of therapeutic in circulation after administration [1]. In many cases, these polymer–drug conjugates undergo phase-1 metabolism to remove the inactive polymer and yield an active drug. A current example of a drug–polymer conjugate is poly(L-glutamic acid) (PG) conjugated to paclitaxel, yielding PG-TXL. Paclitaxel, a potent anticancer agent, is a molecule with poor aqueous solubility and fights cancer by attacking cellular components that control processes such as mitosis, transport, and motility, decreasing growth [2]. While the actions of paclitaxel are ideal for attacking tumors, healthy cells are also susceptible to its actions. Conjugation to PG can increase tumor-selective uptake and reduce adverse side effects resulting from damage to healthy cells.

Polymer conjugation functions to increase the targeting specificity of a particular therapeutic to the desired tissue or region of disease. In addition to polymer alone, receptor-specific ligands can be grafted to either the conjugated polymer or the drug itself, which results in site-specific accumulation of the therapeutic [3]. Known as active targeting, this is an effective method to reduce nonspecific uptake and improve efficacy.

2.6.3　Implantable and Transdermal Drug Delivery Systems

Implantable and transdermal drug delivery devices present methods of prolonged administration with relatively stable dosing patterns. These techniques also benefit from the use of polymers, both degradable and nondegradable. Unlike the colloidal carrier systems discussed in Section 2.6.1, these drug delivery devices have been in use for longer periods and are used more frequently. In general, these devices are used to regulate dosing and increase convenience, rather than improve solubility and stability of the drug molecule itself.

　　Implantable devices must be embedded in the body, typically subcutaneously. Therefore, there are several important factors that must be considered when developing materials for this application. The materials used to construct these devices must be chemically inert, hypoallergenic (as to not invoke an allergic reaction from the immune system), noncarcinogenic, and mechanically stable at the insertion site [4].

2.7　KEY POINTS

- There is a trifecta of issues to be overcome when administering drugs to the body: absorption of the drug into various body compartments, stability of the drug and/or carrier system *in vivo*, and solubility of the drug either *in vivo* or within the carrier system.
- The body contains many membranous boundaries which function as protective barriers, including the epithelium, endothelium, mucosal membranes, and the BBB.
- The stability of the drug and/or its carrier system is an important characteristic to be concerned with.

2.8　HOMEWORK PROBLEMS

1. Describe the different methods by which a drug molecule can cross epithelial barriers.
2. Name and briefly describe the four different cellular junctions.
3. What is the role of CYP 450 3A in oral drug delivery?
4. What distinguishes the capillaries of the BBB from systemic capillaries?
5. Name five chemical and/or physical properties of drug molecules that can affect the way they are transported in the body.
6. What is bioavailability? In the case of oral bioavailability, what other factors play a role?
7. What does EPR stand for, and how does this facilitate passively targeted drug delivery?
8. Name and give a brief description three types of polymeric carrier systems.

REFERENCES

1. Imbuluzqueta E, Carlos G, Ariza J, Blanco-Prieto M. Drug delivery systems for potential treatment of intracellular bacterial infections. Front Biosci 2010;15:397–417.

2. Zuwała-Jagiełło J. Endocytosis mediated by receptors-function and participation in oral drug delivery. Postepy Hig Med Dosw 2003;57:275–291.

3. Ranade V. Drug delivery systems 5A. Oral drug delivery. J Clin Pharmacol 1991;31:2–16.

4. Langer RS, Peppas NA. Present and future applications of biomaterials in controlled drug delivery systems. Biomaterials 1981;2:201–214.

5. Meera George AE. Polyionic hydrocolliods for the intestinal delivery of protein drugs: alginate and chitosan-a review. J Control Release 2006;114:1–14.

6. Wawrezinieick A, Pean JM, Wuthrich P. Oral bioavailiability and drug/carrier particulate systems. Med Sci 2008;24:659–664.

7. Jain K. Strategies and technologies for drug delivery systems. Trends Pharmacol Sci 1998;19:155–157.

8. Smith A. Drug delivery systems in the 20th century: merely scratching the surface. Pharma Sci Technol Today 1999;2:225–227.

9. Rosen H, Thierry A. The rise and rise of drug delivery. Nat Rev Drug Discov 2005;4: 381–385.

10. Edwards D, Abdelaziz B-J, Langer R. Recent advances in pulmonary drug delivery using large, porous, inhaled particles. J Appl Physiol 1998;85:379–385.

11. McConnell E, Fadda H, Basit A. Gut instincts: explorations in intestinal physiology and drug delivery. Int J Pharm 2008;364:213–226.

12. Mustara G, Dinh SM. Approaches to oral delivery for challenging molecules. Clin Rev Ther Drug Carrier Syst 2006;23:111–135.

13. Guy R. Current status and future prospects of transdermal drug delivery. Pharm Res 1996;13:1765–1769.

14. Thies C. Microencapsulation. Ed. Arza Seidel In: Kirk-Othmer Encyclopedia of Chemical Technology. 2005;16: p 438–463.

15. Hoffman A. The origin and evolution of "controlled" drug delivery systems. J Control Release 2008;132:153–163.

16. Venkatraman SS, Ma LL, Natarajan JV, Chattopadhyay S. Front Biosci (Schol Ed) 2010;2:801–814.

17. Weissig V, Cheng SM, D'Souza GG. J Liposome Res 2006;16:249–264.

18. Khuller GK, Kapur M, Sharma S. Liposome technology for drug delivery against mycobacterial infections. Curr Pharm Des 2004;10:3263–3274.

19. Park JW. Liposome-based drug delivery in breast cancer treatment. Breast Cancer Res 2002;4:95–99.

20. Langner M, Kral TE. Pol J Pharmacol 1999;51:211–222.

21. Agoram B, Woltosz WS, Bolger MB. Predicting the impact of physiological and biochemical processes on oral drug bioavailability. Adv Drug Deliv Rev 2001;50:541–567.

22. Madera J. Regulation of the movement of solutes across tight junctions. Annu Rev Physiol 1998;60:143–159.

23. Gabor F, Bogner E, Weissenboeck A, Wirth M. The lectin-cell interaction and its implications to intestinal lectin-mediated drug delivery. Adv Drug Deliv Rev 2004;56:459–480.

24. Jones BA, Gores GJ. Physiology and pathophysiology of apoptosis in epithelial cells of the liver, pancreas, and intestine. Am J Physiol Gastrointest Liver Physiol 1997;273: G1174–G1188.

25. Veltman K, Hummel S, Chichon C, Sonnenborn U, Schmidt M. Identification of specific mrRNAs targeting proteins of the apical junctional complex that stimulate the probiotic effect of E. coli Nissle 1917 on T84 epithelial cells. Int J Biochem Cell Biol 2012;44: 341–349.

26. Whitehead K, Mitragotri S. Mechanistric analysis of chemical permeation enhancers for oral drug delivery. Pharm Res 2008;25:1412–1419.

27. Deli M. Potential use of tight junction modulators to reversibly open membranous barriers and improve drug delivery. Biochim Biophys Acta 2009;1788:892–910.

28. Wang W, Uzzau S, Goldblum SE, Fasano A. Human zonulin, a potential modulator of intestinal tight junctions. J Cell Sci 2000;113:4435–4440.

29. Tavelin S, Hashimoto K, Malkinson J, Lazorova L, Toth I, et al. A new principle for tight junction modulation based on occludin peptides. Mol Pharmacol 2003;64:1530–1540.

30. Benet L, Takashi I, Yuanchao Z, Jeffrey S, Vincent W. Intestinal MDR transport proteins and P-450 enzymes as barriers to oral drug delivery. J Control Release 1999;62:25–31.

31. Clark MA, Hirst BH, Jepson MA. Lectin-mediated mucosal delivery of drugs and microparticles. Adv Drug Deliv Rev 2000;43:207–223.

32. Bonnefille P, Sezgin-Bayindir Z, Belkhelfa H, Arellano C, Gandia P, et al. The use of isolated enterocytes to study Phase I intestinal drug metabolism: validation with rat and pig intestine. Fund Clin Pharmacol 2011;25:104–114.

33. Nursat A, Giry M, Turner JR, Colgan SP. Rho protein regulates tight junctions and perijunctional actin organization in polarized epithelia. Proc Natl Acad Sci USA 1995;92: 10629–10633.

34. Prausnitz MR, Langer R. Transdermal drug delivery. Nat Biotechnol 2008;26:1261–1268.

35. Asbill C, El-Kattan AF, Ayman F, Michniak B. Enhancement of transdermal drug delivery: chemical and physical approaches. Crit Rev Ther Drug Carrier Syst 2000;17:621–658.

36. Kooiman K, Harteveld M, De Jong N, Van Wamel A. Transiently increased endothelial layer permeability by ultrasound-activated microbubbles. IEEE Transactions on Biomedical Engineering. 2006;57: p 529–531.

37. Hajitou A, Pasqualini R, Arap W. Vascular targeting: recent advances and therapeutic perspectives. Trends Cardiovasc Med 2006;16:80–88.

38. Charoenphol P, Mocherla S, Bouis D, Namdee K, Pinsky DJ, et al. Targeting therapeutics to the vascular wall in atherosclerosis-Carrier size matters. Atherosclerosis 2011;217:364–370.

39. Molema G, De Leij LFMH, Meijer DKF. Tumor vascular endothelium: bor target in tumor directed drug delivery and immunotherapy. Pharm Res 1997;14:2–10.

40. Norris D, Puri N, Sinko P. The effect of physical barriers and properties on the oral absorption of particulates. Adv Drug Deliv Rev 1998;34:135–143.

41. Bhat P, Flanagen D, Donovan M. The limiting role of mucus in drug absorption: drug permeation through mucus solution. Int J Pharm 1995;126:179–187.

42. Bhat P, Flanagen D, Donovan M. Drug binding to gastric mucus glycoproteins. Int J Pharm 1996;134:15–25.

43. Hillery A, Lloyd M, Andrew W, Swarbrick J. Drug Delivery and Targeting for Pharmacists and Pharmaceutical Scientists. Boca Raton (FL) Taylor and Francis Publishing Group. 2001. p 2–47.

44. Mahato R, Narang A. Pharmaceutical Dosage Forms and Drug Delivery. 2 ed. Boca Raton (FL): CRC Press; 2012.

45. Jones A, Gumbleton M, Duncan R. Understanding endocytotic pathways and intracellular trafficking: a prerequisite for effective design of advanced drug delivery systems. Adv Drug Deliv Rev 2003;55:1353–1357.

46. Masaoka Y, Tanaka Y, Kataoka M, Sakuma S, Yamashita S. Site of drug absorption after oral administration: assessment of membrane permeability and luminal concentration of drugs in each segment of gastrointestinal tract. Eur J Pharm Sci 2006;29:240–250.

47. Chen Y, Liu L. Modern methods for delivery of drugs across the blood brain barrier. Adv Drug Deliv Rev 2011;63:470–491.

48. Scherrmann JM. Drug delivery to the brain via the blood brain barrier. Vascul Pharmacol 2002;28:349–354.

49. Wolka A, Huber J, Davis T. Pain and the blood brain barrier: obstacles to drug delivery. Adv Drug Deliv Rev 2003;55:987–1006.

50. Abbott J, Romero I. Transporting therapeutics across the blood brain barrier. Mol Med Today 1996;2:106–113.

51. Drees A, Hollnack E, Eisenblatter T, Galla HJ. In: Boer AG, editor. The Multidrug Resistance Protein BMDP/ABCG2: A New and Highly Relevant Efflux Pump at the Blood-Brain Barrier. International Congress Series. 2005;1277: p 154–168.

52. Taylor EM. The impact of efflux transporters in the brain on the development of drugs for CNS disorders. Clin Pharmacokinet 2002;41:81–92.

53. Tsuji A, Tamai I. Blood-brain barrier function of P-glycoprotein. Adv Drug Deliv Rev 1997;25:287–298.

54. Veber D, Johnson S, Hung-Yuan C, Smith B, Ward K, Kopple K. Molecular properties that influence the oral bioavailability of drug candidates. J Med Chem 2002;45:2615–2623.

55. Schmucker DL. Liver function and phase 1 drug metabolism in the elderly: a paradox. Drugs Aging 2001;18:837–851.

56. Liddel C, Stedman C. Hepatic Metabolism of Drugs. Gastroenterol Hepatol 2007;2: 241–249.

57. Park BK, Kitteringham NR, Maggs JL, Pirmohamed M, Williams DP. The role of metabolic activation in drug-induced hepatotoxicity. Annu Rev Pharmacol Toxicol 2005:177–202.

58. Benet L, Chi-Yuan W, Mary H, Vincent W. Intestinal drug metabolism and antitransport processes: a potential paradigm shift in oral drug delivery. J Control Release 1996;39:139–143.

59. Zhang Y, Benet L. The gut as a barrier to drug absorption: the comined forle of Cytochrome P4503A and P-glycoprotein. Clin Pharmacokinet 2001;40:159–168.

60. Zhou S, Chan SY, Goh BC, Chan E, Duan W, et al. Mechanism-based inhibition of cytochrome P450 3A4 by therapeutic drugs. Clin Pharmacokinet 2005;44:279–304.

61. Wacher V, Salphati L, Benet L. Active secretion and enterocytic drug metabolism barriers to drug absorption. Adv Drug Deliv Rev 1996;20:99–112.

62. Kwan KC. Oral bioavailability and first pass effects. Drug Deliv Today 1997;25:1329–1336.

63. Petrak K. Essential properties of drug-targeting delivery systems. Drug Deliv Today 2005;10.

64. Singh R, Matharu P, Lalla JK. A diffusion controlled drug delivery system for theophylline. Drug Dev Ind Pharm 1994;20:1225–1238.

65. Leichty W, Kryscio D, Slaughter B, Peppas N. Polymers for drug delivery systems. Annu Rev Chem Biomed Eng 2010;1:149–173.

66. Berkland C, Kipper M, Narasimhan B, Kim K, Pack D. Microsphere size, precipitation kinetics, and drug distribution control drug releae from biodegradable polyanhydride microspheres. J Control Release 2004;94:129–141.

67. Soppimath KA, Tejraj M, Kulkarni A, Rudzinski W. Biodegradable polymeric nanoparticles as drug delivery devices. J Control Release 2001;70:1–20.

PART II

INJECTABLE POLYMERIC DRUG DELIVERY SYSTEMS

POLYMER–DRUG CONJUGATES

Cristina Fante and Francesca Greco

School of Pharmacy, University of Reading, Reading, UK

3.1 INTRODUCTION

Polymer–drug conjugates are nanosized (1–100 nm) pharmaceuticals in which low molecular weight (MW) drug molecules are *covalently* linked to a polymeric carrier via a biodegradable linker [1–3]. Therefore, the general structure of a polymer–drug conjugate is made of three components: the drug, the polymer, and the linker that connects them (Fig. 3.1). Optionally, a targeting group could also be attached to the polymer to actively direct the system toward a specific biological target.

Conjugation of a drug to a polymer alters both its physicochemical properties (e.g., solubility and stability) and its pharmacokinetics (PK) (including body distribution and cellular uptake), with significant impact on its overall therapeutic performance. This chapter provides an overview on polymer–drug conjugates. First, a historical description of their original conception and development will be provided (Section 3.2); then, an explanation of the biological rationale underpinning this technology will be presented (Section 3.3). The structural features of polymer–drug conjugates, including requirements for system optimization, will be described (Section 3.4). Then, the steps undertaken in the preparation of a conjugate are analyzed (Section 3.5).

Engineering Polymer Systems for Improved Drug Delivery, First Edition.
Edited by Rebecca A. Bader and David A. Putnam.
© 2014 John Wiley & Sons, Inc. Published 2014 by John Wiley & Sons, Inc.

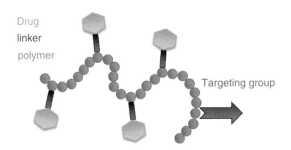

Drug
linker
polymer

Targeting group

Figure 3.1. General structure of a polymer–drug conjugate.

In the final part of the chapter, the current challenges of this field are discussed (Section 3.6).

3.2 HISTORICAL PERSPECTIVE

The concept of polymer–drug conjugates was first introduced in the 1970s, when Helmut Ringsdorf first conceived the therapeutic potential of linking a drug to a polymeric carrier [1]. In particular, Ringsdorf suggested that covalent conjugation of a drug to a water-soluble polymer would improve the solubility of hydrophobic drugs and enhance their stability in body fluids. In addition, he hypothesized that the presence of a targeting group would direct the conjugate toward the target tissue. Here, cellular uptake of the conjugate by endocytosis would allow its internalization and processing (described in more detail in Section 3.3) [4].

Ringsdorf's innovative approach inspired research by the groups led by Ruth Duncan and Jindrich Kopecek, based in Keele and Prague Universities, respectively, which resulted in the conjugation of the anticancer agent doxorubicin (Dox) to a hydroxypropyl metacrylamide (HPMA) copolymer [5]. This HPMA copolymer–Dox conjugate (called PK1 from the initials of Prague and Keele) progressed into clinical evaluation [6]. The HPMA copolymer–Dox conjugate was subsequently modified to promote hepatic targeting in the treatment of primary liver cancer. Such an analog (named PK2) contained galactosamine, an active targeting group able to bind to the asialoglycoprotein receptor present on the hepatocytes membrane [7].

In the same years when these first conjugates were being developed, Hiroshi Maeda and his group at Kumamoto University described the unique features of the tumor vasculature (i.e., discontinuous tumor capillaries and poor lymphatic drainage) that result in the preferential accumulation of macromolecules into the tumor tissue [8, 9]. This phenomenon was named the *enhanced permeability and retention* (EPR) effect and it will be described later in this chapter (Section 3.3.1).

PK1 was the first anticancer conjugate (based on a synthetic polymer) to enter clinical trials in 1994 [6]. Since then, a number of conjugates of different poly-mers (e.g., polyethylene glycol (PEG) and poly(glutamic acid) (PGA)) and anticancer drugs (e.g., paclitaxel, palatinates, camptothecin) have been developed. To date, 16 polymer–anticancer drug conjugates have followed PK1 into clinical investigation (further discussed in Section 3.5.4) [10], with PGA–paclitaxel (OPAXIO®, PPX or CT-2103, previously known as XYOTAX®) now being the leading conjugate in phase III trials for use against advanced lung cancer [11].

3.3 POLYMER–DRUG CONJUGATES: BIOLOGICAL RATIONALE

3.3.1 Changes in Physicochemical Properties

When a drug is covalently attached to a polymer, its physicochemical properties (water solubility and stability) and its biological behavior (PK and pharmacodynamics) change dramatically (Table 3.1).

Water solubility. Water-soluble polymeric carriers extend their hydrophilic character to the conjugated drug, with consequent advantages for the administration of insoluble drugs. For example, the anticancer agent paclitaxel, poorly water-soluble and generally administered as a solution in organic solvents (i.e., Cremophor EL), shows high solubility in water when conjugated to PGA [12].

Drug stability. Polymer conjugation can improve the stability of a drug by protecting it from chemical and/or enzymatic degradation. This is the case for camptothecin, an anticancer drug that gets rapidly deactivated in the blood (hydrolysis of the lactone

TABLE 3.1. Advantages Generally Observed for Polymer–Drug Conjugates over Traditional Chemotherapy

Parameter	Free Drug	Polymer–Drug Conjugate	References
Water solubility	Typically low: makes parenteral administration difficult.	Improved drug solubility	12, 13
Drug stability	Limited stability (e.g., enzymatic instability and/or hydrolysis)	Improved stability (e.g., protection against enzymatic and/or hydrolytic inactivation)	14
Body clearance	Rapid elimination	Prolonged circulation time	15, 16
Selectivity for the tumor tissue	Lack of selectivity (only a fraction of the administered dose reaches the tumor); Side effects	Passive tumor targeting (higher percentage of the dose reaches the tumor); Reduced side effects	6, 15–17
Drug resistance	P-gp-mediated drug resistance	Lysosomotropic delivery: circumvention of drug resistance	1, 4, 18

ring with conversion to the carboxylate form) but protected from degradation when conjugated to PGA [14].

Pharmacokinetics. The conjugate is characterized by a reduced elimination rate and a prolonged circulation time compared to the free drug. This is a consequence of its high MW. The modified pharmacokinetic behavior is beneficial for cancer treatment because it facilitates the accumulation of the drug in the tumor tissue by means of the EPR effect (Section 3.3.1). In addition, the macromolecular size affects the mechanism of cellular internalization of the drug, which is taken up exclusively by endocytosis (lysosomotropic delivery, Section 3.3.2) [15].

Drug resistance. When taken up by the cell through the endocytic pathway, the drug is encapsulated inside the endosome/lysosome compartments. This allows the drug to bypass one of the mechanisms that lead to drug resistance, which is the expulsion of material from the cytosol to the extracellular matrix through membrane efflux pumps (P-glycoprotein) [18].

3.3.2   Passive Tumor Targeting: The EPR Effect

Traditional anticancer drugs are typically low MW molecules able to diffuse through the different body tissues in a nonselective manner (Fig. 3.2). Conversely, polymer–drug conjugates, because of their size, are unable to freely cross biological barriers [8, 16]. Indeed, after intravenous administration, conjugates accumulate in the tumor tissues to a higher extent and for longer than the corresponding free drug [9, 13]. This phenomenon (the EPR effect) is typical of macromolecules and has been shown to originate from two factors:

1. *Enhanced vascular permeability* of the tumor capillaries. Healthy vessels and tumor vessels are structurally very different. Healthy vessels have a tight endothelium, which is permeable to small molecules but *not* to macromolecules.

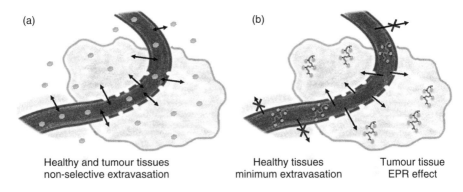

(a)   (b)

Healthy and tumour tissues
non-selective extravasation

Healthy tissues
minimum extravasation

Tumour tissue
EPR effect

Figure 3.2. Schematic representation of the passive tumor targeting of macromolecules. (a) A low molecular weight drug is able to diffuse into both healthy and tumor tissues. (b) Macromolecules extravasate only where the vasculature is discontinuous and accumulate where the lymphatic system is ineffective (i.e., the tumor tissue).

On the other hand, tumor vessels have a defective endothelium, which is permeable to *both* small molecules and macromolecules (for example, up to 800 kDa for HPMA copolymer [19]) (Fig. 3.2). This feature allows the conjugate to preferentially extravasate into the tumor tissue over healthy tissues.

2. *Enhanced retention* of macromolecules in the interstitial space. After extravasation in the tumor tissue, the clearance of small molecules is very different from the clearance of macromolecules. Small molecules can freely diffuse in the interstitial fluids as well as back into the bloodstream. On the other hand, the clearance of macromolecules depends on the lymphatic system. The tumor tissue is characterized by a poor lymphatic drainage, which results in the decreased clearance of macromolecules and their accumulation in the interstitial space (more than 72 h) [20].

3.3.3 Lysosomotropic Delivery

Once the conjugate reaches the tumor tissue, it is internalized by cancer cells. However, polymer conjugation changes the PK of the drug at the cellular level. While low MW drugs can generally reach their intracellular target by diffusing through the cellular membrane, macromolecules are taken up by the cells through endocytosis [4]. This pathway consists of the internalization of the conjugate into the early endosomes, which eventually ends up in the lysosomes (Fig. 3.3). These organelles differ from other intracellular organelles in two main aspects: the low pH (4–5) and the presence of proteolytic enzymes (e.g., cathepsins). Both these features have been exploited as triggers to promote the release of the drug molecules from the conjugate inside

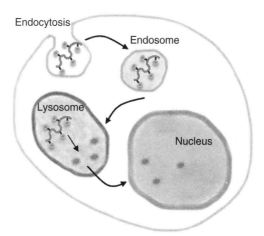

Figure 3.3. Mechanism of endocytic uptake and lysosomotropic delivery of polymer–drug conjugates. Conjugates are designed to release the drug in the lysosomes upon selective activation (typically, enzymatic or hydrolytic cleavage of the linker).

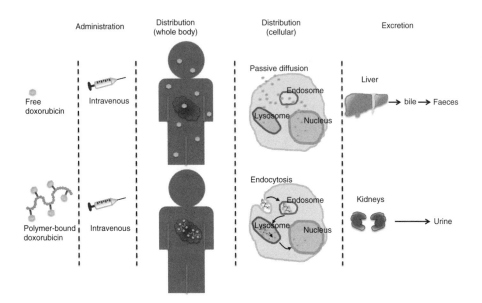

Figure 3.4. Schematic comparison of the fate of HPMA copolymer–doxorubicin and free doxorubicin, from administration to excretion.

the lysosome [21, 22] (Section 3.4.3). The restriction of drug delivery to the endocytic route and the consequent intracellular drug release has two main advantages: (i) circumvention of the mechanism of drug resistance associated with membrane efflux pumps (P-glycoprotein); (ii) intracellular localization, with effective access to the intracellular target.

3.3.4 The Journey of the Drug: HPMA Copolymer–Doxorubicin Compared to Free Doxorubicin

Polymer conjugation impacts heavily on the physicochemical properties and on the biological behavior of a drug. Fig. 3.4 compares the journeys undertaken by free doxorubicin and by HPMA copolymer–doxorubicin from their administration (intravenously for both compounds) to their elimination from the body (in the feces via the bile for doxorubicin and in the urines for HPMA copolymer–doxorubicin).

3.4 STRUCTURAL FEATURES OF POLYMER–DRUG CONJUGATES

Polymer–drug conjugates have a common tripartite structure, represented by the polymer, the drug, and the linker, which connects them (as shown in Fig. 3.1). An optional targeting moiety might be included to direct the conjugate to a specific tissue [1–3]. This section describes essential requirements needed for these components and highlights the parameters that guide their choice.

3.4.1 The Polymer

The choice of an appropriate carrier is a key factor in the development of a clinically useful polymer–drug conjugate, as the physicochemical properties of the polymer determine the pharmacokinetic parameters of the conjugate as a whole. For use in cancer treatment, the polymer must meet several requirements.

Water solubility. The polymer must be soluble in water to increase the water solubility of the conjugated drug in physiological environments. Indeed, traditional anticancer agents (e.g., paclitaxel) are generally poorly soluble compounds, and are difficult to administer. For example, paclitaxel requires coadministration with Cremophor EL, an organic solvent able to solubilize the drug but which can cause anaphylactic reactions. Conjugation to PGA makes paclitaxel highly water soluble [12] and allows faster and safer administration [23].

Safety. The polymer must be nontoxic and unable to stimulate the immune system (nonimmunogenic). These features are essential for safe administration of the conjugate.

Drug-loading capacity. The polymer must provide multiple sites for conjugation of the drug. An adequate drug payload is essential, particularly when the drug is characterized by low potency and therefore administration in higher doses is required.

Biodegradability. After the delivery of the drug, the polymer needs to be eliminated to prevent its accumulation in the body. Biodegradable polymers (i.e., polymers that break down into smaller fragments in biological systems) such as PGA are therefore ideal candidates for use in polymer–drug conjugates. Nonbiodegradable polymers (e.g., PEG and HPMA copolymer) can also be used as polymeric carries, but care should be taken in the choice of their size (see immediately below).

Adequate molecular weight. MW is a key parameter, as it drives the rate and the extent of elimination of the polymer from the body. Polymers are excreted through renal filtration in a size-dependent process. The size threshold above which a polymer cannot be excreted renally is affected by many factors (e.g., level of hydration of the polymer and polymer architecture) and, as such, is unique to each polymer. However, 40 kDa is generally taken as the MW constituting the renal threshold for elimination. Therefore, the MW of a nonbiodegradable polymer must be lower than 40 kDa in order to prevent its accumulation in the body after repeated administrations. In the case of a biodegradable polymer, the renal elimination does not represent an issue in the choice of the MW, as the polymer is broken into smaller fragments.

In addition to polymer elimination, other considerations are required in the choice of an appropriate MW of the polymer. In particular, the MW has to be

- sufficiently high to ensure long circulation and take full advantage of the EPR effect (20–80 kDa is generally accepted as a suitable range for this purpose [19]);
- not too high, so as to avoid preferential macrophage uptake, to allow diffusion of the conjugate in the extracellular space, and to allow internalization into tumor cells by endocytosis [24].

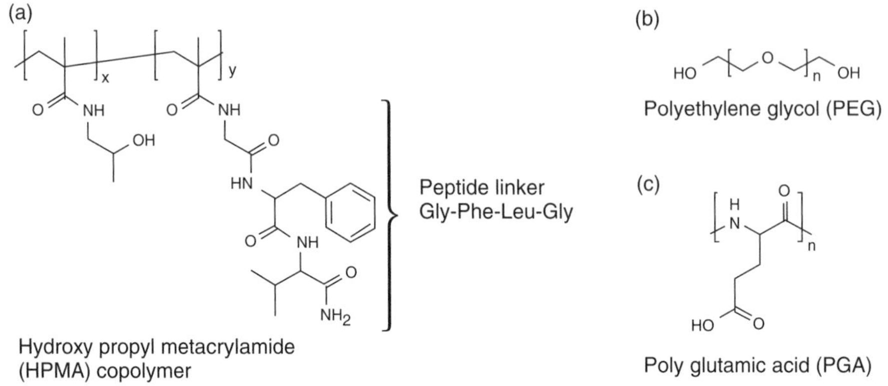

(a)

(b)

Polyethylene glycol (PEG)

Peptide linker
Gly-Phe-Leu-Gly

(c)

Hydroxy propyl metacrylamide
(HPMA) copolymer

Poly glutamic acid (PGA)

Figure 3.5. Structures of the polymers that have been investigated most in the context of polymer–drug conjugation.

The polymers that have been most extensively investigated in the context of polymer–drug conjugation are the HPMA copolymer, PEG, and PGA, and their chemical structures are reported in Fig. 3.5.

3.4.1.1 HPMA Copolymers. HPMA copolymers are the first and most studied synthetic carrier used for drug conjugation. Initial studies concerning drug conjugation focused on an HPMA copolymer as a model polymer [22, 24, 25], and, to date, six HPMA copolymer conjugates have entered clinical evaluation (See Section 3.6.1.1 and Table 3.2).

3.4.1.2 PEG. PEG is a hydrophilic polymer with a good safety profile [28]. In fact, PEG has been widely used for protein conjugation, and four PEG–protein conjugates are now on the market (Oncaspar®, PEG–INTRON®, Pegasys®, and Neulasta®) [29]. However, in the context of polymer conjugation, unmodified PEG has the disadvantage of a low drug-loading capacity because of the possibility to achieve drug conjugation only in correspondence of the two terminal hydroxyl groups. Branched [30] and dendron [31] structures have been designed to overcome this limitation, and three multiarm PEG–drug conjugates are currently in clinical evaluation (NKTR-102, NKTR-105, and EZN-2208) [29]. Among linear PEG–drug conjugates, PEG–camptothecin (Pegamotecan) entered clinical trials and reached Phase II [32]. At this stage, it was discontinued because it showed the same toxicology profile compared with the free drug, probably due to the instability of the ester linkage between the polymer and camptothecin.

3.4.1.3 PGA. PGA has also been used for drug conjugation, and the PGA conjugate of paclitaxel (OPAXIO®) is expected to be the first polymer–drug conjugate to reach the market [11, 23, 26, 33]. PGA has all the qualities required for its parenteral administration: water solubility, nontoxicity, nonimmunogenicity, and good

TABLE 3.2. Examples of Anticancer Drugs Conjugated to Polymers

Drug (functional group)	Limitations of the free drug	Conjugate (polymer)	Effect of conjugation	References
Camptothecin (Alcohol)	Poor water solubility Instability of the lactone ring Side effects (e.g., severe diarrhoea)	CT-2106 (PGA)	Active lactone form Stabilized Enhanced solubility Phase I: well tolerated (Absence of camptothecin related toxixity)	14, 17
Doxorubicin (Amino)	Cardiotoxicity	PK1 (HPMA copolymer)	Clinical evaluation: Fivefold decreased Dox Toxicity (Phase I) Reduced side effects (Phase II)	6, 10
Paclitaxel (Alcohol)	Low solubility (Cremophor EL and ethanol as solubilizing agents)	Opaxio® (PGA)	Enhanced water solubility Decreased toxicity	11, 23, 26, 33
Platinates (Amino)	Nephrotoxicity Neurotoxicity;	ProLindac (HPMA copolymer)	Phase I: improved tolerability	27
TNP-470 (Amino)	Neurotoxicity Short half-life.	Caplostatin (HPMA copolymer)	*In vivo* preclinical studies: No neurotoxicity $t_{1/2}$ Extended to 48 h.	16

drug-loading capacity. In addition, compared to HPMA copolymer or PEG, PGA has the advantage of being biodegradable [34]. Its metabolism is enzymatic, and cathepsin B is the lysosomal protease responsible for such degradation [35]. These properties make PGA an ideal carrier for use in drug delivery.

3.4.2 The Drug

Polymer–drug conjugates have been traditionally designed for use in cancer therapy. Theoretically, the drug carried by the polymer may belong to any class of anticancer agents. However, a number of essential requirements must be met to design an effective conjugate.

Presence of an appropriate functional group. The structure must provide a chemical group that will allow conjugation of the drug to the polymer. To this end, amino groups have been considered ideal because of their ability to form amide bonds when reacted with the carboxylic acids of a polymer (e.g., the pendent chain of PGA or the terminal groups of carboxyPEG). Alcohols are another example of suitable functional group, as they can form ester bonds or acetals with the carboxylic acids of the polymer.

Potency. As the conjugate and the drug are covalently attached together, their administration is strongly connected. For this reason, the drug must be potent enough to ensure that the therapeutic dose can be administered without having to administer excessive amounts of polymer.

Stability. As previously discussed, polymer–drug conjugates are designed to release the drug at the target site. Therefore, it is important that the drug has sufficient stability to resist the environmental conditions of the target site. As drug release typically occurs in the lysosomal compartment (Section 3.3.3), it is important that the chosen drug is stable at low pH and in the presence of proteolytic enzymes.

The drugs that have most frequently been selected for polymer conjugation are listed in Table 3.2. Recently, novel classes of drugs have been conjugated and investigated preclinically (e.g., dopamine [36], dexamethasone [37]; 8-aminoquinoline [38]; also discussed in Section 3.6.1.)

3.4.3 The Linker

The third crucial part in the development of a conjugate is the design of the polymer–drug linker, which must meet some specific requirements.

Stability in the bloodstream. After intravenous injection, the linker must be stable in the bloodstream, as premature release of the drug can result in unwanted toxicity. For example, an HPMA copolymer–camptothecin conjugate (MAG–CPT) that contained an ester bond between the drug and the polymer was evaluated clinically. Phase I clinical trials were discontinued prematurely because of the serious bladder toxicity observed, probably due to the linker's instability in the acidic urinary tract [39]. An ester linkage was also used to conjugate an HPMA copolymer to paclitaxel (PNU166945), and severe neurotoxicity was observed in Phase I trials, proving that the drug was released in the bloodstream [40]. Interestingly, the stability of the linkage depends not only on the type of chemical bond but also on the overall chemical environment (e.g., polymer structure, polymer architecture, and conjugate conformation). For instance, when paclitaxel was conjugated to PGA through an ester linkage, the conjugate was stable during circulation and the linkage was not cleaved by plasma esterase [34].

Selective release. A second requirement is that the linker needs to ensure drug release exclusively in the tumor. The internalization by the endocytic route implies that macromolecules are strictly directed to the lysosomal compartment and exposed both to an acidic environment and to a variety of hydrolytic enzymes. Consequently, pH-sensitive and enzymatically cleavable linkers have been developed to ensure lysosomotropic drug release [41, 42].

N-cis-aconityl and *N*-maleyl linkers were the first pH-sensitive linkers designed for a polymer–drug conjugate (poly-D-lysine–daunomycin [43]). *In vitro* studies demonstrated that the conjugate was internalized by endocytosis, and both linkers liberated the free drug in the lysosomal compartment. In more recent studies, Dox has been attached to HPMA copolymer via a pH-sensitive hydrazone bond [21]. In addition to the *in vitro* Dox release at pH 5 and relative stability of the conjugate at pH 7.4, *in vivo* studies showed a significantly enhanced antitumor activity in comparison with free Dox and PK1 conjugate.

Enzymatically cleavable linkers were designed to exploit the complex enzyme composition of lysosomes to trigger drug delivery. Lysosomal enzymes belong to different classes (e.g., protease, phosphatase, lipase, and nuclease) and are able to degrade most macromolecules entering the cells. The cysteine protease cathepsin B has been shown to be the main enzyme responsible for the cleavage of a range of oligopeptides with potential application as linkers [22, 44]. After extensive studies by Duncan and Kopececk, the tetrapeptide Gly-Phe-Leu-Gly was optimized and used as a linker for the conjugation of doxorubicin to the HPMA copolymer (PK1) [25]. More recently, Shabat's group built on this concept and developed a self-immolative dendritic linker based on the Gly-Phe-Leu-Gly moiety that was able to amplify a single cathepsin B-dependent cleavage event into the release of three molecules of the active drug [45].

It is important to note that the conjugated drug has a substantial effect on the degradation of the linker. The peptidyl spacer Gly-Gly proved nonbiodegradable when used in an HPMA copolymer–doxorubicin conjugate [46], but it was cleaved by lysosomal enzymes when melphalan was conjugated, instead [47].

Cathepsin B is also the enzyme responsible for the metabolism of poly(L-glutamic acid) and for the release of paclitaxel when linked to PGA through an ester linker [48]. However, cathepsin B is not the only enzyme exploited for drug release (Table 3.3). Proteases are overexpressed in malignant tumors, as they play a key role in metastasis progression, degrading basement membranes and the extracellular matrix [54]. Matrix metalloproteases (MMPs) are a particularly interesting class of proteases. They are overexpressed in different tumors (e.g., malignant melanoma), and a specific subtype, MMP-2, has been shown to be involved in metastatic growth and angiogenesis [55]. An albumin-bound doxorubicin conjugate was designed for selective activation by MMP-2

TABLE 3.3. Examples of Enzymes Exploited for Drug Release in Polymer–Drug Conjugates

Enzyme	Linker	Conjugates	References
Cathepsin B	Gly-Phe-Leu-Gly	HPMA copolymer– doxorubicin	25
	Gly-Phe-Leu-Gly-PABC dendrimer	HPMA copolymer–PTX	45
Matrix metalloprotease	Gly-Pro-Leu-Gly-Val	mPEG–Dox	49
	Phe-Val-Gly-Leu-Ile-Gly	DX–MTX	50
	Gly-Pro-Leu-Gly-Ile-Ala-Gly-Gln	Albumin–Dox	51
Collagenase	Gly-Phe-Ala-Leu-	PHEG–MMC	41
	Pro-Leu-Gly-Pro-Gly	PEG–grafted PHEG–PDM	52
Plasmin	D-Val-Leu-Lys	PHEA–Cytarabine	53

and has given interesting preclinical results (antitumor effect with maximum tolerated dose fourfold higher than the free doxorubicin in melanoma models *in vivo* [51]).

3.4.4 Targeting Group

Polymer–drug conjugates are able to passively target the tumor tissue via the EPR effect (described in Section 3.3.2). In addition, targeting groups can be added onto a conjugate to direct it toward the tissue of interest. Such groups selectively bind to tissue-specific markers and are designed to actively drive the conjugate to such tissue. Active targeting relies on a specific recognition, such as that between a ligand and its receptor. A number of targeting groups have been used, including peptides (e.g., melanocytes stimulating hormone [56]), ligands (e.g., folate [57]), and antibodies (e.g., antitransferrin receptor antibody [58]). However, to date, only one conjugate bearing a targeting moiety has been tested clinically. Such a conjugate is PK2, previously mentioned in this chapter as an analog of PK1 (the HPMA copolymer conjugate of doxorubicin) carrying galactosamine to target the hepatocyte galactose receptor [7, 59, 60]. PK2 is now in Phase II clinical trials. Its accumulation in the tumor has been found to be significantly higher than that of the free drug but lower than that of the nontargeted conjugate PK1. This interesting behavior has been attributed to the different conformation that the conjugate might have in presence of the additional component (galactosamine).

3.5 MAKING A POLYMER–DRUG CONJUGATE

3.5.1 In the Chemistry Lab

The preparation of a polymer–drug conjugate starts with the covalent attachment of a drug to the polymeric carrier. This is typically carried out via a conjugation reaction,

TABLE 3.4. Examples of Common Conjugation Strategies

Drug (functional group)	Polymer (functional group)	Reaction[a]	References
Doxorubicin (amino)	HPMA copolymer (activated ester)	Aminolysis[b]	5
Paclitaxel (hydroxyl group)	Poly(glutamic acid) (carboxylic acid)	DCC coupling[b]	13
Camptothecin (hydroxyl group)	Poly(glutamic acid) (carboxylic acid)	Various coupling agents explored[b]	14
Camptothecin (hydroxyl group)	HPMA copolymer (reaction of camptothecin with the activated ester of the Gly of the linker)	Condensation in the presence of DMAP[c]	61

[a] For multistep reactions, the reaction reported refers to one of the following:
[b] The conjugation step in which the drug is linked to the polymeric carrier.
[c] The step in which the drug is attached to the linker, which will be conjugated to the polymer in subsequent steps.

which generally involves an activation of the chemical groups on the polymer and a subsequent coupling with the chosen drug. The exact reaction conditions to be used depend on the functional groups present on the drug and on the polymer (Table 3.4).

After conjugation, purification of the conjugate from residual reagents and thorough characterization of the conjugate have to be carried out. Many techniques have been employed to characterize polymer–drug conjugates, including nuclear magnetic resonance, ultraviolet–visible, and infrared spectroscopy. Table 3.5 summarizes the main information obtained from various analytical techniques. Thorough characterization of a conjugate generally requires a combination of techniques (rather than a single technique).

3.5.2 In the Bio Lab, *in vitro* Studies

3.5.2.1 Cytotoxicity. In vitro cytotoxicity assays are typically one of the first assessments carried out in the biological evaluation of polymer–drug conjugates. These assays measure the cytotoxic activity of a conjugate against cell lines (generally, cancer cell lines). A comparison against the parent free drug is also carried out. It is important to highlight that the conjugates are generally less active than their parent free drugs in this type of experiments (e.g., 25). This is due to the different cellular pharmacokinetics, with the free drug being able to enter and act promptly on a cell. Conversely, the conjugate has a more delayed onset of action due to its multistep cellular PK (internalization, intracellular trafficking, drug release in the lysosomes).

Cytotoxicity assays can be followed by more specific assays that aim to investigate the molecular mechanisms responsible for cell death (e.g., assays to determine apoptosis).

TABLE 3.5. Most Common Techniques used for the Physicochemical Characterization of Polymer–Drug Conjugates

Technique	Characterization
Nuclear magnetic resonance (NMR) spectroscopy	Identity Total drug content
Fourier transform infrared (FTIR) spectroscopy	Identity
Ultraviolet-visible spectroscopy (UV-vis)	Identity Total drug content Free drug content
MALDI-TOF mass spectrometry (MS)	Identity MW/polydispersity
High performance liquid chromatography (HPLC)	Total drug content Free drug content
Gel permeation chromatography (GPC)	MW/polydispersity
Light scattering	MW/polydispersity
Small angle neutron scattering (SANS)	Conformation
Small angle x-ray scattering (SAXS)	Conformation

3.5.2.2 Hemolytic Activity. Polymer–drugs are generally administered intravenously. It is therefore important to ensure that they are biocompatible and nontoxic to blood cells. Hemolysis assays aim at assessing that a conjugate does not disrupt the membrane of red blood cells. These results are also taken more generally as a measurement of compatibility toward healthy cells.

3.5.2.3 Drug Release. Most polymer–drug conjugates are prodrug systems, designed to be stable in transport and to generate the free drug at the target site. Therefore, drug release studies are normally carried out to ensure (i) that the linker is stable while in circulation and (ii) that the drug is released under conditions similar to those found by the conjugate at the target site. For instance, stability of the system is typically assessed by incubating a conjugate with blood plasma and ensuring that no (or negligible) drug release occurs. In a similar manner, drug release at the target is typically assessed by incubating a conjugate under conditions mimicking the clinical scenario (e.g., in a mixture of lysosomal enzymes, if the conjugate is designed for lysosomotropic delivery).

3.5.3 Preclinical

After *in vitro* assessment, the polymer–drug conjugate undergoes preclinical studies in animal models. These studies are aimed at establishing the safety of the polymer–drug conjugate and confirming its activity.

In vivo pharmacokinetics. PK studies are carried out in conjugates to test their body distribution *in vivo*. In particular, these studies look for evidence that the conjugate is able to passively accumulate in the tumor tissue through the EPR effect and that the fraction of drug reaching healthy tissues is reduced [6]. These studies are also aimed at determining other PK parameters such as distribution and excretion half-lives, volume of distribution, and clearance.

3.5.3.1 Antitumor Activity. As polymer–drug conjugates are generally meant for use as anticancer treatment, their ability to reduce tumors *in vivo* needs to be tested. Animal models carrying tumors are administered the polymer–drug conjugate under assessment. The ability of the conjugate to stop tumor growth and even to reduce tumor size is analyzed. Untreated animals and animals injected with the free drug are typically used as comparison.

3.5.3.2 Toxicological Assessment. The increased selectivity of polymer–drug conjugates for the tumor tissue generally results in a better toxicological profile of the drug. As a general parameter, the weight of the animal (in addition to its viability) is monitored, as a decrease of weight is interpreted as a toxic effect. In addition, the ability of the conjugate to reduce the side effects of the free drug is assessed by monitoring key organ functions (e.g., cardiac function for doxorubicin) and comparing their functionality after administration of the free or conjugated drug.

3.5.4 Clinical

After preclinical assessment, polymer–drug conjugates need to be evaluated clinically. The aim of clinical studies on conjugates is to prove their safety and efficacy in patients. As polymer–drug conjugates are generally designed as anticancer treatment, Phase I studies are carried out directly in cancer patients rather than in healthy volunteers. As polymer–drug conjugates are designed for the treatment of solid tumors, Phase I studies are often carried out in patients with a range of malignancies. Subsequent clinical studies are then targeted to the most promising tumor types. For example, Phase I studies for HPMA copolymer–doxorubicin were carried out in various cancer types, including breast, lung and colon cancer [6]. The follow-on Phase II study was limited to lung, colon, and breast cancer, as these cancer types had shown a response to the treatment in Phase I.

In addition to measuring the anticancer activity and the safety of the conjugates, additional information (e.g., PK profile) is collected during clinical studies. To date, a number of conjugates have undergone clinical evaluation (reported in Table 3.6).

3.6 CURRENT CHALLENGES AND FUTURE PERSPECTIVES

3.6.1 Recent Developments

3.6.1.1 New Drugs and Combination Therapy. Classical polymer–drug conjugates carry established anticancer agents such as paclitaxel and doxorubicin. Recent studies have extended the application of polymer–drug conjugates to

TABLE 3.6. Clinical Status of Polymer–Anticancer Drug Conjugates that have Entered Clinical Evaluation

Status	Conjugate	Name	References
Phase III	PGA–paclitaxel	CT-2103; Opaxio®	11, 23, 26, 33
	PEG–irinotecan	NKTR-102	62, 63
Phase II	HPMA–DACH–platinate	AP5346; ProLindac®	27
	HPMA copolymer–doxorubicin	PK1; FCE28068	6, 10
Phase I/II	HPMA copolymer–doxorubicin–galactosamine	PK2; FCE28069	60
	HPMA copolymer–carboplatinate	AP5280	64
	PGA–camptothecin	CT-2106	17
	Cyclodextrin polymer–camptothecin	IT-101	65
Phase I	Carboxymethyldextran–exatecan camptothecin	DE-310	66
	PEG–docetaxel	NKTR-105	67
	PEG–SN38	EZN-2208	68
	PHF–camptothecin	XMT-1001	69
Discontinued	PEG–camptothecin	Pegamotecan	32
	PEG–paclitaxel		70
	HPMA copolymer–camptothecin	MAG–CPT	39
	HPMA copolymer–paclitaxel	PNU166945	40
	Oxidized dextran–doxorubicin	DOX–OXD	71

experimental drugs (e.g., the antiangiogenic drug TNP-470). Furthermore, these versatile systems have been applied to therapeutic areas other than cancer, such as cardiovascular and neurodegenerative disorders (the antiapoptotic PGA–peptoid [1, 3]), rheumatoid arthritis (e.g., PEG–dexametasone [37]; linear cyclodextrin–α-Methylprednisolone [72]), and protozoal infection (HPMA copolymer conjugate of the antileishmanial drug 8-aminoquinoline [38, 73]).

Recent studies have also applied the concept of polymer–drug conjugates to the delivery of more than one drug (i.e., for combination therapy). For instance, an HPMA copolymer carrying both chemotherapy (Dox) and endocrine therapy (aminoglutethimide) displayed markedly increased antitumor activity in breast cancer models compared to the conjugate carrying only Dox (PK1) [74, 75]. Promising preclinical results have also been obtained with a PEG conjugate of epirubicin and nitric oxide, which has been developed to take advantage of the synergistic effect of the two drugs and to counterbalance the cardiotoxicity of epirubicin with the cardioprotective action of nitric oxide [76, 77]. Other drug combinations that have been explored in the context of combination therapy include gemcitabine and doxorubicin [78], doxorubicin and dexamethasone [79], and paclitaxel and alendronate [80].

3.6.1.2 New Polymeric Carriers. In recent years, there has been growing interest in the development of novel polymeric carriers. Size, branching, flexibility, and molecular conformation in solution have been shown to deeply impact the therapeutic performance of the polymer [81]. For instance, it has been shown that branching leads to increased blood circulation time, and the number of branches has been hypothesized to be a key parameter, more important than the MW or the final architecture of the polymer [82]. These findings have important implications for drug delivery, especially if the branched structure offers the possibility of an increased drug-loading capacity [45, 83, 84].

The development of self-immolative polymers is another innovative research trend of recent years [85]. This strategy involves the "domino-like" fragmentation of the polymeric backbone triggered by a specific signal (e.g., the cleavage of a terminal protecting group) [86]. The advantages of these systems are believed to be twofold: (i) the possibility of using high MW polymers that disassemble once their "delivery role" has been accomplished, and (ii) the possibility of translating a single cleavage into the multiple release of drug molecules [45].

New classes of responsive materials that are able to change their conformation upon a specific stimulus and hence facilitate drug delivery are also under development [87]. Such a stimulus might be a mild biological change in pH [88, 89] or temperature [90], but also can be an external trigger such as UV light [91] or IR irradiation [92].

3.6.2 The Future of Polymer–Drug Conjugates

The initial idea of a polymer–drug conjugate dates back to 1975 [1], and an HPMA copolymer–doxorubicin entered clinical evaluation nearly 20 years ago (1994). However, to date, no polymer–drug conjugate has yet reached the market. The PGA–paclitaxel conjugate Opaxio® is the polymer–drug conjugate closest to market authorization. In 2008, three Phase III clinical studies of this conjugate in patients affected by non-small cell lung carcinoma (NSCLC) were completed (Table 3.7) and the main findings were related to:

Safety. The safety profile of paclitaxel was improved by PGA conjugation, as it showed lower incidence of nausea, alopecia, and hypersensitivity reactions (requiring no premedications), and allowed faster infusion time (20–30 min compared to 3.24 h of the free paclitaxel).

Activity. PGA–PTX showed a significant antitumor activity but it did not prove superior to the control arms. An interesting improvement in overall survival was observed in women with premenopausal levels of estrogens (which correlates with higher expression of cathepsin B, the metabolizing enzyme for PGA–PTX). Consequently, a Phase II trial was initiated to investigate whether such an observation was significant. However, the very recent results of this study reported that, despite the fact that the conjugate was well tolerated, the absence of improvement in progression-free survival and overall survival did not warrant any further testing [93]. A number of Phase II studies are also ongoing to investigate the activity of PGA–PTX against a variety of malignancies (e.g., breast, ovarian, esophageal).

TABLE 3.7. Completed Phase III Trials of PGA–PTX (Opaxio®) in NSCLC

Study	Treatment and dosage	Comparator	Patients	Outcome	References
Stellar 2	Second line; monotherapy 175 and 210 mg m^{-2} every 3 wk	Docetaxel	849, PS 0–2	Similar survival Shorter infusion times No hypersensitivity Less frequent neutropenia More common neuropathy	23
Stellar 3	First line with carboplatin 210 mg m^{-2} every 3 wk	PTX + carboplatin	400, PS 2	No superior survival Less frequent alopecia, cardiac Events, myalgias More frequent neurotoxicity	26
Stellar 4	First line; monotherapy 175 or 235 mg m^{-2} every 3 wk	Gemcitabine + vinorelbine	477, PS 2	Active and well tolerated Less frequent neutropenia/anemia Fewer transfusions required More common neuropathy	11
Pioneer	First line; monotherapy 175 mg m^{-2} every 3 wk	PTX	200, PS 2 Women only	Discontinued (High number of deaths in the PGA–PTX arm)	33

The case of Opaxio® prompts some general considerations about the challenges concerning the translation of polymer–drug conjugates from the lab to the market.

3.6.2.1 Complexity of Polymer–Drug Conjugate Technology.
Polymer–drug conjugates are inherently more complex systems than standard small molecules and this has an impact on their development strategy. Polymer–drug conjugates are multicomponent systems (drug, linker, and polymer), generally polydispersed, which require several manufacturing steps. For these reasons, they are developed individually or in small libraries aimed at investigating the influence of a single parameter (e.g., the MW of the polymer or the type of linker) on the overall performance. This differs from the approach undertaken for the development of small molecules, which are generally produced in larger libraries and screened in biological studies. In addition, the performance of polymer–drug conjugates is attributed to the system as a whole (i.e., combination of the chosen polymer, linker, and drug) and not to a specific feature, as the same individual components might have different biological behaviors when used in different conjugates.

3.6.2.2 Choice of an Appropriate Patients Population.
Polymer–drug conjugates are essentially prodrug systems (i.e., designed to release the drug at the site of action). As discussed extensively in Section 4.3, drug release relies on activation from an appropriate biological trigger, typically an enzyme. However, it is not entirely clear to what extent enzyme expression is consistent across tumor types and across different patients. This is a key point, as an insufficient expression of key enzymes would result in insufficient drug release. In a parallel manner, the extent of the EPR effect varies across tumor types. Therefore, prescreening of patients and treatment of appropriate patient populations could potentially lead to higher clinical efficacy.

3.7 KEY POINTS

- Polymer–drug conjugates are a drug delivery technology where a drug is covalently attached to a polymeric carrier.
- Polymer–drug conjugates are constituted by three structural components: a polymeric carrier, drug molecules, and a biodegradable linker. A targeting moiety can also be added to achieve active targeting. Each of these components needs to meet specific requirements.
- Polymer–drug conjugates are able to target the tumor tissue by means of the EPR effect, which produces a passive accumulation of macromolecules in the tumor tissue.
- Internalization of polymer–drug conjugates occurs by endocytosis, and drug release typically occurs in the lysosomes.
- Preparation of the conjugates is a multisteps process, which involves synthesis, characterization, as well as *in vitro*, *in vivo*, and clinical assessment.

3.8   WORKED EXAMPLE

A conjugate contains an active pharmaceutical ingredient (API) content of 1% w/w. The API is normally administered at a dose of 10 mg kg^{-1}. Assuming that the required dose of the API is the same for the conjugated and unconjugated form, calculate how much conjugate needs to be administered. Comment on the feasibility of this system.

Answer:

Step 1. Calculate the dose of API needed.

For a patient of 70 kg, the dose required is

$$(10 \times 70) = 700 \ \text{mg}.$$

Step 2. Calculate the dose of conjugate needed.

As the conjugate contains 1% of API, 100-fold of conjugate need to be administered, that is,
$$700 \ \text{mg} \times 100 = 70,000 \ \text{mg} = 70 \ \text{g}.$$

Step 3. Discuss the feasibility of this approach.

This approach is clearly not feasible, as it would require administration of too large a dose of conjugate (70 g).

This example highlights the importance of selecting potent drugs and polymer carriers that allow high drug loading.

3.9   HOMEWORK PROBLEMS

1. Discuss the possible issues you would encounter if you wanted to conjugate a drug containing two different types of functional groups.

2. A scientist wants to conjugate the anticancer drug paclitaxel to a polymeric carrier to form a polymer–paclitaxel conjugate. For this purpose, he considers two possible carriers: carboxy PEG and PGA. Both carriers have a MW of 30,000 Da. Calculate the maximum theoretical loading that could be achieved with each carrier (express it as % w/w). Which carrier would you think the scientist will favor and why? Note that (i) the MW of paclitaxel is 853.9; (ii) conjugation of each drug molecule results in the loss of a water molecule (one H from the drug and OH from the polymer carrier); (iii) PGA contains approximately 200 monomers per chain.

3. A conjugate was incubated with a mixture of lysosomal enzymes and no drug release was observed in these conditions. The same conjugate was tested for antitumor activity *in vivo* and an anticancer effect was observed. Taking into account the information provided above, hypothesize a possible mechanism of action for this conjugate.

REFERENCES

1. Ringsdorf H. Structure and properties of pharmacologically active polymers. J Polym Sci 1975;51:135–153.
2. Duncan R. Polymer conjugates as anticancer nanomedicines. Nat Rev Cancer 2006;6:688–701.
3. Canal F, Sanchis J, Vicent MJ. Polymer-drug conjugates as nano-sized medicines. Curr Opin Biotechnol 2011;22:894–900.
4. De Duve C, De Barsy T, Poole B, Trouet A, Tulkens P, Van Hoof F. Lysosomotropic agents. Biochem Pharmacol 1974;23:2495–2531.
5. Kopecek J, Rejmanova P, Strohalm J, Ulbrich K, Rihova B, Chytry V, Duncan R, Lloyd JB. Synthetic polymeric drugs 1991. US Patent 5, 037, 883.
6. Vasey PA, Kaye SB, Morrison R, Twelves C, Wilson P, Duncan R, Thomson AH, Murray LS, Hilditch TE, Murray T, Burtles S, Fraier D, Frigerio E, Cassidy J. Phase I clinical and pharmacokinetic study of PK1 [N-(2-hydroxypropyl)methacrylamide copolymer doxorubicin]: first member of a new class of chemotherapeutic agents-drug-polymer conjugates. Clin Cancer Res 1999;5:83–94.
7. Pimm MV, Perkins AC, Duncan R, Ulbrich K. Targeting of N-(2-hydroxypropyl) methacrylamide copolymer-doxorubicin conjugate to the hepatocyte galactose-receptor in mice: visualisation and quantification by gamma scintigraphy as a basis for clinical targeting studies. J Drug Target 1993;1:125–131.
8. Maeda H, Ueda M, Morinaga T, Matsumotu T. Conjugation of poly(styrene-comaleic acid) derivatives to the antitumor protein neocarzinostatin: pronounced improvements in pharmacological proteins. J Med Chem 1985;28:455–461.
9. Matsumura Y, Maeda H. A new concept for macromolecular therapeutics in cancer chemotherapy: mechanism of tumoritropic accumulation of proteins and the antitumor agent SMANCS. Cancer Res 1986;46:6387–6392.
10. Seymour LW, Ferry DR, Kerr DJ, Rea D, Whitlock M, Poiner R, Boivin C, Hesslewood S, Twelves C, Blackie R, Schatzlein A, Jodrell D, Bissett D, Calvert H, Lind M, Robbins A, Burtles S, Duncan R, Cassidy J. Phase II studies of polymer-doxorubicin (PK1, FCE28068) in the treatment of breast, lung and colorectal cancer. Int J Oncol 2009;34:1629–1636.
11. O'Brien MER, Socinski MA, Popovich AY, Bondarenko IN, Tomova A, Bilynskyi BT, Hotko YS, Ganul VL, Kostinsky IY, Eisenfeld AJ, Sandalic L, Oldham FB, Bandstra B, Sandler AB, Singer JW. Randomized phase III trial comparing single-agent paclitaxel poliglumex (CT-2103, PPX) with single-agent gemcitabine or vinorelbine for the treatment of PS 2 patients with chemotherapy-naive advanced non-small cell lung cancer. J Thorac Oncol 2008;3:728–734.
12. Li C, Yu DF, Newman RA, Cabrai F, Stephens LC, Hunter N, Milas L, Wallace S. Complete regression of well-established tumors using a novel water-soluble poly(L-glutamic acid)-paclitaxel conjugate. Cancer Res 1998;58:2404–2409.

13. Li C, Yu D, Inoue T, Yang DJ, Milas L, Hunter NR, Kim EE, Wallace S. Synthesis and evaluation of water-soluble polyethylene glycol-paclitaxel conjugate as a paclitaxel prodrug. Anticancer Drugs 1996;7(6):642–648.

14. Bhatt R, de Vries P, Tulinsky J, Bellamy G, Baker B, Singer JW, Klein P. Synthesis and in vivo antitumor activity of poly(L-glutamic acid) conjugate of 20(S)-camptothecin. J Med Chem 2003;46:190–193.

15. Lammers T, Kühnlein R, Kissel M, Subr V, Etrych T, Pola R, Pechar M, Ulbrich K, Storm G, Huber P, Peschke P. Effect of physicochemical modification on the biodistribution and tumor accumulation of HPMA copolymers. J Control Release 2005;110(1):103–118.

16. Satchi-Fainaro R, Puder M, Davies JW, Tran HT, Sampson DA, Greene A, Corfas G, Folkman J. Targeting angiogenesis with a conjugate of HPMA copolymer and TNP-470. Nat Med 2004;10:255–261.

17. Homsi J, Simon GR, Garret CR, Springett G, De Conti R, Chiappori AA, Munster PN, Burton MK, Stromatt S, Allievi C, Angiuli P, Eisenfeld A, Sullivan DM, Daud AI. Phase I Trial of Poly-L-Glutamate Camptothecin (CT-2106) administered weekly in patients with advanced solid malignancies. Clin Cancer Res 2007;13(19):5855–5861.

18. Minko T, Kopeckova P, Pozharov V, Kopecek J. HPMA copolymer bound adriamycin overcomes MDR1 gene encoded resistance in a human ovarian carcinoma cell line. J Control Release 1998;54:223–233.

19. Seymour LW, Miyamoto Y, Maeda H, Brereton M, Strohalm J, Ulbrich K, Duncan R. Influence of the molecular weight on passive tumor accumulation of a soluble macromolecular drug carrier. Eur J Cancer 1995;31:766–770.

20. Noguchi Y, Wu J, Duncan R, Strohalm J, Ulbrich K, Akaike T, Maeda H. Early phase tumor accumulation of macromolecules: a great difference in clearance rate between tumor and normal tissues. Jpn J Cancer Res 1998;89:307–314.

21. Ulbrich K, Etrych T, Chytila P, Jelinkova M, Rihova B. HPMA copolymers with pH-controlled release of doxorubicin In vitro cytotoxicity and in vivo antitumor activity. J Control Release 2003;87:33–47.

22. Duncan R, Cable HC, Lloyd JB, Rejmanova P, Kopecek J. Polymers containing enzymatically degradable bonds. Design of oligopeptide side chains in poly(N-(2-hydroxypropyl) methacrylamide copolymers to promote efficient degradation by lysosomal enzymes. Macromol Chem 1983;184:1997–2008.

23. Paz-Ares L, Ross H, O'Brien M, Riviere A, Gatzemeier U, Von Pawel J, Kaukel E, Freitag L, Digel W, Bischoff H, Garcìa-Campelo R, Iannotti N, Reiterer P, Bover I, Prendiville J, Eisenfeld AJ, Oldham FB, Bandstra B, Singer JW, Bonomi P. Phase III trial comparing paclitaxel poliglumex vs docetaxel in the second-line treatment of non-small-cell lung cancer. Br J Cancer 2008;98:1608–1613.

24. Duncan R, Rejmanova P, Kopecek J, Lloyd JB. Pinocytic uptake and intracellular degradation of N-(2-hydroxypropyl)methacrylamide copolymers: a potential drug delivery system. Biochim Biophys Acta 1981;678:143–150.

25. Duncan R, Seymour LW, O'Hare KB, Flanagan PA, Wedge S, Hume IC, Ulbrich K, Strohalm J, Subr V, Spreafico F, Grandi M, Ripamonti M, Farao M, Suarato A. Preclinical evaluation of polymer-bound doxorubicin. J Control Release 1992;19:331–346.

26. Langer CJ, O'Byrne KJ, Socinski MA, Mikhailov SM, Lesniewski-Kmak K, Smakal M, Ciuleanu TE, Orlov SV, Dediu M, Heigener D, Eisenfeld AJ, Sandalic L, Oldham FB, Singer JW, Ross HJ. Phase III trial comparing paclitaxel poliglumex (CT-2103,PPX) in combination with carboplatin versus standard paclitaxel and carboplatin in the treatment

of PS 2 patients with chemotherapy-naive advanced non-small cell lung cancer. J Thorac Oncol 2008;3:623–630.

27. Campone M, Rademaker-Lakhai JM, Bennouna J, Howell SB, Nowotnik DP, Beijnen JH, Schellens JHM. Phase I and pharmacokinetic trial of AP5346, a DACH–platinum–polymer conjugate, administered weekly for three out of every 4 weeks to advanced solid tumor patients. Cancer Chemother Pharmacol 2007;60:523–533.

28. Webster R, Didier E, Harris P, Siegel N, Stadler J, Tilbury L, Smith D. PEGylated proteins: evaluation of their safety in the absence of definitive metabolism studies. Drug Metab Dispos 2007;35:9–16.

29. Pasut G, Veronese FM. PEG conjugates in clinical development or use as anticancer agents: an overview. Adv Drug Deliv Rev 2009;61:1177–1188.

30. Pasut G, Scaramuzza S, Schiavon O, Mendichi R, Veronese FM. PEG-epirubicin conjugates with high loading. J Bioact Compat Polym 2005;20:213–230.

31. Berna M, Dalzoppo D, Pasut G, Manunta M, Izzo L, Jones AT, Duncan R, Veronese F. Novel monodisperse PEG-dendrons as new tools for targeted drug delivery: synthesis, characterization and cellular uptake. Biomacromolecules 2006;7:146–153.

32. Scott LC, Yao JC, Benson AB, Thomas AL, Falk S, Mena RR, Picus J, Wright J, Mulcahy MF, Ajani JA, Evans TRJ. A phase II study of pegylated-camptothecin (pegamotecan) in the treatment of locally advanced and metastatic gastric and gastro-oesophageal junction adenocarcinoma. Cancer Chemother Pharmacol 2009;63:363–370.

33. Albain KS, Belani CP, Bonomi P, O'Byrne KJ, Schiller JH, Socinski M. PIONEER: a phase III randomized trial of paclitaxel poliglumex versus paclitaxel in chemotherapy-naïve women with advanced-stage non-small-cell lung cancer and performance status of II. Clin Lung Cancer 2006;7:417–419.

34. Singer JW, Baker B, De Vries P, Kumar A, Shaffer S, Vawter E, Bolton M, Garzone P. Poly-(L)-glutamic acid-paclitaxel (CT-2103) [XYOTAX], a biodegradable polymeric drug conjugate: characterization, preclinical pharmacology, and preliminary clinical data. Adv Exp Med Biol 2003;519:81–99.

35. Shaffer SA, Baker-Lee C, Kennedy J, Lai MS, de Vries P, Buhler K, Singer JW. In vitro and in vivo metabolism of paclitaxel polyglumex: identification of metabolites and active protease. Cancer Chemother Pharmacol 2007;59:537–548.

36. Fante C, Eldar-Boock A, Satchi-Fainaro R, Osborn HMI, Greco F. Synthesis and biological evaluation of a polyglutamic acid dopamine conjugate: a new antiangiogenic agent. J Med Chem 2011;54(14):5255–5259.

37. Liu XM, Quan LD, Tian J, Laquer FC, Ciborowski P, Wang D. Synthesis of click PEG-dexamethasone conjugates for the treatment of rheumatoid arthritis. Biomacromolecules 2010;11:2621–2628.

38. Nan A, Croft SL, Yardley V, Ghandehari H. Targetable watersoluble polymer-drug conjugates for the treatment of visceral leishmaniasis. J Control Release 2004;94:115–127.

39. Schoemaker NE, van Kesteren C, Rosing H, Jansen S, Swart M, Lieverst J, Fraier D, Breda M, Pellizzoni C, Spinelli R, Porro MG, Beijnen JH, Schellens JHM, Bokkel Huinink WW. A phase I and pharmacokinetic study of MAG-CPT, a water-soluble polymer conjugate of camptothecin. Br J Cancer 2002;87:608–614.

40. Meerum Terwogt JM, ten Bokkel Huinink WW, Schellens JH, Schot M, Mandjes IA, Zurlo MG, Rocchetti M, Rosing H, Koopman FJ, Beijnen JH. Phase I clinical and pharmacokinetic

study of PNU166945, a novel water-soluble polymer-conjugated prodrug of paclitaxel. Anticancer Drugs 2001;12:315–323.

41. Soyez H, Schacht E, Jelinkova M, Rihova B. Biological evaluation of mitomycin C bound to a biodegradable polymeric carrier. J Control Release 1997;47:71–80.

42. Ulbrich K, Subr V. Polymeric anticancer drugs with pH-controlled activation. Adv Drug Deliv Rev 2004;56:1023–1050.

43. Shen WC, Ryser HJP. Cis-aconityl spacer between daunomycin and macromolecular carriers: a model of pH-sensitive linkage releasing drug from a lysosomotropic conjugate. Biochem Biophys Res Commun 1981;102:1048–1054.

44. Duncan R, Lloyd JB, Kopecek J. Degradation of side chains of N-(2-hydroxypropyl)methacrylamide copolymers by lysosomal enzymes. Biochem Biophys Res Commun 1980;94: 284–290.

45. Erez R, Segal E, Miller K, Satchi-Fainaro R, Shabat D. Enhanced cytotoxicity of a polymer-drug conjugate with triple payload of paclitaxel. Bioorg Med Chem 2009;17(13): 4327–4335.

46. Duncan R, Hume IC, Kopeckova P, Ulbrich K, Strohalm J, Kopecek J. Anticancer agents coupled to N-(2-hydroxypropyl) methacrylamide copolymers. Evaluation of adriamycin conjugates against mouse leukemia L1210 in vivo. J Control Release 1989;10:51–63.

47. Duncan R, Hume IC, Yardley HJ, Flanagan PA, Ulbrich K, Subr V, Strohalm J. Macromolecular prodrugs for use in targeted cancer chemotherapy: melphalan covalently coupled to N- (2-hydroxypropyl)methacrylamide copolymers. J Control Release 1991;16:121–136.

48. Auzenne E, Donato NJ, Li C, Leroux E, Price RE, Farquhar D, Klostergaard J. Superior therapeutic profile of poly-L-glutamic acid-paclitaxel copolymer compared with taxol in xenogeneic compartmental models of human ovarian carcinoma. Clin Cancer Res 2002;8: 573–581.

49. Bae M, Cho S, Song J, Lee GY, Kim K, Yang J, Cho K, Kim SY, Byun Y. Metalloprotease-specific poly(ethylene glycol) methyl ether-peptide-doxorubicin conjugate for targeting anticancer drug delivery based on angiogenesis. Drugs Exp Clin Res 2003;29:15–23.

50. Chau Y, Padera RF, Dang NM, Langer R. Antitumor efficacy of a novel polymer–peptide–drug conjugate in human tumor xenograft models. Int J Cancer 2006;118: 1519–1526.

51. Mansour AM, Drevs J, Esser N, Hamada FM, Badary OA, Unger C, Fichtner I, Kratz F. A new approach for the treatment of malignant melanoma: enhanced antitumor efficacy of an albumin-binding doxorubicine prodrug that is cleaved by matrix metalloproteinase 2. Cancer Res 2003;63:4062–4066.

52. De Winne K, Seymourb LW, Schachta EH. Synthesis and in vitro evaluation of macromolecular antitumour derivatives based on phenylenediamine mustard. Eur J Pharm Sci 2005;24:159–168.

53. Cavallaro G, Pitarresi G, Licciardi M, Giammona G. Polymeric prodrug for release of an antitumoral agent by specific enzymes. Bioconjug Chem 2001;12:143–151.

54. Sloane BF, Yan S, Podgorski I, Linebaugh BE, Cher ML, Mai J, Cavallo-Medved D, Sameni M, Dosescu J, Moin K. Cathepsin B and tumor proteolysis: contribution of the tumor microenvironment. Semin Cancer Biol 2005;15:149–157.

55. Hofmann UB, Westphal JR, Waas ET, Zendman AJW, Cornelissen IMHA, Ruiter DJ, van Muijen GNP. Matrix metalloproteinases in human melanoma cell lines and xenografts:

increased expression of activated matrix metalloproteinase-2 (MMP-2) correlates with melanoma progression. Br J Cancer 1999;81(5):774–782.

56. O'Hare KB, Duncan R, Strohalm J, Ulbrich K, Kopeckova P. Polymeric drug-carriers containing doxorubicin and melanocyte-stimulating hormone: in vitro and in vivo evaluation against murine melanoma. J Drug Target 1993;1(3):217–229.

57. Canal F, Vicent MJ, Pasut G, Schiavon O. Relevance of folic acid/polymer ratio in targeted PEG-epirubicin conjugates. J Control Release 2010;146(3):388–399.

58. Flanagan PA, Kopecková P, Kopecek J, Duncan R. Evaluation of protein-N-(2-hydroxypropyl)methacrylamide copolymer conjugates as targetable drug carriers. 1. Binding, pinocytic uptake and intracellular distribution of transferrin and anti-transferrin receptor antibody conjugates. Biochim Biophys Acta 1989;993(1):83–91.

59. Seymour LW, Ulbrich K, Wedge SR, Hume IC, Strohalm J, Duncan R. N-(2-hydroxypropyl)methacrylamide copolymers targeted to the hepatocyte galactose-receptor: pharmacokinetics in DBA2 mice. Br J Cancer 1991;63:859–866.

60. Seymour LW, Ferry DR, Anderson D, Hesslewood S, Julyan PJ, Poyner R, Doran J, Young AM, Burtles S, Kerr DJ. Hepatic drug targeting: phase I evaluation of polymer-bound doxorubicin. J Clin Oncol 2002;20:1668–1676.

61. Caiolfa VR, Zamai M, Fiorino A, Frigerio E, Pellizzoni C, d'Argy R, Ghiglieri A, Castelli MG, Farao M, Pesenti E, Gigli M, Angelucci F. Polymer-bound camptothecin: initial biodistribution and antitumour activity studies. J Control Release 2000;65:105–119.

62. Hamm JT, Richards D, Ramanathan RK, Becerra C, Jameson G, Walling J, Gribben D, Dhar S, Eldon M, Von Hoff D. Dose-finding study of NKTR-102 in combination with cetuximab. J Clin Oncol 2009;27abstr 13503.

63. Borad MJ, Hamm JT, Rosen LS, Jameson GS, Utz J, Mulay M, Eldon M, Dhar S, Acosta L, Von Hoff DD. Phase I dose finding and pharmacokinetic study of NKTR-102 (PEGylated irinotecan): early evidence of anti-tumor activity. J Clin Oncol 2008;26abstr 13518.

64. Rademaker-Lakhai JM, Terret C, Howell SB, Baud CM, de Boer RF, Pluim D, Beijnen JH, Schellens JHM, Droz JP. A phase I and pharmacological study of the platinum polymer AP5280 given as an intravenous infusion once every 3 weeks in patients with solid tumors. Clin Cancer Res 2004;10:3386–3395.

65. Oliver JC, Yen Y, Synold TW, Schluep T, Davis M. A dose-finding pharmacokinetic study of IT-101, the first de novo designed nanoparticle therapeutic in refractory solid tumors. J Clin Oncol 2008;26abstr 14538.

66. Soepenberg O, de Jonge MJA, Sparreboom A, de Bruin P, Eskens F, de Heus G, Wanders J, Cheverton P, Ducharme MP, Verweij J. Phase I and pharmacokinetic study of DE-310 in patients with advanced solid tumors. Clin Cancer Res 2005;11:703–711.

67. Calvo E, Hoch U, Maslyar DJ. Tolcher AW Dose-escalation phase I study of NKTR-105, a novel pegylated form of docetaxel. J Clin Oncol 2010;28TPS160.

68. Guo Z, Wheler JJ, Naing A, Mani S, Goel S, Mulcahy M, Gamza F, Longley C, Buchbinder A, Kurzrock R. Clinical pharmacokinetics (PK) of EZN-2208, a novel anticancer agent, in patients with advanced malignancies: a phase I, first-in-human, dose-escalation study. J Clin Oncol 2008;26:2556.

69. Sausville EA, Garbo LE, Weiss GJ, Shkolny D, Yurkovetskiy AV, Bethune C, Ramanathan RK, Fram RJ. Phase I study of XMT-1001 given IV every 3 weeks to patients with advanced solid tumors. J Clin Oncol 2010;28:13121.

70. Beeram M, Rowinsky EK, Hammond LA, Patnaik A, Schwartz GH, de Bono JS, Forero L, Forouzesh B, Berg KE, Rubin EH, Beers S, Killian A, Kwiatek J, McGuire J, Spivey L, Takimoto CH. A phase I and pharmacokinetic (PK) study of PEG-paclitaxel in patients with advanced solid tumors. Proc Am Soc Clin Oncol 2002;21:405.

71. Danhauser-Riedl S, Hausmann E, Schick HD, Bender R, Dietzfelbinger H, Rastetter J, Hanauske AR. Phase I clinical and pharmacokinetic trial of dextran conjugated doxorubicin (AD-70, DOX-OXD). Invest New Drugs 1993;11:187–195.

72. Hwang J, Rodgers K, Oliver JC, Schluep T. α-Methylprednisolone conjugated cyclodextrin polymer-based nanoparticles for rheumatoid arthritis therapy. Int J Nanomedicine 2008;3(3):359–372.

73. Roy P, Das S, Auddy RG, Mukherjee A. Biological targeting and drug delivery in control of Leishmaniasis. J Cell Anim Biol 2012;6:73–87.

74. Vicent MJ, Greco F, Nicholson RI, Paul A, Griffiths PC, Duncan R. Polymer therapeutics designed for a combination therapy of hormone-dependent cancer. Angew Chem Int Ed 2005;44:4061–4066.

75. Greco F, Vicent MJ, Gee S, Jones AT, Gee J, Nicholson RI, Duncan R. Investigating the mechanism of enhanced cytotoxicity of HPMA copolymer-Dox-AGM in breast cancer cells. J Control Release 2007;117(1):28–39.

76. Santucci L, Mencarelli A, Renga B, Pasut G, Veronese F, Zacheo A, Germani A, Fiorucci S. Nitric oxide modulates proapoptotic and antiapoptotic properties of chemotherapy agents: the case of NO-pegylated epirubicin. FASEB J 2006;20:765–767.

77. Pasut G, Greco F, Mero A, Mendichi R, Fante C, Green RJ, Veronese FM. Polymer-drug conjugates for combination anticancer therapy: investigating the mechanism of action. J Med Chem 2009;52:6499–6502.

78. Lammers T, Subr V, Ulbrich K, Peschke P, Huber PE, Hennink WE, Storm G. Simultaneous delivery of doxorubicin and gemcitabine to tumors in vivo using prototypic polymeric drug carriers. Biomaterials 2009;30(20):3466–3475.

79. Kostkova H, Etrych T, Rihova B, Ulbrich K. Synergistic effect of HPMA copolymer-bound doxorubicin and dexamethasone in vivo on mouse lymphomas. J Bioact Compat Polym 2011;26(3):270–286.

80. Clementi C, Miller K, Mero A, Satchi-Fainaro R, Pasut G. Dendritic poly(ethylene glycol) bearing paclitaxel and alendronate for targeting bone neoplasms. Mol Pharm 2011;8:1063–1072.

81. Fox ME, Szoka FC, Frechet JMJ. Soluble polymer carriers for the treatment of cancer: the importance of molecular architecture. Acc Chem Res 2009a;42:1141–1151.

82. Lim J, Guo Y, Rostollan CL, Stanfield J, Hsieh JT, Sun X, Simanek EE. The role of the size and number of polyethylene glycol chains in the biodistribution and tumor localization of triazine dendrimers. Mol Pharm 2008;5:540–547.

83. Perumal O, Khandare J, Kolhe P, Kannan S, Lieh-Lai M, Kannan RM. Effects of branching architecture and linker on the activity of hyperbranched polymer-drug conjugates. Bioconjug Chem 2009;20:842–846.

84. Fox ME, Guillaudeu S, Frechet JMJ, Jerger K, Macaraeg N, Szoka FC. Synthesis and in vivo antitumor efficacy of PEGylated poly(L-lysine) dendrimer-camptothecin conjugates. Mol Pharm 2009b;6:1562–1572.

85. Blencowe CA, Russell A, Greco F, Hayes W, Thornthwaite DW. Self-immolative linkers in polymeric delivery systems. Polym Chem 2011;2:773–790.

86. Sagi A, Weinstain R, Karton N, Shabat D. Self-immolative polymers. J Am Chem Soc 2008;130:5434–5435.

87. Heath F, Haria P, Alexander C. Varying polymer architecture to deliver drugs. AAPS J 2007;9:235–240.

88. Henry SM, El-Sayed MEH, Pirie CM, Hoffman AS, Stayton PS. pH-responsive poly(styrene-alt-maleic anhydride) alkylamide copolymers for intracellular drug delivery. Biomacromolecules 2006;7:2407–2414.

89. Heath F, Saeed AO, Pennadam SS, Thurecht KJ, Alexander C. 'Isothermal' phase transitions and supramolecular architecture changes in thermoresponsive polymers via acid-labile side-chains. Polym Chem 2010;1:1252–1262.

90. You YZ, Oupický D. Synthesis of temperature-responsive heterobifunctional block copolymers of poly(ethylene glycol) and poly(N-isopropylacrylamide). Biomacromolecules 2007;8:98–105.

91. Shamay Y, Adar L, Ashkenasy G, David A. Light induced drug delivery into cancer cells. Biomaterials 2011;32:1377–1386.

92. Hribar KC, Lee MH, Lee D, Burdick JA. Enhanced release of small molecules from near-infrared light responsive polymer-nanorod composites. ACS Nano 2011;5:2948–2956.

93. Batus M, Mohajer R, Pach D, Basu S, Fidler MJ, Bonomi PD. Phase II trial of pacli-taxel poliglumex (CT-2103) in pre- and post-menopausal women on hormonal replacement therapy (HRT) with non-small cell lung cancer (NSCLC). J Clin Oncol 2011;29:18047.

4

POLYMERIC MICROPARTICLES

Noelle K. Comolli and Colleen E. Clark

Department of Chemical Engineering, Villanova University, Philadelphia, PA, USA

4.1 INTRODUCTION

"Medicine, is a collection of uncertain prescriptions, the result of which, taken collectively, are more fatal than useful to mankind."

Napoleon Bonaparte

One may think starting this chapter with this quote from Napoleon is a bit pessimistic, but taken in a different light it can be used as inspiration. Napoleon warns us that medicine is uncertain, which is true because it is a science in which new discoveries are constantly changing our perspective. The second part of the quote is what is critical in this chapter, when not careful, medicine can be deadly. How, you are wondering does this relate to polymer microparticles? Simple, it all comes down to the correct dosage. When medicines are delivered at too high a dosage, things become toxic, and too low, there is no therapeutic effect. Dosage to the wrong area can also be harmful. So how does one control that dosage to get it exactly where they want, without having to use too much? Exactly, microparticles! Ok, it is not always that simple, but microparticles can be a step in the right direction.

Engineering Polymer Systems for Improved Drug Delivery, First Edition.
Edited by Rebecca A. Bader and David A. Putnam.
© 2014 John Wiley & Sons, Inc. Published 2014 by John Wiley & Sons, Inc.

As introduced in Chapter 1, polymeric microparticles have been widely researched for controlled drug delivery for many years. This is because coating the drug in a protective polymer layer is often done to allow for higher dosage delivery of a potent drug to a specific area or to protect a drug from degradation before reaching its target. Microparticles have also been designed to extend the time between dosages by controlling their release rate, thus making it easier for patients to take. The best analogy for these particles is that they are like an M&M® candy. However, instead of using a coating to make the chocolate "melt in your mouth, not in your hand" [1], they are making the drug release in your intestine not your stomach, for example.

In this chapter, you will see how encapsulating drugs into a polymeric microparticle can increase the circulation time of the drug, decrease systemic clearance, protect the drug from enzymatic or acidic degradation, control the rate of rate of drug release, and provide targeting to a specific area. This chapter will also review the basic principles of polymeric microparticle design, synthesis and characterization methods.

4.2   THE RATIONALE FOR MICROPARTICLES

Controlled release is a key design goal of any drug delivery device for increased patient compliance, increased efficacy, and decreased unwanted side effects from repeated uncontrolled dosages. Other chapters in this text provide sufficient evidence to the benefits of encapsulating drugs in polymer-based materials to control delivery including nanoparticles and hydrogels, however, this chapter focuses specifically on *microparticles*. The first goal of this chapter is to define polymer microparticles and explain why the *micrometer* size range is desirable for particulate drug delivery.

4.2.1   What is a Microparticle?

Before going much further, it is important to actually define a polymeric microparticle. To be considered a *microparticle*, the individual particle must have an effective diameter on the order of $1-1000$ μm. However, in most cases, the microparticles are less than 100 μm in diameter, and those in the small micrometer $(0.5-10$ μm) range are often referred to as *nanoparticles* (despite their micrometer size) [2–4]. The polymeric part is the actual solid vehicle itself, in which the drug is either physically entrapped (solid microparticles, Fig. 4.1a) or dissolved in a liquid which is encapsulated by the polymer (liquid-filled microparticles, Fig. 4.1b). There are benefits and challenges to both types of microparticles, however, the reason for picking one over the other is largely dependent on the drug itself. Drugs that are hydrophobic are more easily incorporated into solid-filled particles, as they are able to codissolve in the same phase as the polymer. On the other hand, hydrophilic drugs (most proteins, peptides, biologics) are more readily encapsulated into a liquid-filled capsule because they do not codissolve with the polymer phase.

The polymer itself is what controls the drug delivery rate and provides the protection (from pH, enzyme, water, heat, etc). The polymer can control the release via several mechanisms, for example, swelling (via temperature [5–7] or response

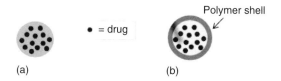

Figure 4.1. Schematic of solid (a) versus liquid-filled (b) polymeric microparticles.

to pH [8, 9]), diffusion (solid microparticles [2, 10, 11]), or controlled degradation (biodegradable polymers [2, 10–12]). Therefore, the choice of the polymer is critical in the design of a successful microparticle for a particular application.

4.2.2 The Benefits of Particulate Drug Delivery

Incorporation of therapeutics, particularly proteins, into biodegradable polymeric particles is beneficial for multiple reasons. Polymeric particles protect the protein from proteolysis and denaturation (loss of the three-dimensional structure and thereby function), as well as enhance the therapeutic efficacy and prolong the release of the protein [4, 13–16]. The release rate of the protein from these polymeric particles has been found to be related to the protein loading and polymer degradation rate and proportional to the size of the particle [3, 11]. This allows particles to be designed in such a way that a controlled, sustained release of drug can be achieved.

4.2.3 Why Micro?

Or maybe the question you are thinking is why not nano? The simple answer is: smaller is not always better. Although cellular uptake has been shown to be size-dependent (0.1 μm > 1 μm > 10 μm [17, 16]), with a preference for smaller size, too small a size can lead to uptake by too many cells. For example, too small a size in lung delivery (optimal is 4–6 μm) can lead to systemic delivery via blood vessels rather than targeting of the lung mucosa.

Larger particles also lead to higher drug loading [18] and longer control of release (shift in the release profile) [3]. Nanoparticles, on average, release on the order of hours to days, whereas microparticles provide on the order of weeks of controlled delivery.

Table 4.1 gives relative sizes of different structures in the human body, giving an idea of the range of sizes necessary for delivery. The choice of micro- versus nano-sized polymeric particles really comes down to location—it is decided by where you need that particle to go and how long you want the delivery controlled.

4.3 DEFINING THE DESIGN CRITERIA

In engineering, it is always best to first define the problem: that is, list the knowns, unknowns, and desired outcome. The first question is simple: what is the desired

TABLE 4.1. Relative Size Comparison of Biological Components

Name	Diameter	References
Staphylococcus aureus	1 μm	19
Red blood cell	7.8 μm	20
White blood cells (monocytes, leukocytes, neutrophils)	12–18 μm	20
IgG antibody	14.8 nm	21
Tumor vasculature	200 nm–1.2 μm	22
Aorta	25 mm	20
Capillaries	8 μm	20

outcome (i.e., the goal of using the microparticle)? As mentioned above, this could be for many reasons, including protecting the drug, extending release time, and/or controlling the release location. In order to define what is known and unknown for the design, more questions need to be answered, such as, What is the target area? What is the desired delivery route? What is the time frame of drug release? Answering these questions will define what polymer, what type of microparticle, and which synthesis method is best suited for that particular design.

4.3.1   Desired Route of Delivery

One of the first design choices is the determination of the route of delivery for the microparticles. Is the delivery route oral, inhaled, injection (subcutaneous, intravenous (IV), intramuscular (IM))? What are the physical and chemical barriers between the delivery site and the target location? As discussed in Chapter 2, these include, but are not limited to, pH changes, enzymes, mucus, the vascular system, the immune system (including white blood cells and immune proteins), and fluid and mechanical forces. Changes in the chemical environment can be taken advantage of in triggering the swelling behaviour or stimulating biodegradation. The amount of travel time to reach the target release site can also affect the delivery route of choice. If immediate activity is desired, the delivery method chosen may be a direct delivery route, such as, IM injection. However, if slow activity is desired, oral delivery would be preferred [16, 19].

4.3.2   Local Tissue Environment

The chemical and physical properties of the environment of the target tissue will determine the polymers ability to respond (degrade, swell, collapse, etc). Every tissue/cell has its own environmental factors, which include the local vascular structure and the presence of fluid convection (mucus, cerebrospinal fluid, extracellular fluid, blood) at the site. These will determine not only the characteristics of the microparticle needed (size, shape) but also the polymer selection because of the need for stability in that environment. For example, changes in local vascular or tissue structure can be advantageous in trapping microparticles for extended local release. The presence of certain cell surface receptors can be used as a mechanism for cellular uptake of the microparticle and/or drug release. Designs such as these rely on a strong understanding of the cellular physiology, and the biochemical environment at the target site.

4.3.3   Time Frame for Drug Release

The most critical factor in choosing a polymer is the desired rate of drug release. Drug release can be controlled by either the biodegradation time of the polymer or the response of the polymer to the local tissue environment (pH, temperature) or external forces (magnetic). Time frames for microparticle delivery can range from weeks to months, depending on the polymer and size of the microparticle. The long-term delivery achieved by microparticles is a great advantage over nanoparticles which usually release drugs over shorter time frames.

4.4   POLYMER SELECTION

Selecting the right polymer is the most important decision to make when designing a microparticle delivery system. The choice of the polymer will determine both the mechanism of drug release and the length of the release time. It also plays a role in selecting the synthesis method best suited for the manufacture of these microparticles. The choice usually depends on the location, extent of delivery time needed, and the drug itself. For example, a protein-based therapeutic targeting the colon may be delivered orally by a pH-responsive polymer because the polymer would protect the protein through the low pH of the stomach and release it by swelling at the higher pH of the colon. However, the same pH-responsive polymer would not be beneficial for pulmonary delivery of a therapeutic targeting the lungs where there is no pH shift to cause the release of the drug.

4.4.1   Synthetic Biodegradable Polymers

In order to be biodegradable, the polymers must gradually degrade over time into materials that can be metabolized or excreted from the body. These biodegradable particles release their drug via some combination of erosion and diffusion. Erosion is the physical dissolution of the polymer resulting from degradation and is most commonly seen as hydrolysis. As the water penetrates the polymer it hydrolyzes the polymer (bulk erosion) but if the polymer is highly hydrophobic it must degrade from the surface only (surface erosion). In most real systems, the polymerization is a combination of these two and an initial burst is seen where surface erosion dominates before bulk erosion can occur. Another method for release of the drug is diffusion controlled by the concentration gradient of the drug in the microparticle. This diffusion process, in combination with bulk erosion and surface erosion, is commonly seen in biodegradable devices [12, 20].

Polymers widely used in these applications include poly(lactic acid) (PLA), poly(glycolic acid) (PGA) and their copolymer poly(lactic-co-glycolic acid) (PLGA) [11, 21–25]. It has been shown that microparticles made from PLA with diameter of 30 μm or less have approximately a homogeneous degradation rate throughout the entire particle [22]. The biocompatibility of PLA is evident in its frequent use in drug delivery, and only a mild inflammatory response results when PLA microparticles are injected into tissue [22]. The PLA microparticles when injected into tissue alone can lead to fibrous encapsulation of the entire microparticle area. Incorporation of these microparticles into a nondegradable polymeric hydrogel could protect the particles from this cellular response. The incorporation of the microparticles within the hydrogel could also serve to further localize the delivery, minimizing unwanted side effects.

4.4.2   Polysaccharides: Natural Biodegradable Polymers

Natural polymers (polysaccharides) are long chains of sugars (mono saccharides) that are both abundant and inexpensive. They have been shown to be biocompatible and biodegradable. The ability of these polysaccharides to be degraded by the natural bacteria present in the human colon makes them an ideal candidate for delivering drugs to the colon. In order to do this, most polysaccharides will need to be coated with an enteric coating to protect their cargo (especially if a protein or peptide) from the acidic environment of the stomach and upper gastrointestinal tract. Once the polysaccharide microparticle reaches the colon, it can be degraded by bacteria for releasing the drug for local use or for adsorption to systemic delivery.

Polysaccharides are found naturally occurring in algae, bacteria, animals, and plants. Some of the most common examples used in drug delivery designs are based on alignates, chitosan, and chondroitin sulfate.

4.4.3   Responsive Polymers

As discussed in depth in Chapter 12, microparticles that can "sense" their environment to trigger release rely upon polymers that respond to either changes in pH or temperature, or other stimuli. The response of the polymer can vary from phase separation, chemical, swelling behavior and surface changes. These responses are most often the result of changes in Vander Waals interactions, hydrogen bonding, or hydrophobic interactions with the polymer and its solvent. The most common types of polymers used in this application are pH-responsive polymers because the pH in the body varies from approximately 2 in the stomach to approximately 8 in parts of the small intestine. Therefore, a polymer whose swelling can be controlled to protect a drug at low pH and release it at higher pH would be ideal for oral delivery techniques. Polymers that have been proposed to do just that include polyacrylic and polymethacrylic acids. Some of the drugs that have been attempted to be delivered with these pH-responsive polymers include insulin [26–29], caffeine, and lysozyme. Other pH responsive polymers used in drug delivery include poly(maleic anhydride), poly(N,N-dimethylaminoethyl methacrylate), and poly(amidoamine)s.

Temperature-sensitive polymers have also been proposed in drug delivery applications, meaning they exhibit either a lower critical solution temperature (LCST) or an upper critical solution temperature (UCST). Polymers that fall out of solution upon heating exhibit an LCST (the temperature where this phase separation occurs), and conversely, those that go into solution upon heating exhibit a UCST. Taking advantage of these phase separations can trigger the release of the drug from the polymer or its entrapment in the polymer. Polymers that exhibit an LCST within the physiological range include poly-*N*-isopropylacrylamide (PNIPAM), poly(*N*,*N*-diethyl acrylamide) (PDEAM) and poly(methyl vinyl ether) (PMVE). As for polymers exhibiting UCST within the physiological range, networks of poly(acrylic acid), and poly(acrylamide) have been studied, however, most designs use an LCST responsive polymer.

4.4.4 Polyethylene Glycol

Polyethylene glycol (PEG) is one of the most common biomaterials. PEG exhibits two key properties that make it different from many other polymers. First and foremost, PEG is a *hydrophilic* polymer whereas most other polymers are *hydrophobic*. This *hydropholicity* increases PEG's ability to prevent protein and cellular adhesion (i.e., creating a nonfouling surface). This is because PEG preferentially binds to water on its surface, preventing proteins from adhering. The ability to strongly bind water also allows PEG to maintain its 3-D shape. Therefore, PEG coating on microparticles hinders engulfment by cells (such as macrophages and lymphocytes).

Another important property of PEG is that it is not biodegradable. Therefore, PEG alone is rarely used in microparticle design, but rather as a copolymer with a biodegradable or responsive polymer. PEG is added sometimes as a spacer between various functional groups because it is biocompatible and relatively inert. PEG can also be added to increase the hydropholicity of a microparticle (especially in a micelle or liposomal type design), or simply to aid in the prevention of macrophage uptake during systemic circulation [30, 31, 15].

4.5 MICROPARTICLE SYNTHESIS

4.5.1 Emulsions

Many microparticle synthesis methods take advantage of emulsions, either single or double. The emulsion can be formed spontaneously, in the case of liposomes or micelles, or more commonly with the addition of mechanical force (stirring, sonication, homogenization). The two most common techniques are based on using an oil phase (organic solvent) to dissolve the polymer and emulsifying this phase into micrometer-sized beads using mechanical force. The drug can be incorporated either with the polymer in the oil phase or as a second emulsion within the oil phase. The choice of which phase to incorporate the drug into depends on its hydrophobicity.

Single-emulsion (oil-in-water, O/W) microparticles are the simplest to make, but this technique requires the drug to be hydrophobic so it can codissolve with the polymer in the organic (oil) phase. Once dissolved, the oil phase is added to a larger volume of water (usually at minimum 10 times the volume of the oil phase) and thoroughly mixed. This mixture is similar to an oil-and-vinegar salad dressing; the more the mixing, the smaller the oil phase beads are in the water phase. If the agitation is removed, the mixture will eventually settle again into two separate continuous phases. The input of energy in emulsion methods is usually provided by sonication or through a homogenizer. Once the emulsification is complete, the solvent needs to be removed, which allows the polymer to harden into solid microparticles with the drug evenly dispersed throughout. Solvent removal can often be done by simply allowing it to evaporate; however, this must be done under continuous mixing to prevent phase separation. The longer the solvent takes to remove, the greater the chance for the drug to diffuse out of the oil phase and into the water phase, so in some cases a secondary solvent may be added to the water phase to help extract the primary solvent from the polymer. The single-emulsion method tends to yield a higher drug loading than to the double-emulsion method because the drug entropically favors the hydrophobic (oil) phase over the water phase.

The double-emulsion technique is commonly referred to as the water-in-oil-in-water (W/O/W) method and is illustrated in Fig. 4.2.

The basic process involves dissolving the chosen polymer in a solvent (the oil phase). The therapeutic protein or drug is then dissolved in an aqueous phase, and then

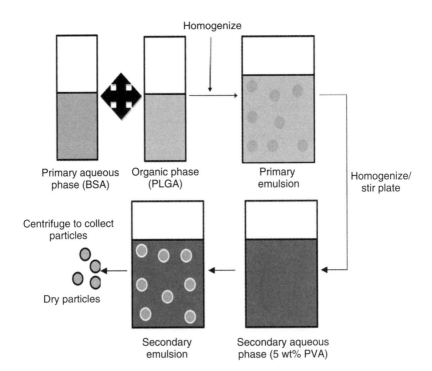

Figure 4.2. Water-in-oil-in-water double emulsion method for microparticle synthesis.

emulsified with the oil phase. In order to physically entrap these water-phase beads within the polymer, the emulsion is quickly added to a second larger water phase. The emulsion creates a shell of polymer/oil phase around the inner aqueous phase beads. This double emulsion, however, is just as unstable as the primary emulsion and requires mixing (either using a homogenizer or a magnetic stir bar) to maintain it. The secondary water phase also usually includes a surfactant of some kind to help stabilize the emulsion. The oil-phase solvent slowly evaporates, leaving a hardened polymer shell around the water-phase drug. The double-emulsion method can be obviously used only for drugs that are hydrophilic and stable in aqueous environments. Double-emulsion particles have been used to entrap many different protein therapeutics such as insulin, albumin, human growth hormone, and basic fibroblast growth factor (reviewed in Cleland (1997) [4], Soppimath et al. (2001) [32], Putney (1998) [33], and Brannon-Peppas (1995) [34]).

One of the prime limiting factors to microparticle design for protein therapeutics is the use of hazardous organic solvents for the oil phase. These solvents, especially at the phase boundary of the primary aqueous-oil emulsion, can denature the therapeutic protein by damaging their secondary and tertiary structures, leaving them inactive [35, 36]. The choice of organic solvent is not so simple. The solvent must have a low miscibility with water but also be a good solvent for the polymer chosen. If the solvent is at all miscible with water, the protein can easily be lost to this mixing, especially during the hardening step in the secondary water phase, which in most cases will last several for hours. The solvent also must be readily evaporated because organic extracts from the compounds would not be acceptable for clinical applications.

Birnbaum et al. performed a thorough study of the effect of using either ethyl acetate, dichloromethane, or a dichloromethane–methanol mixture on the formulation and release of β-estradiol from PLGA microparticles [37]. The investigators concluded that the microparticles made from ethyl acetate had the most homogeneous distribution of β-estradiol and that the release from these microparticles as well as those prepared from the dichloromethane–methanol mixture was more optimal than those microparticles fabricated using dichloromethane alone [37]. Studies by other research groups have confirmed that when proteins are encapsulated in W/O/W particles with ethyl acetate as solvent, there is more stable protein remaining than with dichloromethane [4, 36].

4.5.2 Preventing Agglomeration

Polymer microparticles made via emulsion techniques are prone to agglomeration (sticking together). This can be disastrous because the desired micrometer size will be lost when large amounts of microparticles stick together. In order to prevent agglomeration, surface-active agents (surfactants) are commonly added during the hardening phase. These surfactants increase the surface tension, by coating the polymer surface. The most commonly used surfactant is poly(vinyl alcohol) (PVA), and also others including polaxamer, tween, and pluronic. This approach prevents adhesion of other polymer microparticles. Although the surfactant is often hard to remove after processing [38], recent studies have found that coating with certain surfactants can increase the microparticles' cellular uptake and their ability to kill cancer cells (when loaded with a chemotherapeutic) over those not treated with the surfactant [39]. This indicates that the complete removal of the surfactant may not always be necessary; on the other hand, it will most likely have an effect on the resulting microparticles' biocompatibility.

4.5.3 Collection and Drying

No matter what synthesis method is used, microparticles need to be collected from their liquid suspension and sterilized. The two main methods for collecting these microparticles are centrifugation or extrusion. When particles are allowed to spin overtime and harden in solution, centrifugation is most often used to collect them. Centrifugation requires high speeds ($\sim$10,000g) and often long times to collect all the microparticles in the pellet. The disadvantage of centrifugation is that the pellet can also collect the surfactant (especially when the surfactant is PVA). The pellet can be "washed" by resuspending it in distilled water and centrifuging again to form the pellet. This "wash" process may be repeated once or twice. An advantage to centrifugation is that the supernatant can be saved for confirming drug loading. Also, centrifugation can be used to help narrow the size distribution. Starting at a lower speed, larger microparticles can be collected and removed via the pellet. Increasing the speed for the next spin for the supernatant will then collect smaller microparticles. This step can be repeated until the desired size range is collected.

Many times, these microparticles are also dried prior to use via lyopholization in order to get an exact weight for dosages and for stability during storage. If the microparticle is to be stored in an aqueous solution, the drug would most likely be lost via degradation of the microparticle or swelling. This makes drying seem critical; however, sometimes in the drying process itself, the drug and/or the polymer can be damaged [40]. Images of dried microparticles show the cracking of and surface damage to the polymer shell. However, the long-term storage issues, as well as the need to measure an exact dosage of microparticles (by weight) most often outweighs issues with drying.

Extrusion refers to sending the dissolved polymer in solution through a needle-like device either into a drying environment (spray dryers) for immediate hardening or into a complexation solution for gelation (common for polysaccharides). Spray drying uses either a single or double emulsion and, instead of allowing the microparticle to harden in solution before collecting and drying, sprays the solution through a small nozzle, aerosolizing it into small droplets (micrometer size) that rapidly dry in a collection chamber [41, 42]. These devices are commonly used in both food and pharmaceutical industries.

Polysaccharide microparticles are most often formed by spraying the dissolved polymer into a complexation solution (often calcium chloride) where the solution is exposed to a droplet generator (high voltage electric pulse) [43]. The polymer forms gel-like beads because of ionic interactions with the solution. These beads are then transferred to a cationic solution to form solid microcapsules. The positively charged surfaces can be counteracted with the addition of alginate [43]. This method

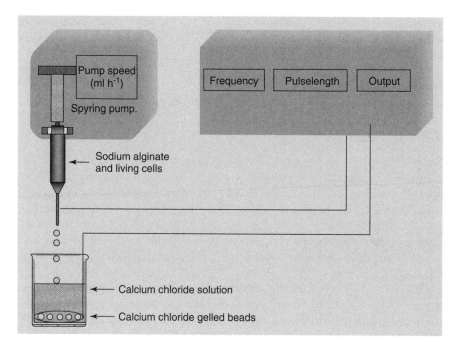

Figure 4.3. Complexation of polysaccharides to form microparticles. Reproduced with the permission of the Royal Society of Chemistry [43].

is summarized in Fig. 4.3. Extrusion techniques are the most reliable for controlling the size of the microparticles. This is because the size of particle is dependent upon the size of the needle-like tip used and can be easily altered by changing the tip.

4.5.4 Sterilization

A major drawback to the use of microparticles for delivery of therapeutics is the difficulty in sterilizing the polymer. As many of the microparticles are meant to biodegrade in the presence of an aqueous solution, washing the particles with ethanol:water mixtures is not advisable, as it may lead to loss of some of the entrapped drug during washing. The common sterilization techniques of electron beams and steam (autoclave) application are likely to melt the polymer as well as denature the entrapped protein.

A novel solution that has been evaluated by several researchers is the use of supercritical fluids for the sterilization and processing of the microparticles. Processing of microparticles using supercritical fluids, most commonly supercritical CO_2, has been successfully done using several techniques [44, 45]. A common technique used is known as the rapid expansion method, where the polymer and drug are codissolved in the supercritical fluid. The supercritical fluid is then rapidly expanded, allowing the transition into a tri-phase region where the polymer and drug are no longer in solution, and facilitating formation of micrometer- or submicrometer-sized composite particles [46, 47]. The idea that the supercritical fluid itself could sterilize the polymer was first suggested by Dillow et al. [48].

4.6 MICROPARTICLE CHARACTERIZATION METHODS

4.6.1 Morphology

Microparticle morphology is most often assumed to be spherical, but this is not always the case. Some polymer microparticles look more like a red blood cell (a disk shape) than a sphere. Therefore, it is critical to always confirm the shape of the microparticles from a specific synthesis method. Microparticle morphology is most easily confirmed using electron microscopy—scanning electron microscopy (SEM) or environmental scanning electron microscopy (ESEM). SEM and ESEM are based on high energy electron beams and, therefore, require the surface to be conductive. In traditional SEM, the sample must be dry and conductive and, therefore, for polymers, a metal coating is usually sprayed onto the sample to enhance imaging. Care must be taken to not overcoat the sample, however, because the resulting image could be misinterpreted for what is sample and what is coating. More advanced humidity chambers available on ESEMs allow samples to be imaged while "wet." This does not mean that the sample can be immersed in solution, but rather, the polymer does not need to be completely dried. This allows visualization of the microparticle in what would be the more "natural" state because *in vivo* it will be wet. Transmission electron microscopy (TEM) is often used for smaller size (nano-sized) imaging, but can also provide useful morphological images of microparticles (Fig. 4.4).

Although electron microscopy gives an excellent visualization of what the polymer microparticle looks like, it cannot confirm the location of the polymer or the drug within the microparticle. For this confirmation, using fluorescent imaging either with regular fluorescent microscopy or confocal microscopy is preferred. This methodology can also be helpful in confirming the availability of ligands on the surface of a microparticle (Fig. 4.5).

4.6.2 Size and Polydispersity

SEM and other forms of microscopy can show the size range of the particles and often even have tools to measure individual particle sizes within their software. However, microscopy often can be skewed, usually unintentionally, by where the sample is viewed. The best way to get a more accurate size estimate, including the polydispersity (size range) of a microparticle sample, is to use dynamic light scattering (DLS). DLS views a dilute solution of microparticles by reading the amount of blocked light (adsorption) through Beer's law to determine how many particles there are and what their particle sizes are. Most DLS instruments will give you not only the average particle size in a sample but also a plot of the range of sizes and the polydispersity index (PDI). The PDI gives you an idea of how narrow or wide the bell-shaped

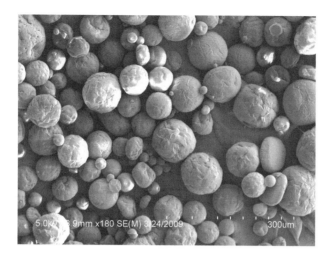

Figure 4.4. A representative SEM image of PLGA microparticles. This large field view gives an idea of the range of sizes exhibited from the standard W/O/W method of synthesis. The rough surfaces are typical to see after drying of the samples for visualization. The collapsed red blood cell-like microparticles are not a typical geometry.

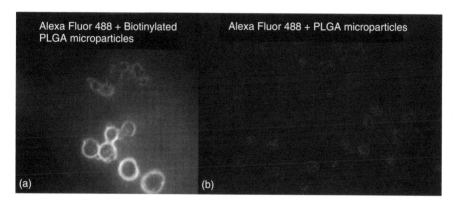

Figure 4.5. Flourescent microscopy was used to show the attachment of Alexa Fluor-488-tagged avidin to a biotinylated PLGA microparticle, hence confirming the biotin is available for binding while on the PLGA microparticle (a). (b) The image confirms the binding is specific to the biotin and not the PLGA.

curve spreads around that average size. The smaller the PDI, the narrower the "bell," meaning you have better control during your synthesis method. A small PDI is desired for most clinical applications and can be achieved through either altering the synthesis method or by serial centrifugation during collection.

4.6.3 Drug Encapsulation Efficiency

An important design element of microparticle drug delivery is optimizing the encapsulation efficiency. The encapsulation efficiency is determined using either a direct measure of the amount of drug encapsulated ($M_{\text{drug encapsulated}}$) or an indirect measure using the amount lost to estimate the amount of drug actually encapsulated (Eq. 4.1). This number should not be confused with the percentage of microparticles, that is drug (the drug loading, Eq. 4.2).

$$\text{Encapsulation efficiency (\%)} = \left(\frac{M_{\text{drug encapsulated}}}{M_{\text{drug used}}} \right) \times 100 \qquad (4.1)$$

$$\text{Drug loading (\%)} = \left(\frac{M_{\text{drug encapsulated}}}{M_{\text{microparticles}}} \right) \times 100 \qquad (4.2)$$

Estimating the encapsulation efficiency, that is how much of the drug load makes it into the microparticles, is a difficult task. Many researchers use the basic assumption that the microparticle can be dissolved in a solvent and the drug can be separated from the polymer and quantified. If the drug is water soluble, it can be extracted into water by simple mixing. However, as the timescale is not always the same for these methods, it is uncertain how fast the equilibrium of these phases will be reached. It is also unclear whether there is any partitioning effect of the drug between the solvent and the water phase. Similar problems may occur when separating the drug from the polymer using two different organic solvents. Despite the complications with the extraction method, the measurement of the extracted water phase's concentration of drug appears to be the standard method for direct determination of the encapsulation efficiency [49]. Other indirect methods based upon measurement of the loss of drug to the secondary water phase have also been attempted. These methods, however, might be underestimating the amount of protein lost, as they account for loss only in the final step of the process.

Because of these varied measurement methods, the encapsulation efficiency estimated varies over a wide range, usually dependent directly upon the processing factors [4]. In most cases, there is a large loss of drug, which when using therapeutic proteins and tropic factors, can be a highly expensive loss. Many researchers have focused on methods to increase the encapsulation efficiency of the W/O/W emulsion method by removing one of the water phases to prevent loss of the hydrophilic drug across the gradient created between the small, concentrated internal phase and the large, empty external phase. These methods have included solid emulsions in O/W [50, 51], solid-in-O/O emulsions, as well as spray drying [23, 52, 53]. The results of using solid emulsions of proteins within organic solvents have shown that the biochemical/physical stability of the protein is greater than when dissolved at the interface of the water–oil phase boundary [54].

Another method proposed to reduce the effect of the concentration gradient created is to saturate the secondary water phase with the drug, thus driving the gradient in the direction of the particle [55]. However, when dealing with expensive proteins, saturating the secondary phase is often impractical and therefore not recommended. Other factors that have been shown to affect the encapsulation in PLA/PLGA-based microparticles are the concentration of the polymer in the organic phase and the concentration of the protein in the aqueous phase; however, the results vary depending upon each polymer–drug interaction [14, 34, 56–58].

Other methods for increased protein stability and encapsulation that have been proposed include the use of PLA–PEG blends. The idea is that the inclusion of a hydrophilic block on the polymer will help to retain the protein and stabilize the emulsion during solidification. Previous research has shown great success at entrapping model proteins [30, 31] and enzymes [15] within PLA–PEG particles.

4.6.4 Protein Stability During Encapsulation

Many therapeutics are protein- or peptide-based, making it a challenge to maintain their stability during delivery to the desired area of the body. In order to evaluate protein stability during encapsulation and release, the term stability needs to be defined first. The first level of protein stability is the chemical stability or, simply, the retention of the primary structure of the amino acid sequence. However, activity of these proteins depends upon retaining their three-dimensional structure that is created by the secondary and sometimes tertiary and quaternary structures of these amino acid chains [49]. Physical and biochemical stability of the protein requires that it retains its three-dimensional structure and also the primary amino acid sequence. This level of stability can be assessed by basic biological assays for antibody recognition (e.g., enzyme-linked immunosorbent assay (ELISA), Western blotting) and size and shape (circular dichroism, sodium dodecyl sulfate polyacrylamide gel electrophoresis (SDS PAGE)). Loss of the three-dimensional structure of a protein is commonly referred to as denaturing of the protein. The unfolding of the protein can easily occur in the presence of high or low temperatures, exposure to organic solvents, and changes in pH (as experienced in the gastrointestinal tract). The denaturing can sometimes be reversed, while aggregation and precipitation of the protein is not so easily reversed and can be caused by similar conditions [49].

The final level of protein stability is the assessment of biological activity. The only way to determine the biological activity is to test whether the pharmaceutical efficacy of the protein remains functional [49]. In many applications, this test is not easy to accomplish, so only biochemical or physical stability is assessed. It should be remembered, though, that the physical stability of the protein, while a necessary condition for biological activity, does not guarantee biological activity.

Many have proposed that the entrapment of protein-based therapeutics can protect them from degradation and unfolding in the body. However, several stages in the processing of microparticles can lead to the loss of function or physical instability of a peptide- or protein-based therapeutic. These include the exposure of the protein to organic solvents at the phase boundary of both the primary and secondary emulsions, as well as mechanical shearing from the sonication or homogenization [49]. It has been shown that the primary loss of protein stability takes place via aggregation at the interface of the primary W/O emulsion boundary. The protein usually unfolds as its hydrophobic core is drawn to the organic side of the interface [35]. As it turns out, the choice of the solvent itself is critical in maintaining the stability of the protein.

In an attempt to improve the protein stability during encapsulation, a few researchers have looked into adding different stabilizers to the primary aqueous phase. The most common and effective stabilizer used is serum albumins (either human or bovine; HSA or BSA) [59–61]. It is believed that the serum albumins act as sacrificial proteins at interfaces by preferentially aggregating themselves at the interface, instead of the entrapped protein therapeutic [62].

4.7 DRUG RELEASE FROM MICROPARTICLES

4.7.1 Theory

Drug release from particles is primarily dependent upon what the particles are made of and the system the particles are in. There are many different ways a particle can release its encapsulated drug ranging from degradation to environmentally controlled swelling. The type of polymer, the polymer's molecular weight, the copolymer composition, the nature of excipients added to the particle, and the size of the particle, all have a direct impact on the delivery rate of the drug from polymeric particles [63]. For particles that release drug through a swelling mechanism, environmental factors play a major role in their release.

4.7.1.1 Polymer Controlled Release. The three main mechanisms that allow for the release of encapsulated drug from polymer microparticles are diffusion, polymer degradation, or a combination of both. Diffusional release is rooted in mass transfer of the drug into the surrounding area. The concentration of drug is the highest within or on the surface of the microparticles and diffuses away from the particles over time at a certain flux.

Polymer degradation can occur through enzymatic degradation, hydrolysis, or a combination of both. Using the body's natural enzymes as a partial degradation technique can be beneficial, but can also have harmful effects on the overall delivery of the drug. The body may degrade the particles prior to their reaching their target area, leading to a potential loss of therapeutic efficacy.

Hydrolysis, or the cleavage of chemical bonds in the presence of water, degrades polymer in two ways—surface erosion and bulk erosion. Surface erosion occurs on the exterior surface of the microparticles where it interacts with the surrounding solution. In this instance, the polymer will degrade from the outside to the inside. The underlying polymer will not begin to degrade until the surface polymer has been completely degraded. When bulk erosion occurs, degradation occurs through the entire polymer evenly. Here, both the surface and the interior of the polymer degrade at the same rate. Surface and bulk erosion often collaboratively degrade microparticles.

Release of drug is generally a combination of surface erosion, bulk erosion, and diffusion. Release from polymers utilizing both diffusional and degradation release can be broken down into two to three main steps—induction, or burst phase, followed by a short lag phase, and then a longer diffusional phase. A burst phase is often seen at the beginning of drug release over a 24–48 h time period. During this burst phase, an initial release of drug is seen as a result of desorption of proteins from the surface of mesopores on the outer surface of the particles. Following this phase, there is occasionally a short lag phase leading into a longer diffusional phase. During the diffusion phase, diffusional release dominates, while erosion continues to participate in drug release. The drug diffuses out of the polymer shell through the pores formed during the degradation of the polymer. Occasionally, there is a final quick release phase where the polymer shell is severely degraded and the remaining drug is released [63].

4.7.1.2 *Swelling Controlled Release Particles.* Swelling is another release method used by certain types of particles. Polymers used for swelling release mechanisms are often pH or temperature-responsive. As the environment the particle is in changes, the particle begins to swell, which allows for the drug to be released. These particles are often useful when attempting an oral delivery method because of the extreme changes in pH throughout the digestive system.

Hydrogels are an example of a type of polymer particle that is extremely dependent upon environmental conditions for drug release. Hydrogels are comprised of hydrophilic polymeric networks containing chemical or physical cross-links. These types of particles swell as they take on and retain large volumes of water. Like other polymeric particles, the drug can be enclosed or immersed within the hydrogel. There are four main kinds of systems that are used to control the release of drug from hydrogels—diffusion-controlled, swelling-controlled, chemically controlled, and environmentally controlled.

Diffusion-controlled release can be broken down into two categories—reservoir systems and matrix systems. Reservoir systems consist of a drug that is enclosed within the core of the polymer (Fig. 4.1a). Because the drug is concentrated within the core of the particle, it can evenly diffuse out at a steady rate. Matrix systems incorporate a drug that is dispersed evenly throughout the hydrogel (Fig. 4.1b). Here, drug release occurs through the mesh in the hydrogel and through water-filled pores.

Swelling-controlled release systems encapsulate the drug within a glassy polymer which is used as a matrix device. When the particles come into contact with a solvent, they begin to swell as they take on water. A transition from a glassy state to a rubbery state occurs, which allows the drug to seep out of the polymer. The same method can be applied to chemical or other environmental triggers such as chemical, temperature, or pH changes.

4.7.2 Release Kinetics and Effecting Factors

The polymer type or copolymer composition, particle morphology, and excipients present in the system all play a role in the type and speed of release from particles. Different polymers degrade at different rates in a controlled system. The rate of hydrolysis of the polymer's functional groups affects the rate at which it degrades [63]. The type of polymer also affects the kind of erosion that occurs. For example, PLG is a bulk-eroding polymer. Bulk-eroding polymers readily allow for the permeation of water into the matrix and throughout the entire microparticle [63]. Surface-eroding polymers, such as polyanhydrides, are comprised of hydrophobic monomers linked by labile bonds. These monomers and their linkage mechanism resist water penetration into the bulk polymer, while the outer shell of the polymer quickly degrades through hydrolysis [63]. Similarly, the copolymer composition can affect the degradation rate. For example, PLA degrades more slowly than PGA. By using a combination of both these polymers (PLGA), the rate of drug release can be controlled by the ratio of the lactic to glycolic acid used.

The polymer's molecular weight can also have an effect on drug release. Increase in the molecular weight of a polymer will decrease its diffusivity. In lower molecular weight substances, pores are formed more readily in the polymer, allowing more drug to be released faster. The decrease in molecular weight corresponding to a faster release holds true for most small molecules, peptides, and proteins [64, 65]. In contrast to this, surface-eroding polyanhydride particles' release rates seem to be independent of the molecular weight [66, 67].

Excipients may be added to the particles to stabilize the drug during fabrication or transportation of the particles. These excipients may affect the rate at which the drug is released from the particles. One example of this is seen in the use of PVA to stabilize the primary emulsion during BSA particle formation. The result of this stabilization was a more uniform distribution of BSA in the particles [68]. Increasing the concentration of PVA resulted in a decreased burst phase and a decrease in the overall release rate of the drug [68].

Finally, the size and morphology of the microparticle will play a major role in its degradation. As the size of the particle decreases, the surface area-to-volume ratio of the particle increases, allowing more degradation based on the overall size of the particle over time. The rate at which the drug is released from smaller particles will be more than from larger particles. Smaller particles will also undergo hydrolysis and water penetration at a more rapid pace than larger particles.

Constant, or linear, release is highly desirable for many pharmaceutical therapeutic treatments. Often times, when using a polymeric microparticle, the initial burst phase of drug will release as much as 50% of the encapsulated drug [69]. Researchers have found that decreasing the overall size of microparticles tends to alter the release kinetics from a zero-order mechanism to a Fickian diffusion-controlled process [70]. Some researchers have suggested mixing particles of different sizes or different natures for a more controlled release [71]. By using particles that are of different sizes, the release rate has the potential to become more linear because of the range of degradation rates. This idea holds true for using particles constructed of different materials as well. The use of a polymer that degrades slowly in conjunction with one that degrades more rapidly will allow variable degradation rates among the particles and therefore has the potential for a more linear release.

4.7.3 Experiment

Before drug delivery from the particles can be tested *in vivo*, release of the particles should be tested in a system similar to the target area. Factors to be taken into account when testing particles *in vitro* are the temperature of the target area (i.e., body temperature for most pharmaceutical applications), pH, fluid movement, fluid replacement, contact with shear forces, and any other factors that may affect the release or identity of the particles within the system. It is especially important to maintain conditions and changes when using a polymer that is dependent on environmental conditions.

Once all system factors have been taken into account, an experiment can be conducted at these desired conditions. For polymeric particles, this is often done by placing microparticles within a dialysis bag, which is then placed at the bottom of a liquid-filled container. In order to stimulate body-like conditions, often times, the container is constantly stirred or mixed using a paddle or stir bar. This mimics the continuous movement of fluids throughout the body. Other methods for *in vitro* testing involve placing the particles in a small container or in glass tubes mimicking a body-like environment. Often times, this system is kept in an incubator to maintain the temperature of the system. Before placing the particles in solution, they should be weighed for release analysis. A buffer solution, usually phosphate buffer solution (PBS), is used to mimic body-like conditions. Samples should be taken at small intervals upon particle introduction into the system to allow researchers to view a potential burst phase. Once the first 24–48 h has past, samples should be taken at regular intervals over the remainder of the desired release period. Occasionally, to prevent loss of particles within samples, suspensions are centrifuged before sample removal. Maintaining the volume of the system is critical so that there is no spike in concentration due to a smaller volume at the end of the study. Experiments can also be done to simulate potential changes in the system, such as an increase in temperature during fever conditions.

For particles that rely on pH or temperature for release, experiments need to be altered slightly. At desired time frames, the factor that the release is dependent upon needs to be changed. For example, when testing pH-sensitive particles moving through the digestive tract, the pH of the system needs to be changed within the normal time frame that it would take particles to move through the system. pH of the system may start around 1.2 for a period of 2 h and then increase at set intervals over the next few hours to a higher pH [72].

Once data is gathered, it can be analyzed through various methods depending on the drug that was encapsulated. If the encapsulated entity has the nature of protein, a simple protein assay can be done to show the release profile of the particles over the allotted timeframe. If the entity is not of protein nature, other methods to analyze the samples are high performance liquid chromatography (HPLC) and UV-spectrophotometry.

After proof that the drug releases at the desired rate has been obtained *in vitro, in vivo* studies can be conducted. A major hurtle of *in vivo* studies is the ability to get sterile microparticles to the target area of interest without too much degradation. Particles and all components of the particles need to be sterilized before being subjected to the *in vivo* model. This is sometimes done through the use of ethylene oxide [73]. It is necessary to be cautious when sterilizing particles because it is very easy to harm the integrity of particles or the encapsulated drug. In the case of injectable microparticles, the particles are often delivered in combination with a buffer (PBS) and water mixture. Particles should be injected close to the target area to gain the best efficiency. There are different methods to ascertain whether the particles have reached their desired area and are performing properly. The use of a radiolabeled drug is one method to confirm that the drug is being released from the particles [73].

4.7.4 Modeling of Drug Release

Many different techniques can be used to model data gathered from release studies of microparticles. The induction, or burst phase, is the initial burst of drug that is released as a result of due to desorption of proteins from the surface of mesopores on the outer surface of the particles. This can be seen in the release profile as an initial spike before the inflection point. The second phase, as stated previously, is the diffusion phase. This is the phase where the polymer shell begins to degrade and form small pores. As the polymer degrades, the pores allow the drug to diffuse out of the polymer shell and into the surrounding area. Drug desorption rate determines the dynamics of the initial drug burst and the diffusion rate determines the subsequent release of drug over the allotted period.

One example of a common model used can be seen in Eq. 4.3 where the first segment of the equation is the burst phase and the second is the diffusion phase. The fraction of drug released ($f_{release}$) is predicted using Eq. 4.3. The unknown parameters (ϕ_d^{burst}, k_d, D_d^*, and t_d) are determined by fitting the experimental data to Eq. 4.3 using a nonlinear least-squares approach. ϕ^{burst} and drug induction time are determined from the inflection point in the experimental data. The inflection point indicates a switch from the induction phase to the diffusion phase. The drug desorption rate constant (k_d) and the effective drug diffusivity are determined through the nonlinear least-squares approach using a modeling program. In this approach, the objective function, the sum-of-square error, is minimized over N measurements of the differences between experimental data and the model-predicted output. This can be seen in Eq. 4.4.

$$f_{release} = \phi_d^{burst}(1 - e^{-k_d t}) + (1 - \phi_d^{burst})\left(1 - \frac{6}{\pi^2}\sum_{j=1}^{\infty}\frac{-e^{-j^2\pi^2\overline{D}_d^*(t-t^d)/r_0^2}}{j^2}\right) \quad (4.3)$$

where

ϕ_d^{burst} = the mass fraction of drug involved in the burst phase.
k_d = drug desorption rate constant.
D_d^* = effective drug diffusivity.
t_d = drug induction time (time for micropores to form).
r_0 = initial microparticle radius.

$$\underset{k_d, D_d}{\text{Min}} \sum_{i=1}^{N} [F_{release}(i) - f_{release}(i)]^2 \quad (4.4)$$

where

$f_{release}$ = mass fraction of released drug (from data).

Another example of a similar modeling method was derived in an attempt to characterize the release of a drug from biodegradable polymer blends. This model goes a step further to incorporate a three-phase release profile—the burst phase, degradative drug dissolution release, and diffusional release [74]. In general, it is easier to model drug release from surface-eroding systems because the drug is released layer by layer. With new technologies, however, this is not the primary way a drug is released from particles. Mathematical models for bulk erosion systems mainly stem from the Higuchi model. This model was altered slightly, adding a time-dependent constant, as can be seen in Eq. 4.5.

$$D_t = D_o \times \exp(k \times t) \qquad (4.5)$$

where

D_t = time dependent diffusion coefficient
D_o = constant diffusion coefficient
k = degradation constant
t = time

This model, though, is primarily used for single-step drug release. A biphasic release model was proposed by Batycky et al. for polymer microspheres. This new model takes into account an initial burst and a diffusion period. The induction phase, or burst, was estimated through visual analysis.

Research has shown that the best way to model release from some particles is in a three-step sequence. The three steps are (i) a solvent penetration to the mix, (ii) a degradation-dependent "relaxation of the network" that creates more free volume for drug dissolution, and (iii) drug removal to the surrounding medium through diffusion [74]. The release profile is dependent upon several factors, such as the nature of the drug (hydrophobic/hydrophilic), polymer degradation rate, water permeability, and drug–polymer interactions.

Research on the slowly degrading polymer polycaprolactone (PCL) has found that degradation does not play a major role in drug release because only a very mild degradation in molecular weight occurred over a period of a 1 month. However, PCL has a low glass transition temperature and because the studies were run at human body temperature, the PCL chains were highly flexible and rubbery. This allows for free volume to form within the matrix of polymer, which means that the step where the polymer relaxes and creates more free volume is not the rate-limiting step. Instead, after the initial burst and water penetration, the drug release profile proceeded straight to diffusion. Because diffusion was the main mechanism of release, Fick's law under nonsteady-state conditions was applied (Eq. 4.6)

$$\frac{\partial C}{\partial t} = D \times \frac{\partial^2 C}{\partial x^2} \qquad (4.6)$$

The following three boundary conditions were applied to the partial differential equation. Each boundary ($x = 1$ and $x = -1$) is zero and the initial concentration is C_0. The solution to the differential equation is given by Eq. 4.7.

$$\left\{\frac{M_t}{M_\infty}\right\} \text{diff} = 1 - \sum_{n=0}^{\infty} \frac{8}{(2n+1)^2 \times \Pi^2} \times \exp\left(-D(2n+1)^2 \times \Pi^2 \times \frac{t}{4l^2}\right) \quad (4.7)$$

The kinetics of the initial burst follows an exponential relationship [75] and is often dictated by the drug desorption rate shown in Eq. 4.8 (where k_b is the kinetic rate constant for the burst phase):

$$\left\{\frac{M_t}{M_\infty}\right\}_{\text{Burst}} = 1 - \exp(-k_b \times t) \quad (4.8)$$

We combine the models for burst and Fickian diffusion results in Eq. 4.9 [74].

$$\left\{\frac{M_t}{M_\infty}\right\}_{\text{PCL}} = \varnothing_{b,\text{PCL}}(1 - \exp(-k_{b,\text{PCL}}t)) + \varnothing_{d,\text{PCL}}\left(1 - \sum_{n=0}^{\infty} \frac{8}{(2n+1)^2 * \pi^2}\right.$$
$$\left. \times \exp\left(-D_{\text{PCL}}(2n+1)^2 \times \pi^2 \times (t - t_{b,\text{PCL}})/(4 \times l^2)\right)\right) \quad (4.9)$$

where $t_{b,\text{PCL}}$ is an initial burst, within the first few days of release study, $\varnothing_{b,\text{PCL}}$ is a fraction released within the burst phase, $k_{b,\text{PCL}}$ is a burst constant, $\varnothing_{d,\text{PCL}}$ is a fraction of drug released due to diffusion, and D_{PCL} is the drug's diffusion coefficient. Experimental data can be fitted to the model using computational methods. From the model, PCL undergoes a fast initial burst, with up to 24% of drug released within the first 2 days [74].

Similar research has been conducted using PLGA. PLGA has a higher T_g (40–45 °C), and therefore, there is very limited free volume for taxol, the drug of interest, to be transported at physiological temperature. This is very different from the PCL used before. The PLGA particles need to rely more on degradation to break long polymer chains and to create a more open network. This indicates that the degradation-dependent relaxation of the polymer chains plays an important role in the release of drug from the PLGA shell. All three steps stated earlier were taken into account for the PLGA model (Eq. 4.10). The total mass fraction of the drug that was released is a summation of the burst release, relaxation-induced drug dissolution release, and diffusion-controlled release.

$$\left\{\frac{M_t}{M_\infty}\right\}_{\text{PLGA}} = \varnothing_{b,\text{PLGA}}(1 - \exp(-k_{b,\text{PLGA}}t)) + \varnothing_{r,\text{PLGA}}\{\exp[k_{r,\text{PLGA}}(t - t_{b,\text{PLGA}})] - 1\}$$
$$+ \varnothing_{d,\text{PLGA}}\left(1 - \sum_{n=0}^{\infty} \frac{8}{(2n+1)^2 \times \pi^2} \times \exp(-D_{\text{PLGA}}(2n+1)^2 \times \pi^2\right.$$
$$\left. \times \frac{t - t_{r,\text{PLGA}}}{4l^2}\right) \quad (4.10)$$

where

$\varnothing_{r,PLGA}$ = coefficient of relaxational release
$t_{r,PLGA}$ = the end of relaxation-induced release
$k_{r,PLGA}$ = PLGA degradative relaxation constant

When the experimental data was analyzed, it was seen that after very little burst, the burst phase was the limiting release factor. Because taxol is hydrophobic and has very low aqueous solubility, limited water penetration worked to inhibit release. The authors termed this period the "latent period" and it was given the symbol $t_{b,PLGA}$). The second term in Eq. 4.10 represents the drug release induced by polymer relaxation, which creates more free volume. As polymer chains are hydrolyzed, they become shorter, allowing for the degree of entanglement to decrease. This allows for the drug to seep out of the polymer. Matlab was used to fit the data gathered to the model. Very little burst phase was found, followed by a long induction-burst period. Once the polymer reached the point where water absorption became significant, the second stage of the drug release started.

Drug release from hydrogels needs to be modeled in a different manner. For example, certain hydrogels are made from a triblock copolymer—PEG–PLGA–PEG. The polymer is free-flowing at room temperature but, when injected at body temperature, it becomes gel-like [76]. Drug release from hydrogels can be affected by parameters including the size of pores, degradability of the hydrogel, size, hydrophobicity, concentration of the drug, and the presence of specific interactions between the hydrogels and the drug used [76]. Typically, release is diffusion-controlled at an initial stage and then there is a combination of a diffusion and degradation phase at a later stage. A two-stage release model has been created through experimentation using BSA as a model drug and a PLLA–PEO–PLLA triblock polymer.

The diffusional drug release using slab geometry yields Eq. 4.11 [76].

$$\frac{M_t}{M_\infty} = 1 - \sum 8 \exp \left[\frac{-D(2n+1)^2 \times \pi^2 \times \frac{t}{l^2}}{(2n+1)^2 \times \pi^2} \right] \tag{4.11}$$

where

M_t/M_∞ = fraction of drug released
D = diffusion coefficient
l = thickness of device

It was estimated that the early time approximation holds up for about 60% of release and the late time approximation holds for 40–100% of the diffusion profile. First-order kinetics was assumed and the Higuchi equation was used (Eq. 4.12) [76].

$$\frac{dM_t}{dt} = \left(\frac{A}{2} \right) \times \left(2 \times C_0 \times P_0 \times \frac{(\exp(kt))}{t} \right)^{1/2} \tag{4.12}$$

where

A = surface area of the device
C_0 = initial concentration of drug
P_0 = permeability of the drug in the absence of degradation of polymer
k = first-order rate constant of permeability

Two drugs with different hydrophobicities were examined, both in the PEG–PLGA–PEG triblock copolymer complex. As a result, two different model possibilities were created. In the first model possibility, the release profile was given simply as the Heller release equation (Eq. 4.13).

$$\frac{dM_t}{dt} = C \left(\frac{\exp(kt)}{t} \right)^{1/2}$$ (4.13)

The second model examined was a modified Higuchi model. The modified version was created assuming that the drug release was mainly from the hydrophilic domain of the triblock polymer, which can be explained by a diffusion equation. The hydrophobic domain can be described through a modified Higuchi equation. This can be seen in Eq. 4.14. The model for release of one of the studied drugs, spironolactone, can be a linear combination of these two parts of the equation.

$$\frac{dM_t}{dt} = B \exp(-kt) + C \left(\frac{\exp(k't)}{t} \right)^{1/2}$$ (4.14)

where

B = unknown parameter, function of Co
k = unknown parameter, function of Co
D = diffusion coefficient
P_0 = permeability coefficient of the drug in absence of degradation
k' = related to degradation rate of the polymer

Figure 4.6 shows the release over time of spironolactone from PEG–PLGA–PEG triblock copolymer [76]. Hydrophilic drug release from homogeneous matrices is diffusion-dominant, while the release of hydrophobic drugs is initially diffusion-dominant, but followed by a degradation-dominant release at later stages.

4.8 MICROPARTICLE DESIGN EXAMPLES

In today's pharmaceutical industry, more efficient and effective ways of treating various diseases are needed. Researchers are looking to microparticles as a new method for treating many diseases ranging from simple treatments such as vaccines to more complex treatments for diseases such as cancer.

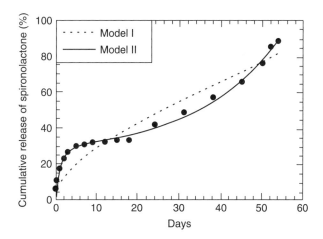

Figure 4.6. Comparison of modeling spironolactone release from a triblock copolymer with the Heller model (Model I) and a modified Higuchi model (Model II). Reprinted from Reference 76, Copyright (2000), with permission from Elsevier.

4.8.1 Cancer Research

Cancer is a broad group of diseases involving uncontrolled cell growth and the spread of abnormal cells. Cancer cells grow in masses and form tumors, which can spread throughout the body, causing great damage. Current treatments for cancer include surgery, chemotherapy, radiation therapy, targeted therapy, gene therapy, and many others. Side effects of most of these treatments include nausea, vomiting, fatigue, and anemia; and most methods result in damage to healthy cells. Researchers have been finding new ways to more effectively treat cancer through the use of microparticles. A major disadvantage of cancer drugs is their lack of selectivity. Microparticles are being looked into as a means to more effectively target and treat cancer. The use of an extremely toxic drug is advantageous if the treatment method can be targeted to specifically the cancer cells and not normal cells.

4.8.2 Vaccine Applications

Throughout history, vaccines have been extremely pertinent in the treatment and eradication of many deadly diseases. There is a growing need for a new method of treating diseases such as acquired immunodeficiency syndrome (AIDS), hepatitis B, anthrax, and severe acute respiratory syndrome (SARS) [77]. One problem that researchers are running into is the need for repeated injections. Through the use of slow-releasing particles, the need for multiple injections could be eradicated. For example, the current anthrax vaccine requires five booster shots over the course of a year and a half following the first inoculation [77]. The concept of a booster shot could be discarded through the use of slow-releasing injectable microparticles.

4.8.3 Oral Drug Delivery and Gastrointestinal Delivery

The potential that pH-responsive polymers have in oral and gastrointestinal drug delivery is immense. Because of the pH differences within the body, the ability of a polymer particle to swell and contract at varying pH levels can be taken advantage of. For example, Eudragit-S100 is a copolymer that has been approved by the US Food and Drug Administration (FDA) for drug delivery use [78]. This polymer is insoluble in acid media and dissolves at pH 6.5–7.0 [78]. These characteristics make this polymer an excellent option when attempting for drug release in the last portion of the intestine. Work has been done with this polymer and polymers like this to create an ideal dosage and release timeframe for certain drugs.

4.9 KEY POINTS

- Before starting microparticle design, one must establish the target, time frame of delivery, and method of delivery desired.
- Polymer selection is critical in the design of a successful microparticle drug delivery system.
- Synthesis depends upon the polymer selected and must be tailored for the specific drug (model drugs will not interact the same with the polymer).
- Characterization techniques for size, polydispersity, morphology, and protein stability (if protein-based drug) are well established.
- Release from the microparticle depends upon the type of microparticle (liquid-filled reservoirs vs. solid dispersed) as well as the response of the polymer to the environment (swelling, diffusion, and/or degradation).
- Many mathematical models have been developed to describe the experimental results seen for drug release from microparticles based on a combination of Fickian diffusion and burst release effects.

4.10 WORKED EXAMPLE

Assuming that the release of a hydrophobic, evenly dispersed drug from a polymeric microparticle of radius R is controlled by pure Fickian diffusion, provide the starting equation, boundary and initial conditions, and the graphical solution for drug concentration versus r. Assume the initial drug concentration is C_0, and the surface concentration is C_d.

Solution

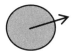

$$D_{drug} \frac{1}{r^2} \frac{\partial}{\partial r} \left(r^2 \frac{\partial C_{drug}}{\partial r} \right) = \frac{\partial C_{drug}}{\partial t}$$

Initial condition: $C_{drug}(r, 0) = C_0$ for all $r > R$
Boundary conditions:

$$\text{At } r = R, \quad C_{drug}(R, t) = C_S$$
$$\text{At } r = \infty, \quad C_{drug}(\infty, t) = 0$$

Graphically, this should look like as shown:

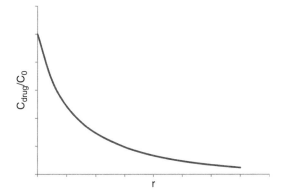

where the actual solution can be found using a pseudo-steady state approach (Higuchi):
$$\frac{C_{drug}}{C_0} = \sqrt{C_s \times (2C_0 - C_s) \times D_{drug} \times t}$$

4.11 HOMEWORK PROBLEMS

1. A new water-soluble drug is proposed for encapsulation in PLA microparticles. What type of synthesis should be used to make this system? If this drug is actually a protein, what steps in the synthesis could be hazardous to the protein's stability?

2. PEGylating the outside of a microparticle has been proposed to increase the systemic ciruculation of microparticles by decreasing macrophage uptake.
   a. What issues could PEG have when coated on a chitosan microparticle? How might it affect drug encapsulation?
   b. What if the microparticle was made from PCL?
3. Biotin has been added to the surface of PLGA microparticles in an effort to help target specific cells. The addition of biotin on the encapsulation of a model protein (BSA) was tested using a direct measurement method. Using the following data, answer the questions below.

PLGA-Biotin		PLGA	
Absorbance	0.7620	Absorbance	0.4220
Concentration	110.32 $\mu g\,ml^{-1}$	Concentration	53.65 $\mu g\,ml^{-1}$
PLGA	22.6 mg	PLGA	20.4 mg
BSA	6.5 mg	BASA	6.5 mg
Particle	29.1 mg	Particle	16.9 mg
Encapsulated BSA	1.65 mg	Ecapsulated BSA	0.80 mg

   a. What is the encapsulation efficiency of the biotinylated and nonbiotinylated microparticles?
   b. What is the percent loading of the two microparticles?
   c. Why do you think there is the difference in encapsulation?
4. While studying the release kinetics of a microparticle system, you realize you are running into an issue with burst release. Which model would help you determine the burst effect? What parameter would best represent this?

REFERENCES

1. "History Timeline." About Mars. Mars Incorporated, n.d. Web. 27 Jan. 2012 Incorporated, M. History of M & M's. 2012.
2. Anderson JM, Shive MS. *Biodegradation and biocompatibility of PLA and PLGA microspheres.* Adv Drug Deliv Rev 2012;64:72–82.
3. Berkland C et al. *Precise control of PLG microsphere size provides enhanced control of drug release rate.* J Control Release 2002;82(1):137–147.
4. Cleland JL. Protein Delivery from biodegradable microspheres. In: Sanders L, editor. Protein Delivery Physical Systems. Hingham, MA: Kluwer Academic Publishers; 1997. p 1–25.
5. Kim SY, Ha JC, Lee YM. Poly(ethylene oxide)-poly(propylene oxide)-poly(ethylene oxide)/poly(ε-caprolactone) (PCL) amphiphilic block copolymeric nanospheres: II. Thermo-responsive drug release behaviors. J Control Release 2000;65(3):345–358.

6. Upadhyay D et al. Magnetised thermo responsive lipid vehicles for targeted and controlled lung drug delivery. Pharm Res 2012;29(9):2456–2467.

7. Alarcon CDLH, Pennadam S, Alexander C. Stimuli responsive polymers for biomedical applications. Chem Soc Rev 2005;34(3):276–285.

8. Schoener CA, Hutson HN, Peppas NA. pH-responsive hydrogels with dispersed hydrophobic nanoparticles for the delivery of hydrophobic therapeutic agents. Polym Int 2012;61(6):874–879.

9. Schoener CA, Hutson HN, Peppas NA. pH-responsive hydrogels with dispersed hydrophobic nanoparticles for the oral delivery of chemotherapeutics. J Biomed Mater Res Part A 2013;101A:2229–2236.

10. Saltzman WM. Drug delivery: engineering principles for drug therapy. In: Gubbins KE, editor. Topics in Chemical Engineering. New York: Oxford University Press; 2001 p. 271–273.

11. Cao X, Shoichet MS. Biodegradation and biocompatibility of PLA and PLGA microspheres. Biomaterials 1998;20:329–339.

12. Heller J, Himmelstein K. Poly(ortho ester) biodegradable polymer systems. Methods Enzymol 1985;112:422–436.

13. Jiang W, Schwendeman SP. Stabilization and controlled release of bovine serum albumin encapsulated in poly(D, L-lactide) and poly(ethylene glycol) microsphere blends. Pharm Res 2001;18(6):878–885.

14. Brayden DJ. Controlled release technologies for drug delivery. Drug Discov Today 2003;8(21):976–978.

15. Dziubla TD, Karim A, Muzykantov VR. Polymer nanocarriers protecting active enzyme cargo against proteolysis. J Control Release 2005;102(2):427–439.

16. Desai MP et al. Gastrointestinal uptake of biodegradable microparticles: effect of particle size. Pharm Res 1996;13(12):1838–1845.

17. Desai MP et al. The mechanism of uptake of biodegradable microparticles in caco-2 cells is size dependent. Pharm Res 1997;14(11):1568–1573.

18. Siepmann J et al. Effect of the size of biodegradable microparticles on drug release: experiment and theory. J Control Release 2004;96(1):123–134.

19. Chen J, Jo S, Park K. Polysaccharide hydrogels for protein drug delivery. Carbohydr Polym 1995;28(1):69–76.

20. Huang X, Brazel C. On the importance and mechanisms of burst release in matrix-controlled drug delivery systems. J Control Release 2001;73(2–3):121–136.

21. Sharif S, O'Hagen D. A comparison of alternative methods for the determination of the levels of proteins entrapped in poly(lactide-co-glycolide) microparticles. Int J Pharm 1995;115(2):259–263.

22. Anderson JM, Shive MS. Biodegradation and biocompatibility of PLA and PLGA microspheres. Adv Drug Deliv Rev 1997;28(1):5–24.

23. Witschi C, Doekler E. Influence of the microencapsulation method and peptide loading on the poly(lactic acid) and poly(lactic co glycolic acid) degradation during in vitro testing. J Control Release 1998;51:327–341.

24. Panyam J, Dali MM, Sahoo SK, Ma W, Chakravarthi SS, Amidon GL, Levy RJ, Labhasetwar V. Polymer degradation and in vitro release of a model protein from poly(D,L-lactide-co-glycolide) nano- and microparticles. J Control Release 2003;92(1–2): 173–187.

25. Uchida T, Yoshida K, Ninomiya A, Goto S. Optimization of preparative conditions for polylactide (PLA) microspheres containing ovalbumin. Chem Pharm Bull (Tokyo) 1995;43(9):1569–1573.

26. Lowman A et al. Oral delivery of insulin using pH-responsive complexation gels. J Pharm Sci 1999;88(9):933–937.

27. Lowman A, Peppas N. Solute transport analysis in pH-responsive, complexing hydrogels of poly(methacrylic acid-g-ethylene glycol). J Biomater Sci Polym Ed 1999;10(9):999–1009.

28. Morishita M et al. Elucidation of the mechanism of incorporation of insulin in controlled release systems based on complexation polymers. J Control Release 2002;81(1):25–32.

29. Nakamura K et al. Oral insulin delivery using P (MAA-g-EG) hydrogels: effects of network morphology on insulin delivery characteristics. J Control Release 2004;95(3):589–599.

30. Garcia-Fuentes M, Prego C, Torres D, Alonso MJ. A comparative study of the potential of solid triglyceride nanostructures coated with chitosan or polyethylene glycol as carriers for oral calcitonin delivery. Eur J Pharm Sci 2005;25:133–143.

31. Vila A, Sanchez A, Evora C, Soriano I, MCCallion O, Alonso MJ. PLA-PEG particles as nasal protein carriers: the influence of the particle size. Int J Pharm 2005;292:43–52.

32. Soppimath KS, Aminabhavi TM, Kuliarni AR, Rudzinski WE. Biodegradable polymeric nanoparticles as drug delivery devices. J Control Release 2000;70:1–20.

33. Putney S. Encapsulation of proteins for improved delivery. Curr Opin Chem Biol 1998;2:548–552.

34. Brannon-Peppas L. Recent advances on the use of biodegradable microparticles and nanoparticles in controlled drug delivery. Int J Pharm 1995;116(1):1–9.

35. Raghuvanshi R, Goyal S, Singh O, Panda AK. Stabilization of dichloromethane induced protein denaturation during microencapsulation. Pharm Dev Technol 1998;3:211–222.

36. Li X, Zhang Y, Yan R, Jia W, Yuan M, Deng X, Huang Z. Influence of process parameters on the protein stability encapsulated in poly-DL-lactide-poly(ethylene glycol) microspheres. J Control Release 2000;68:41–52.

37. Birnbaum DT et al. Controlled release of [beta]-estradiol from PLAGA microparticles:the effect of organic phase solvent on encapsulation and release. J Control Release 2000;65(3):375–387.

38. Coccoli V et al. Engineering of poly(ε-caprolactone) microcarriers to modulate protein encapsulation capability and release kinetic. J Mater Sci Mater Med 2008;19(4):1703–1711.

39. Menon JU et al. Effects of surfactants on the properties of PLGA nanoparticles. J Biomed Mater Res A 2012;100(8):1998–2005.

40. Heller MC, Carpenter JF, Randolph TW. Protein formulation and lyophilization cycle design: prevention of damage due to freeze-concentration induced phase separation. Biotechnol Bioeng 1999;63(2):166–174.

41. Bodmeier R, Chen H. Preparation of biodegradable poly($\pm$)lactide microparticles using a spray-drying technique. J Pharm Pharmacol 1988;40(11):754–757.

42. Rattes ALR, Oliveira WP. Spray drying conditions and encapsulating composition effects on formation and properties of sodium diclofenac microparticles. Powder Technol 2007;171(1):7–14.

43. Wang W et al. Microencapsulation using natural polysaccharides for drug delivery and cell implantation. J Mater Chem 2006;16(32):3252–3267.

44. Tomasko D, Li H, Liu D, Han X, Wingert MJ, Lee LJ, Koelling W. A review of CO_2 applications in the processing of polymers. Ind Eng Chem Res 2003;42:6431–6456.

45. Yeo S-D, Kiran E. Formation of polymer particles with supercritical fluids: a review. J Supercrit Fluids 2005;34:287–308.

46. Meziani M, Pathak P, Desai T, Sun YP. Supercritical fluid processing of nanoscale particles from biodegradable and biocompatible polymers. Ind Eng Chem Res 2006;45:3420–3424.

47. Turk M, Upper G, Hils P. Formation of composite drug-polymer particles by coprecipitation during the rapid expansion of supercritical fluids. J Supercrit Fluids 2006;39:253–263.

48. Dillow AK, Dehghani F, Hrkach JS, Foster NR, Langer R. Bacterial Inactivation by using near- and supercrical carbon dioxide. Proc Natl Acad Sci U S A 1999;96(18):10344–10348.

49. Bilati U, Allemann E, Doekler E. Strategic approaches for overcoming peptide and protein instability within biodegradable nano and microparticles. Eur J Pharm BioPharm 2005;59:375–388.

50. Morita T et al. Evaluation of in vivo release characteristics of protein-loaded biodegradable microspheres in rats and severe combined immunodeficiency disease mice. J Control Release 2001;73(2–3):213–221.

51. Morita T, Sakamura Y, Horikiri Y, Suzuki T, Yoshino H. Protein encapsulation into biodegradable microspheres by a novel S/O/W emulsion method using poly (ethylene glycol) as a protein micronization adjuvant. J Control Release 2000;69:435–444.

52. Baras B, Benoit MA, Gillard J. Parameters influencing the antigen release from spray dried poly (DL-lactide) microparticles. Int J Pharm 2000;200:133–145.

53. Baras B, Benoit MA, Poulain-Godefroy O, Schacht AM, Capron A, Gillard J, Riveau G. Vacine properties of antigens entrapped in miroparticles produced by spray drying techniques and using various polyester polymers. Vaccine 2000;18:1495–1505.

54. Griebenow K, Klibanov AM. On protein denaturation in aqueous organic mixtures but not pure organic solvents. J Am Chem Soc 1996;118:11695–11700.

55. Hans ML, Lowman AM. Synthesis, Characterization, and Application of Biodegradable Polymeric Prodrug Micelles for Long-Term Drug Delivery. Philadelphia, PA: Drexel University; 2006. p xii 177 leaves.

56. Fu K, Harrell R, Zinski K, Um C, Jaklenec A, Frazier J, Lotan N, Burke P, Klibanov A, Langer R. A potential approach for decreasing the burst effect of protein from PLGA microspheres. J Pharm Sci 2003;92(8):1582–1591.

57. Brannon-Peppas L. Design and mathematical analysis of controlled release from microsphere-containing polymeric implants. J Control Release 1992;20(3):201–207.

58. Brannon-Peppas L, Blanchette JO. Nanoparticle and targeted systems for cancer therapy. Adv Drug Deliv Rev 2004;56(11):1649–1659.

59. Quintanar-Guerrero D, Allemann E, Fessi H, Doekler E. Applications of the ion-pairing concept to hydrophilic substances, with special emphasis on peptides. Pharm Res 1997;14(2):119–127.

60. Zamboux M, Bonneaux F, Gref R, Dellacherie E, Vigneron C. Preparation and characterization of protein C loaded PLA nanoparticles. J Control Release 1999;60:179–188.

61. Sanchez A, Villimayor B, Guo Y, McIver J, Alonso MJ. Formulations for the stabilization of tetanus toxoid in poly (lactide-co-glycolide) microspheres. Int J Pharm 1999;185:255–266.

62. van de Weert M, Hoechstetter J, Hennink WE, Crommelin DJ. The effect of water/organic solvent interface on the structural stability of lysozyme. J Control Release 2000;8:351–359.

63. Kim KK, Pack DW. "Microspheres for Drug Delivery". In: *BioMEMS and Biomedical Nanotechnology Volume 1: Biological and Biomedical Nanotechnology*, (Ferrari M, Lee AP, and Lee LJ, Eds.), pp. 19–50, Springer, New York; 2006.

64. Alonso MJ, Blanco D. Protein encapsulation and release from poly(lactide-co-glycolide) microspheres. Effect of the protein and polymer properties and of the co-encapsulation of surfactants. Eur J Pharm BioPharm 1998;45(3):285–294.

65. Metha RC, Thanoo BC, DeLuca PP. Peptide containing microspheres from low molecular weight and hydrophilic poly(D,L-lactide-co-glycolide). J Control Release 1996;41(3):249–257.

66. Hanes J, Chiba M, Langer R. Synthesis and characterization of degradable anhydride-co-imideter polymers containing trimellitylimido-L-typrosine: novel polymers for drug delivery. Macromolecules 1996;29:5279–5287.

67. Langer R, Tabata Y. Polyanhydride microspheres that display near-constant release of water-soluble model drug compounds. Pharm Res 1993;10(3):391–399.

68. Yang YY, Chung TS, Ng NP. Morphology, drug distribution, and in vitro release profiles of biodegradable polymeric microspheres containing protein fabricated by double-emulsion solvent extrac- tion/evaporation method. Biomaterials 2001;22(3):231–241.

69. McGinty JW, O'Donnell PB. Preparation of microspheres by the solvent vaporation technique. Adv Drug Deliv Rev 1997;28:25–42.

70. Bezemer JM, Radersma R, Grijpma DW, Dijkstra PJ, van Blitterswijk CA, Feijen J. Microspheres for protein delivery prepared from amphiphilic multiblock copolymers 2. Modulation of release rate. J Control Release 2000;67:249–260.

71. Ravivarapu HB, Burton K, DeLuca PP. Polymer and microsphere blending to alter the release of a peptide from PLGA microspheres. Eur J Pharm 2000;50:263–270.

72. Aamir MN, Ahmad M, Akhtar N, Murtaza G, Khan SA, Zaman S, Nokhodchi A. Development and in vitro-in vivo relationship of controlled-release microparticles loaded with tramadol hydrochloride. Int J Pharm 2011.

73. Patel ZS, Ueda H, Yamamoto M, Yasuhiko T, Mikos AG. In vitro and in vivo release of vascular endothelial growth factor from gelatin microparticles and biodegradable composite scaffolds. Pharm Res 2008;25.

74. Lao LL, Venkatraman SS, Peppas NA. Modeling of drug release from biodegradable polymer blends. Eur J Pharm Biopharm 2008;70(3):796–803.

75. Batycky RP et al. A theoretical model of erosion and macromolecular drug release from biodegrading microspheres. J Pharm Sci 1997;86(12):1464–1477.

76. Jeong B, Bae YH, Kim SW. Drug release from biodegradable injectable thermosensitive hydrogel of PEG–PLGA–PEG triblock copolymers. J Control Release 2000; 63(1–2):155–163.

77. Shagufta K, Tripti T, Neha R, Amit J, Bal Krishna D. Microspheres: a review. World J Pharm Pharm Sci 2012;1(1):125–145.

78. Natalia H, Zifei D, Gonul K, Derek JH. Fabrication of pH-sensitive microparticles for drug delivery applications using soft lithography techniques. Mater Res Soc Symp Proc 2008;1095.

5

POLYMERIC NANOPARTICLES

Andrew L. Vasilakes and Thomas D. Dziubla

Department of Chemical and Materials Engineering, University of Kentucky, Lexington, KY, USA

Paritosh P. Wattamwar

Teva Pharmaceutical Industries Ltd., West Chester, PA, USA

5.1 INTRODUCTION

The central goal of drug delivery is the optimization of the pharmacokinetics/pharmocodynamics (PK/PD) for a specific medicinal application. To this end, nanoparticles have become one of the most promising drug delivery technologies, as they are capable of greatly altering the PK/PD of a drug, potentially giving new life to active agents once thought to be unusable. As the PK/PD is determined by the nanoparticle, it is of utmost importance to define what these properties are, requiring highly specific tuning of the carrier system. One class of nanoparticles that provides the greatest flexibility in tuning, and hence the largest class of nanoparticle studied, is polymeric nanoparticles (PNPs) [1–5].

Engineering Polymer Systems for Improved Drug Delivery, First Edition.
Edited by Rebecca A. Bader and David A. Putnam.
© 2014 John Wiley & Sons, Inc. Published 2014 by John Wiley & Sons, Inc.

Importantly, when considering PNPs, it is important to understand what one means by a nanoparticle. According to the National Institute of Health National Cancer Institute, a nanoparticle is any carrier structure that has an aspect ratio less than 100 nm but greater than 1 nm. This narrow definition has turned out to be quite important for the field of tumor targeting and therapy, but is somewhat limiting considering the range of diseases that must be addressed. For this reason, many researchers have adopted a definition of nanoparticle as a system whose length scale is less than 1 μm, but most commonly will include particles in the range of 100–400 nm in size.

PNPs can come in various shapes, compositions, and conformations, which can be used for a variety of approaches including solubility enhancement, immunogenic masking, and controlled release and retention time [5]. Furthermore, PNPs may exhibit unique properties that can allow the particles to flow through vasculature while protecting the active drug until reaching the specific target [6], which can reduce the amount of systemic release and increase local release, allowing the total amount of PNPs and drug administered to be smaller [7, 8].

These advantageous properties can allow simple drug carriers to provide an enhanced delivery effect in comparison to administration of the free drug. Assuming no change in bioavailability, but a simple decrease in drug release rate, the advantage of drug delivery via nanoparticles is depicted in Fig. 5.1 as a comparison between a hypothetical situation involving intravenous (IV) injection of the free drug versus the drug in a slow releasing PNP carrier.

Using IV injection of the free drug, total plasma exposure of the drug for a given dose (as depicted by shaded area under the curve) is limited because of elimination of the drug. This area under the curve can be maximized by encapsulating the drug in a stealth (longer circulating) nanoparticle, which allows for controlled release. For applications requiring repeated IV injection, the use of nanoparticles can greatly reduce both the number and frequency of injections necessary to maintain a therapeutic level of the drug in the serum. These generalized results are typical in encapsulated drug delivery and give a sample of the great potential PNPs provide.

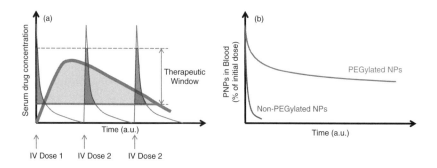

Figure 5.1. (a) Schematic of serum drug concentration after IV administration of either free drug or drug encapsulated in PNPs. (b) Schematic representing the effect of PEGylation on particle circulation.

5.1.1 Why Polymer-Based Nanoparticles?

In order to understand the advantages offered by polymer-based nanoparticles, it is necessary to understand various design criteria that determine the success of any nanoparticle-based therapy. Some of the important design features of nanoparticles are size, surface functionalization, mechanical properties, loading efficiency, encapsulated drug-to-carrier ratio, degradation mechanism, and biocompatibility of the polymer. While the exact structure–function relationships are still being identified, Table 5.1 summarizes the design features that are known to have an impact upon drug delivery parameters.

5.1.1.1 Material Selection (Biocompatibility and Biodegradability).
PNPs can be formed from a vast array of polymers with a variety of properties, including biodegradability, pH sensitivity, temperature responsiveness, reactivity, etc. (Chapter 12 describes in much further detail temperature and pH sensitive polymers), and choosing the correct polymer and configuration for the PNP application desired may be a challenge. Table 5.2 provides a summary of commonly used polymers in PNP design. Note that this table only summarizes homopolymers and common random copolymers. Any of these polymers can be combined into block copolymers for PNPs with properties not possible with the homopolymer.

Owing to their size, nanoparticles are under intense scrutiny regarding their ability to be eliminated from the body. While recent studies have suggested that inert nanoparticles (e.g., gold) are able to be eliminated through the billiary excretion mechanism, it is not certain how ubiquitous this effect is. As such, biodegradability of PNPs, which circumvents the bioaccumulation concerns, is one of the important properties that set them apart from other systems. Typically, biodegradable polymers will degrade via either hydrolysis or enzymatic degradation. For instance, poly(lactic-co-glycolic acid) (PLGA) degrades into both lactic and glycolic acids [57] mainly via hydrolysis of ester bonds [57], and chitosan degrades in biological systems predominantly through presence of lysozyme and bacterial enzymes in the colon [58] into amino sugars [59].

TABLE 5.1. PNP Properties That Affect Pharmacological Outcomes

Design features	Pharmacological Outcomes				
	Localization circulation	Tissue/Cellular	Subcellular	Duration of therapy	Total delivered amount
Surface chemistry	X	X	X	—	—
Responsiveness	X	X	X	X	X
Size	X	X	X	—	X
Shape	X	X	X	X	X
Mechanical properties	X	—	X	—	—
Loading capacity	—	—	—	X	X
Degradation	X	X	X	X	X

TABLE 5.2. Classic Polymers Used in PNPs Synthesis

Common PNP polymers	Material class	Degradation time	Responsiveness	T_g (°C)	FDA approved	Particle examples	References
PNIPAAm	Polyacrylamide	Nonbio-degradable	Thermal swelling	135	Yes	Nanosphere, nanogel	9, 10
PMMA	Polyacrylate	Nonbio-degradable	Organic swelling	95	Yes	Nanosphere	11–13
pHEMA	Polyacrylate	Nonbio-degradable	Hydrolytic swelling	100	Yes	Nanosphere	14, 15
PACA	Polyacrylate	Hours to months	Hydrolysis ion pairing	195	No	Nanosphere	16–20
PAMAM	Polyamide	Nonbio-degradable	pH conformational change	−10 to 25	No	Dendrimer	21–26
PVP	Polyamide	Nonbio-degradable	—	180	Yes	Nanosphere	27, 28
PSA, PCP, etc.	Polyanhydride	Hours to weeks	Hydrolysis (surface erosion)	—	Yes	Nanosphere	29, 30
—	Poly(β-amino ester)	Hours to years	Hydrolysis, pH swelling	—	No	Nanosphere, micelle, nanogel	31–35
PLA	Polyester	Months to years	Hydrolysis	40–60	Yes	Nanosphere	36–41

				T_g	FDA approved		
PLGA	Polyester	Weeks to months	Hydrolysis	40–50	Yes	Nanosphere, Micelle, polymersome, nanocapsule	42–46
PCL	Polyester	Months to years	Hydrolysis	−60	Yes	Nanosphere	39, 47, 48
PEG	Polyether	Nonbiodegradable	—	−70 (400MW) −22 (4000MW)	Yes	—	49–52
PEI, PEG–PEI, PLGA–PEI	Polyethylenimine	Nonbiodegradable	—	−25	—	Nanosphere, nanogel	53, 54
PS	Polystyrene	Nonbiodegradable	—	105	Yes	Nanosphere	55, 56

Glass transition temperatures (T_g) vary depending on molecular weight.

Note: "FDA approved" indicates whether the polymer has been approved for any biomedical application, not just nanomedicine.

PNIPAAm, poly(N-isopropylacrylamide); PMMA, poly(methyl methacrylate); pHEMA, poly(2-hydroxyethyl methacrylate); PACA, poly(alkylcyano acrylate); PAMAM, polyamidoamine; PVP, polyvinylpyrrolidone; PSA, poly(sebacic acid); PCP, poly(carboxyphenoxy propane); PLA, poly(lactic acid); PLGA, poly(lactic-co-glycolic acid); PCL, polycaprolactone; PEG, poly(ethylene glycol); PEI, polyethylenimine; PS, polystyrene.

Given the simple degradation products of PLGA, it is a popular component polymer for a variety of nanospheres, micelles, polymersomes, and nanocapsule systems [43–47] and has already been approved for human use [60, 61]. Poly(β-amino ester) (PBAE) is an new and exciting class of biodegradable polymer. On the basis of the Michael addition reaction of amines and acrylates, a wide variety of available monomers exist [62] that can be applied to form polymers in this class. The resulting polyester has a pH sensitive hydrolysis [32, 34, 35], allowing for a variety of particle delivery systems, including gene delivery [63]. The flexibility and versatility of PBAEs are very promising, yet given their more recent development, no current PBAE formulations have received the U.S. Food and Drug Administration (FDA) approval.

Besides degradation, mechanical properties of certain polymers provide unique advantages over other systems. For instance, the FDA-approved biodegradable polyester, polycapralactone (PCL), is interesting because of its relatively low glass transition temperature, $-60\,^{\circ}$C, giving PCL high molecular deformity at body temperature, ease of synthesis, and extended degradation times due to its hydrophobicity [39, 47, 48]. Other groups of polymers used in PNPs can allow interesting effects, such as the thermally induced swelling and shrinking of nonbiodegradable poly(N-isopropylacrylamide) (PNIPAAm) [9, 10, 64].

While the above-mentioned polymers provide a control over degradation rate, they do not have any therapeutic value. The carrier polymers are desired to be inert, but recent data suggest that degradation products of biodegradable polymers can induce immunogenic response from host cells/tissue, raising questions about their biocompatibility [65–67]. One of the approaches to improve biocompatibility of polymers is to conjugate anti-inflammatory drugs (e.g., aspirin, small-molecule antioxidants) to the polymer or incorporate these drugs into the polymer backbone.

Various small-molecule antioxidants (which have anti-inflammatory properties), such as superoxide dismutase mimetics, vitamin E, gallic acid, catechin, vitamin C, and glutathione, have been conjugated to ultrahigh molecular weight (MW) poly(ethylene), poly(acrylic acid), gelatin, poly(methyl methacrylate), and poly(ethylene glycol), respectively [68–72]. PolyAspirin™ is class of polymers incorporating salicylic acid, a nonsteroidal anti-inflammatory drug (NSAID), into the polymer backbone [73]. We have created a biodegradable antioxidant and antimicrobial PBAE with tunable degradation time and properties [62]. We have also synthesized a biodegradable polyester of trolox, a water-soluble analog of vitamin E, consisting of 100% polymerized trolox [74]. Poly(trolox ester) and the antioxidant PBAE have shown to suppress cellular oxidative stress [75], which is linked to inflammatory response from host cell/tissue [68]. Replacing inert carrier polymers with such functional polymers for formulation of PNPs would reduce polymer-induced inflammation in drug delivery applications.

5.1.1.2 *PNP Surface Chemistry: "Stealth" Considerations.* PNPs, as any nanoparticle system, gain their unique properties from the physiochemical effects at their surface. In order to design particles with unique functional surfaces (e.g., active targeting; Section 5.4.2.), it is first important to understand what the natural response to the "basic" particle configurations is. In general, nanoparticles administered into

blood are rapidly cleared by mononuclear phagocyte system (MPS). This response is a result of both size effects (e.g., filtration, impaction, and occlusion) and surface recognition which is characterized by the accumulation of serum proteins and factors onto the particle surface. The amount and type of proteins adsorbed depend on hydrophobicity and surface charge of the particles, with positively charged nanoparticles being cleared much more rapidly as compared to their negatively charged and neutral counterparts [76]. In fact, by developing surfaces that resist protein deposition and factor accumulation, it is possible to have a nanoparticle that is no longer readily recognized by the MPS and thereby possesses extended circulation times [77, 78]. This "stealth" property is classically seen in hydrophilic neutral polymers that do not possess hydrogen bonding donors. Poly(ethylene glycol) (PEG) is the most common polymer used to achieve this stealth capacity, an effect utilized (as depicted in Fig. 5.1b) for over 40 years [79]. PEG coating forms a hydrophilic layer around PNPs, which allows them to resist recognition by opsonins, thereby circumventing immune response from macrophages [80]. PEG brush density also has an effect upon circulation time; typically, with greater density comes greater circulation time [81], unless the greater density causes other adverse effects such as increased instability [80]. Recently, there have been other PNP polymer coatings using polysaccharides that have no natural receptors [82].

Importantly, there are limitations to the use of PEG, which has increased the demand for alternative stealth polymers. For instance, as PEG is a nonbiodegradable polymer, there are restrictions as to the maximum MW that can be used. Currently, one of the largest in-market PEG molecules being used is in PEGASYS®, which is a PEGylated interferon with a PEG chain weight of 40 kDa to increase retention in blood circulation [83]. The restriction is due to the kidney's maximum size restriction in clearing molecules in the blood stream of around 60 kDa, thereby avoiding the concern of bioaccumulation [79]. Further, as PEG is limited in the number of conjugation sites and mechanical properties, these additional polymer systems increase the flexibility of PNP design available to the formulator without having to sacrifice circulation potential.

5.1.1.3 Size, Shape, and Mechanical Properties.
Circulation of nanoparticles also depends on their size and shape. Depending on the stealth properties of particles, spherical nanoparticles with sizes less than approximately 8 nm result in rapid urinary excretion, whereas spherical particles with sizes in excess of 1 μm result in rapid clearance due to filtration effects in the microvasculature. While there exists some degree of controversy in the literature regarding the exact size cutoffs, a more inclusive statement is that particles with sizes between 20 nm and 1 μm possess prolonged circulation times [84]. The exact extent of the prolonged circulation times is still being elucidated, with much of these results discussed in the passive targeting section (Section 5.4.1). Particle shape also has a profound effect on the circulation life, cell attachment, and cellular uptake [85]. A great example of this is given by the PEG-containing diblock copolymer filomicelles, which have a circulation half-life approaching approximately 1 week [86]. Filomicelles, which are flexible, elongated polymeric micelles, because of their ability to align with blood flow, avoid vascular collisions, extravasation, and phagocytosis. Geng et al. showed that, under flow

conditions, spherical and short filomicelles were readily phagocytosed compared to longer filomicelles [86]. Rigidity of the particles also affects their phagocytosis; rigid particles are readily phagocytosed compared to soft particles [87].

As polymers can be composed from a wide variety of chemistries and can be processed into a variety of shapes and forms, each of the above-mentioned design criteria can be tuned for specific applications. This flexibility in polymer synthesis and nanoparticle formulation methods have made PNPs one of the most widely studied drug delivery methods. This chapter emphasizes the understanding of different types of PNPs, routes of targeting, and biodistribution, and how to measure the different pertinent effects PNPs exhibit.

5.2 PNP DESIGN

Given the extensive array of chemistries and mechanical properties available in polymers, there is conceptually no limit to the forms and designs of PNPs that can be made. In this section, a summary of the approaches that have been developed and their relative advantages and disadvantages will be discussed. While it may not be initially clear which structure of PNP should be chosen for a given application, this overview should help the reader gain an intuitive sense of the breadth of benefits and downfalls of different PNP structures (Table 5.3).

5.2.1 Polymeric Nanospheres and Nanocapsules

Polymeric nanospheres, nanocapsules, and polymersomes are composed of polymers that can collapse on themselves or assemble in solution, and have the unique geometry described in Fig. 5.2.

The categories of nanocapsules and nanospheres differ in that nanospheres are generally solid to the core, where as nanocapsules will usually have a cross-linked surface with a vacant interior that is formed by polymerization in solution [102, 103]. This means that nanospheres can have the drug loaded throughout the particle matrix, whereas nanocapsules generally encapsulate the drug within the interior vacancy. Depending upon the route of synthesis for these PNPs, a drug can also be attached to each nanoparticle's outer matrix [104]. Many of these nanospheres

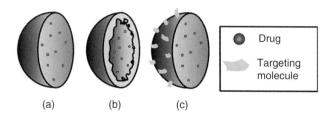

(a)   (b)   (c)

Figure 5.2. Cross-section structural examples of a drug-containing (a) nanosphere, (b) nanocapsule or polymersome, and (c) nanosphere with active targeting.

TABLE 5.3. Examples of PNP Configurations *In Vivo*

Particle type	Shape	Material	Size range	Carrier $t_{1/2}$	Drug $t_{1/2}$	Drug	Formulation	References
Micelle	Sphere	mPEG-PLA	30–60 nm	<1 h (human)	12 h (human)	Paclitaxel	Ring-opening polymerization	88, 89
Micelle	Sphere	PBLA-polyester-PEG	80 nm	2 h (mouse)	9 h (mouse)	Paclitaxel	Nano-precipitation	90
Micelle	Sphere	PEG-poly(aspartic acid)–DOX	40 nm	—	73 h (human), 98 h (mouse)	Doxorubicin	Ring-opening polymerization	91, 92
Polymersome	Hollow sphere	PEG-polybutadiene	100 nm	28 h (mouse)	—	—	Film rehydration	93
Nanocapsule	Hollow sphere	PMMA in HPMC	350 nm–10 μm	—	9 hr (rat)	Tacrolimus	Emulsion, spray drying	94, 95
Nanosphere	Sphere	PEG-chitosan	150 nm	63 h (mouse)	—	—	Double emulsion	96
Nanosphere	Sphere	PEG-PVA	130 nm	1 h (mouse)	—	—	Double emulsion	96
Nanogel	Cross-linked	Polysaccharide-PEG	145 nm	18 h (mouse)	—	—	Nano-precipitation/Michael addition	97, 98
Dendrimer	Branched sphere	PEG-polyester–DOX	22,550 Da	72 min (mouse)	—	Doxorubicin	Divergent polymerization	99, 100
Print	Sphere	PEG	200 nm	3.3 h (mouse)	—	—	PRINT	101

are formed using amphiphilic diblock copolymers, which allows loading of hydrophobic drugs into the core for increased bioavailability.

Pulmonary drug and gene delivery is an application in which PNPs are promising. Some of the difficulties in pulmonary drug delivery are the natural clearance mechanisms, phagocytosis by deep lung macrophages, as well as the variable thickness of the mucin layer. Interestingly, as inert PEG PNP surfaces are known to enhance vascular circulation times, PEGylation of PNPs also enhances their mucopenetration properties [105]. Composition, size, and surface charge are important in the efficacy of drug deposition and cytotoxicity [106]. PLGA chains covalently modified onto poly(vinyl alcohol) (PVA) backbones can produce polymeric nanospheres which have tunable properties, such as a fast or slow degradation rate to deliver drugs appropriately depending on the pathophysiology.

5.2.2 Polymeric Micelles

Polymeric micelles consist of self-assembled amphiphilic polymers and differ from nanocapsules in that their structure is generally formed purely from hydrophobic effects [102, 103]. Polymeric micelles are widely used because of their excellent ability to carry and stabilize hydrophobic molecules in an aqueous environment [7, 8, 107, 108], a useful prospect as many drugs are hydrophobic or lipophilic. Direct injection of free hydrophobic molecules may show very limited uptake by target tissues and organs due to limited solubility. Further, simple free drug injection also may cause greater interaction with the immune system due to direct contact, and thus only small concentrations of the drug may be administered to avoid an immune response [7, 8]. In comparison, because of polymeric micelles' amphiphilic nature, they can harbor the drug molecules in their interior while being less immunogenic to the host [7, 8, 109]. Figure 5.3 is an example cross-section of a drug loaded polymeric micelle with a coating for active targeting.

5.2.3 Polymersomes

Polymersomes (or polymer vesicles), which are synthetic polymer-based analogs of phospholipid liposomes and similar to nanocapsules, are composed of self-assembled di/triblock copolymers (e.g., PEG-poly(lactic acid) (PLA), PEG-polybutadiene (PBD), PEG-poly(propylene sulfide)-PEG) [110, 111] (for detailed review, see Ref. [112]). Like liposomes, polymersomes have a large internal aqueous domain that can be used for loading hydrophilic drugs. The thicker membrane of polymersomes ($\sim$9–22 nm as compared to $\sim$3–4 nm for liposomes) makes them a more robust carrier that can resist membrane deformation forces which commonly disrupt liposomes [110]. Also, owing to the higher PEGylation density of the polymersome surface, polymersomes have a twofold higher circulation life (20–30 h in rats) compared to liposomes [93]. Polymersomes have been used to load significant amounts of hydrophilic and hydrophobic anticancer drugs into the aqueous core and membrane, respectively [52, 113, 114]. Polymersomes can also be used for the simultaneous loading of both water-soluble and water-insoluble small-molecule drugs [115]. Micelles and polymersomes are discussed in depth in Chapter 3.

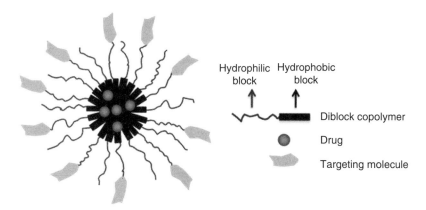

Figure 5.3. Structure of a micelle with loaded drug and active target coating in an aqueous environment.

5.2.4 Polymeric Nanogels

Aspects of both hydrogels [116] and nanoparticles make polymeric nanogels a very exciting and promising drug delivery system. Through variation of the cross-linked structure, size, and material selection, a multitude of options and effects are possible [97, 117–121]. The biggest difference between nanogels and other PNPs is that their structure is cross-linked either physically or chemically and will hydrolytically swell, and, depending on the polymers and cross-linking chemistry used, degradation can be pH responsive which has been extensively utilized as a passive targeting technique [120, 122]. This swelling force, when in an aqueous environment, can be produced through protonation/deprotonation, which will increase the mesh size until equilibrium is met with the cross-links' tension force. There are also nanogels that are temperature sensitive, such as those formed from poly(N-vinylcaprolactam) (VCL) [123], PNIPAAm [64], or poly(oligo(ethylene glycol methacrylate)) (POEGMA) [124]. Figure 5.4 shows the structure of a surface modified spherical nanogel.

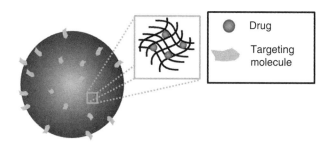

Figure 5.4. Structure of a nanogel, with a zoomed in section showing cross-linking.

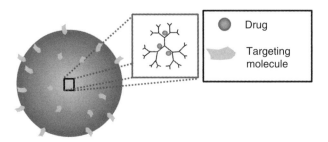

Figure 5.5. Structure of a dendrimer, zoomed in to show generational branching.

5.2.5   Polymeric Dendrimers

Dendritic polymers, called *dendrimers*, have unique characteristics that are elemental to their structure; these molecules are treelike branched structures which can harbor hydrophobic or hydrophilic drugs and shield them from the environment via the dendritic channels extending from the core. Their high monodispersity, compact structure and modifiable surface make dendrimers favorable for drug delivery [125]. Figure 5.5 shows an idealized structure of a dendrimer.

Dendrimers have applications in several different areas, such as ocular drug delivery. Spatero [126] specifically designed phosphorus-containing dendrimers that can react with carteolol, an anti-glaucoma drug. The most widely used dendrimers, poly(amido amine) (PAMAM) [126], have shown promise as an oral drug delivery vehicle because of their ability to penetrate the epithelial lining of the intestine; properties of the dendrimer's generation number and surface charge are key to this effect occurring [22]. There have been concerns with dendrimers and toxicity, but modification with lauric acid or PEG has been shown to improve both biocompatibility and pharmacokinetics. Further, conjugation with cationic amino acids can improve transport permeability of these dendrimers through tight junctions [22].

5.3   PNP FORMULATION METHODS AND TARGETING

In this section, a review of several formulation techniques for PNPs is presented. These techniques can be combined and interchanged to form a variety of PNP structures.

5.3.1   Nano-Precipitation

There are a several different routes of synthesis to prepare nanospheres and nanocapsules, as well as different methods and results of drug loading and targeting. The simplest approach for nanoparticle formulation is through nano-precipitation [127]. Generally, the polymer and drug are dissolved in an organic solvent. This solution is then added to an aqueous solution which is stirred vigorously so that the organic solvent is either quickly evaporated or is extracted into the aqueous phase, which acts as an anti-solvent for the polymer and drug. The polymer then precipitates rapidly, creating nanoparticulates [37, 46]. These particulates are then stabilized either by surfactants in the solution or through charge repulsion on the nanoparticle surface. As particles are formed directly by the rate of solvent removal and polymer aggregation, initial polymer solution viscosity, polymer MW, and concentration greatly impact the final size of the precipitated particles.

As an organic system is used, it is important to ensure that complete removal of the solvent phase is achieved. To remove the organic solvent present, which would be toxic to humans, solvent extraction can be performed, for instance, through evaporating the solvent in a vacuum or freeze-drier. To prevent PNP aggregation, surfactants are commonly added to the aqueous solution. However, this adds an extra step of removing the excess surfactants.

Nano-precipitation approaches can be used to modify surface chemistry to allow target group addition. As an example synthesis utilizing active targeting, compared to unmodified nanospheres composed of nanoprecipitated PEG-PLGA [128], arginine-glycine-aspartic acid (RGD) peptide and peptidomimetic RGD ligand-modified nanospheres were shown to be more effective in mice *in vivo*, exhibiting enhanced cellular uptake and targeting, which resulted in an increased survival [129]. The method that was used to add the RGD peptide sequence to the poly(ε-caprolactone)-*b*-PEG diblock copolymer was through washing the solvent-evaporated polymer with RGD solution after ultraviolet (UV)-irradiation photografting.

5.3.2 Interfacial Polymerization

Interfacial polymerization (or cross-linking) requires two immiscible solvents, one organic and the other aqueous. In this system, the monomers are dissolved in the aqueous phase with the initiator in the organic phase or vice versa. Alternatively, for polycondensation reactions, each co-monomer is dissolved in its appropriate phase. Most commonly, the monomer (or macromer) and drug will be dissolved in the organic phase, and then slowly added dropwise to the aqueous phase, under vigorous stirring. A benefit of using this process is good drug encapsulation into the core of the nanoparticle, rather than just the surface, if using a drug soluble in the organic phase, whereas a disadvantage is that, because of the intense stirring rate, proteins and peptides can be denatured [130].

Lee [103] performed an oil-in-water interfacial polymerization to form nanocapsules, with a cross-linked albumin shell encapsulating paclitaxel. This method required dissolution of a polymer with reactive groups in a water-immiscible organic solvent with the drug already dissolved, which was then added slowly to an aqueous solution of a protein. The organic solvent in the emulsion was then evaporated to produce nanocapsules with a protein–polymer shell with an inner core holding the drug. This procedure used *N*-hydroxysuccinimide-conjugated PEG as the polymer dissolved in dichloromethane with human serum albumin as the protein shell which denatures and cross-links with the PEG to form nanocapsules containing paclitaxel. This can also be described as denaturation polymerization.

5.3.3 Emulsion Polymerization

Emulsion polymerization has been used for decades as the preeminent approach for the synthesis of colloids, including latex paints and coatings. Emulsion polymerization involves a surfactant-laden continuous phase containing micelles. Within the micelles, the monomer and the drug are contained in discrete droplets. To initiate polymerization, an initiator is added to the continuous phase, which diffuses into the micellar domain. Typically, either a free-radical-forming compound is used, or the solution is irradiated with UV or higher energy. The residual monomer requires removal by centrifugation, evaporation, or tangential flow filtration. The benefits of this approach are that it is readily scalable, polymerization proceeds quickly, and additional stabilizer is not required. However, because of the aggressive reaction system, labile compound (e.g., proteins and peptides) are not readily amendable to this approach [130].

A method of forming chemically cross-linked nanogels is through inverse emulsion polymerization using a surfactant and UV irradiation. In an aqueous solution, both the polymer and the cross-linking molecules are dissolved before being added to a surfactant-containing organic solution. This produces inversed polymeric micelles, and then, through irradiation, polymerization is initiated and chemically cross-linked nanogels are formed [120].

5.3.4 Polymeric Micelle Synthesis

Gaucher et al. [131] outlined five different methods for forming drug loaded PNPs, including dialysis, solvent casting, and one-step lyophilization. Typically, polymeric micelles are formed with either amphiphilic or ionic block copolymers. There are a variety of polymers to choose from, with PEG [7, 131] and various polyesters such as PLA [132] being the most common hydrophilic and hydrophobic blocks, respectively. While diblock copolymers are more common, there are some examples of higher order block copolymers as well [131, 133]. Chain lengths of the hydrophilic and hydrophobic blocks can play a large part in the shape of the micelle formed. For instance, hydrophilic chains longer than hydrophobic chains will typically lead to spherical micelles, but the opposite can lead to lamellae and rods [125].

A technique that can attain exceptionally high drug encapsulation efficiency, as well as increased effectiveness of drug delivery [108], is micelle formation using an amphiphilic macromer with a hydrophilic polymer such as PEG and an active drug bonded to the hydrophobic polymer with a biodegradable linker. Employing this method, Yoo et al. [108] created a polymeric micelle in which a triblock copolymer consisting of hydrophilic PEG, hydrophobic PLA, and hydrophobic doxorubicin (DOX) was used. DOX was attached via a hydrazone bond to PLA to form DOX-PLA-PEG. As hydrazone bonds are acid-cleavable, this route was predicted to be effective for specific targeting in cancer therapy. The group previously created a similar micelle with physically associated DOX using PEG-PLA. Comparatively, the chemically conjugated DOX-PLA-PEG had much higher encapsulation efficiency than PEG-PLA with physically associated DOX [134]. The chemical conjugation also allowed the drug to be released more slowly, resulting in a fivefold greater cytotoxicity than physically absorbed DOX, likely due to increased concentration of DOX-containing micelles penetrating into cells through the lysosomal pathway [134]. More on this topic of drug–polymer conjugation is described in Chapter 3.

5.3.5 Nanogel Synthesis

Synthesis of nanogels typically includes cross-linking polymer chains in an already formed PNP [118] through a technique such as emulsion polymerization [120]. For physically cross-linked nanogels, one can perform nano-precipitation [119], which physically binds polymer strands together. Physical cross-linking can be fairly simple, as Nagahama [119] has shown. Briefly, they formed a macromer in dimethyl sulfoxide (DMSO) of PLA and dextran, and then dropwise added water with dissolved protein to this solution under fast mixing to precipitate the polymer into a physically cross-linked nanogel. Physical cross-linking is dependent upon the material selection; some diblock polymers will form micelles, others will form nanogels. As an example, Nowak [135] used polypeptides to form nanogels and showed that chain conformations (α-helix, β-sheet, or random) of the hydrophobic portion of the amphiphilic block copolymer, as well as the use of a diblock or random block copolymer, make a difference as to whether a micelle or nanogel is formed through physical interactions.

Drug loading can be performed through different methods. A simple technique is to soak the formed nanogels in a drug dissolved solution, which will cause the nanogels to swell and increase their mesh size. Drying will effectively collapse the nanogels and encapsulate the drug. Another method is that of direct addition of the drug in solution before the nanogels polymerize. For the technique previously described in Shidhaye [120], one can add drug to the aqueous phase with the polymers before initiating polymerization.

5.3.6 Dendrimer Synthesis

A repeated reaction involving two steps, namely, activation and then growth, is typically utilized to form dendrimers in a convergent or divergent synthesis scheme [25]. In convergent synthesis, monomers add chains from the exterior to the interior. Convergent strategies allow for the synthesis of "janus" particles, where spatially separated domains on the surface of the dendrimer can have distinct functional groups. More commonly used, however, is divergent synthesis, where polymerization of the dendrimer occurs from a central point. The divergent method is common in forming PAMAM polymeric dendrimers, whereas the convergent method originally was developed for poly(aryl ether) dendrimers. While there are a myriad of different bonding moieties for polymeric dendrimers, PAMAM dendrimers can be synthesized stepwise through Michael addition of an amine to methyl acrylate, followed by reaction with ethylenediamine to add more amine groups for further Michael addition. Drug loading of dendrimers may occur through utilizing a covalently linked functional material in the stepwise reaction [126], through using the highly branched polymer network for physical entrapment of drug, or via affinity actions between the drug in solution and the polymer backbone during dendrimer synthesis [25].

5.3.7 Particle Replication in Nonwetting Templates (PRINT) Synthesis

Unlike the synthesis of micelles, vesicles and dendrimers, which represent kinetically and/or thermodynamically driven "bottom-up" approach to control nanoparticle characteristics (e.g., shape, size, surface and mechanical properties), synthesis of nanoparticles by PRINT is a "top-down" method for achieving particles of a variety of shapes. PRINT uses an imprint lithography technique to fabricate monodispersed particles ranging from 80 nm to 20 μm with a variety of shapes.

PRINT is a soft lithography technique based on molds of perfluorinated polyether elastomers. This material has very low surface energy, which prevents wetting of the mold and results in discrete particles. As shown in Fig. 5.6, PRINT process consists of three steps: (i) casting of "delivery sheet," (ii) particle fabrication, and (iii) particle harvesting. The process starts with casting a solution in the form of a film. This solution consists of the drug dissolved in an organic solvent with either a polymer [136] or reactive monomers [137]. The solvent is evaporated from the cast film by heat to result in a solid state solution film called *delivery sheet*, which delivers the

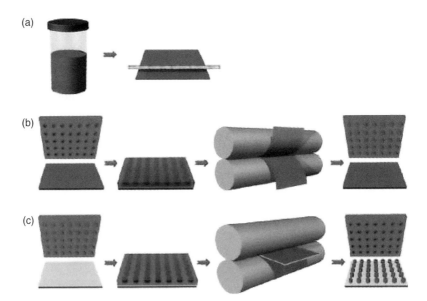

Figure 5.6. (a) Casting of a delivery sheet. A solution of drug and polymer/monomer in organic solvent is drawn as a film onto a PET substrate using a mayer rod. (b) Particle fabrication. The delivery sheet is brought into contact with a perfluoropolyether elastomeric mold using a nip and split. The nip can be heated if required. (c) Particle harvesting. The filled mold is brought into contact with a high-energy film using a heated nip without splitting. After cooling, the mold is separated from the high-energy film or excipient layer which has an array of particles on its surface. Reprinted from Nano Letters [136]. Copyright (1996) American Chemical Society.

composition to the mold. The delivery sheet is then laminated on the patterned side of the mold. Depending on the composition of delivery sheet, either a phase transition or solvent evaporation method is employed to fill the mold. For example, a melt solidification transition can be used to fill the mold by briefly heating the polymer film when in contact with the mold. As the polymer melts, it rises into the mold cavities by capillary action and then solidifies as the polymer film cools down. When the delivery sheet is composed of reactive monomers, the filled mold can be exposed to conditions that initiate the polymerization reaction (e.g., exposing to UV light for photoinitiated reactions). For harvesting particles from the mold, a high-energy film or excipient layer is hot-laminated with a filled mold. Once the mold has cooled down, the excipient film is removed from the mold, with an array of particles on it.

Depending on the shape of the cavity in the mold, monodispersed nanoparticles with a variety of shapes (e.g., spheres, cylinders, cubes, and trapezoids) and aspect ratios can be fabricated [138]. Drugs can be incorporated into the particle matrix to give encapsulation efficiencies as high as 100% [136]. Docetaxel-loaded PLGA nanoparticles with up to 40 wt% drug loading were generated using the PRINT process. Surface properties of PRINT nanoparticles can be tuned either by matrix composition or by post-synthesis functionalization to have ligands and PEG on the surface of the particles. Long circulating PEGylated hydrogel nanoparticles were fabricated using a continuous PRINT process [137].

5.4 NANOPARTICLE TARGETING OVERVIEW

For enhanced selectivity and function in nanoparticle drug delivery, surface modification with specific targeting molecules is becoming very popular [139–141] and provides a means to further decrease the amount of drug administered and reduce toxic side effects of the drug that does not reach the intended target. The following sections will exemplify the different possibilities of using different configurations of PNPs with different compositions and targeting techniques.

The two main categories of targeting PNPs to a specific location for drug delivery are passive and active targeting. Passive targeting is the use of natural shape/size to determine the localization of PNPs. Active targeting involves the use of an affinity-based recognition sequence (e.g., ligand/receptor and antigen/antibody) to determine the distribution of PNPs. In this section, both approaches and considerations are presented.

5.4.1 Passive Targeting

Currently, passive targeting has been the only FDA-approved approach to nanoparticle drug delivery. Most commonly, passive targeting involves utilizing the effects of passive transport principles to reach the desired location. The best example of this is the enhanced permeation and retention (EPR) effect. In areas of high vascular permeability (e.g., sites of inflammation and some tumors), nanoparticles that are long circulating can slowly accumulate in the interstitial space. Ideally, extravasated particles can be taken up by the local cells and the active drug can be delivered. Size is an important factor in EPR passive targeting of PNPs administered via systemic drug delivery, as it impacts the effective biodistribution throughout the body. If nanoparticles are being used for the treatment of solid tumors, then the size range for the nanoparticles used should be around 10–500 nm [142], with the most effective average size being between 50 and 200 nm [142]. Tight junctions between healthy endothelial cells will not allow nanoparticles around 10 nm and up to pass through, but in tumor tissues nanoparticles can typically fenestrate between the loose junctions up to around 500 nm. In general, though, sizes of 5–250 nm have the potential for most drug delivery applications [143, 144].

Another example of the passive targeting mechanism is that of pH responsiveness in anticancer treatment and other pH sensitive applications where the polymer carrier releases the drug at a higher rate either through degradation or via cationic repulsion effects. For instance, in the treatment of colitis, PLGA/methacrylate copolymer nanospheres were loaded with budesonide, a corticosteroid, and delivered to a murine model. In comparison to conventional enteric microparticles, the nanospheres released the drug with a strong pH dependence in the colon and showed superior colon targeting with greater concentration in both noninflamed and inflamed tissue [145].

Micelles sensitive to pH are particularly popular for anticancer drug delivery in which the lowered pH of tumors is utilized with passive targeting and the EPR effect [8, 107, 108]. An example of a method that involves passive targeting via pH sensitivity through polymer design is the use of an amphiphilic diblock copolymer with a hydrophobic PBAE [146] or another acid-sensitive group [7, 8, 107, 147] as the micelle core in combination with a hydrophilic head group. Another example of pH sensitive targeting is by harnessing increased hydrogen bonding at lower pH to extend molecules via repulsion in the corona, which may help release the carried drug more readily [107].

5.4.2 Active Targeting

Active targeting presents an opportunity to further deliver the drug to the desired target tissue. Contrary to passive targeting mechanisms, these coatings can prevent the drug carriers from being swept away from the active site by simple passive transport. This is due to site-specific interactions of the targeting molecule, which can promote endocytosis of the nanoparticles and allow cytoplasmic drug delivery. The production cost of peptides and antibodies, however, increases the cost of the engineered drug delivery system.

As with passive targeting, active targeting can occur either with a single level of targeting or with multiple levels of targeting. Advantages to multilevel active targeting are that you can target more surface area by attacking multiple levels simultaneously, and you have the option of having one drug delivery vehicle being able to treat multiple diseases either separately or together. The addition of targeting groups for both tumor cells and vessels with a tumor-penetrating peptide allows for much greater tumor area to be covered in comparison to passively targeted nanoparticles.

5.4.2.1 Peptide Ligands. A benefit of using a peptide-modified drug carrier over a peptide-conjugated drug is the multimerization of ligand binding, which dramatically increases cell affinity and the drug payload [148]. One of the most thoroughly investigated peptides for cancer cell targeting is the peptide RGD [149]. RGD is part of the recognition sequence for integrin receptors, a protein that plays an important role in angiogenesis. Other peptide sequences are used as well, such as asparagine-glycine-arginine (NGR) [150] and leucine-aspartic acid-valine (LDV) [151]. There are also peptidomimetic versions of peptides, as shown in Fig. 5.7. Using a peptidomimetic RGD peptide that contains tyrosine can actually increase specificity toward integrins $\alpha v \beta 1$ and 3 compared to the RGD peptide [152].

Because of high levels of vasculature formation in cancer, $\alpha v \beta 3$ integrin, to which RGD peptides can attach, is more greatly expressed by endothelial cells in tumors than

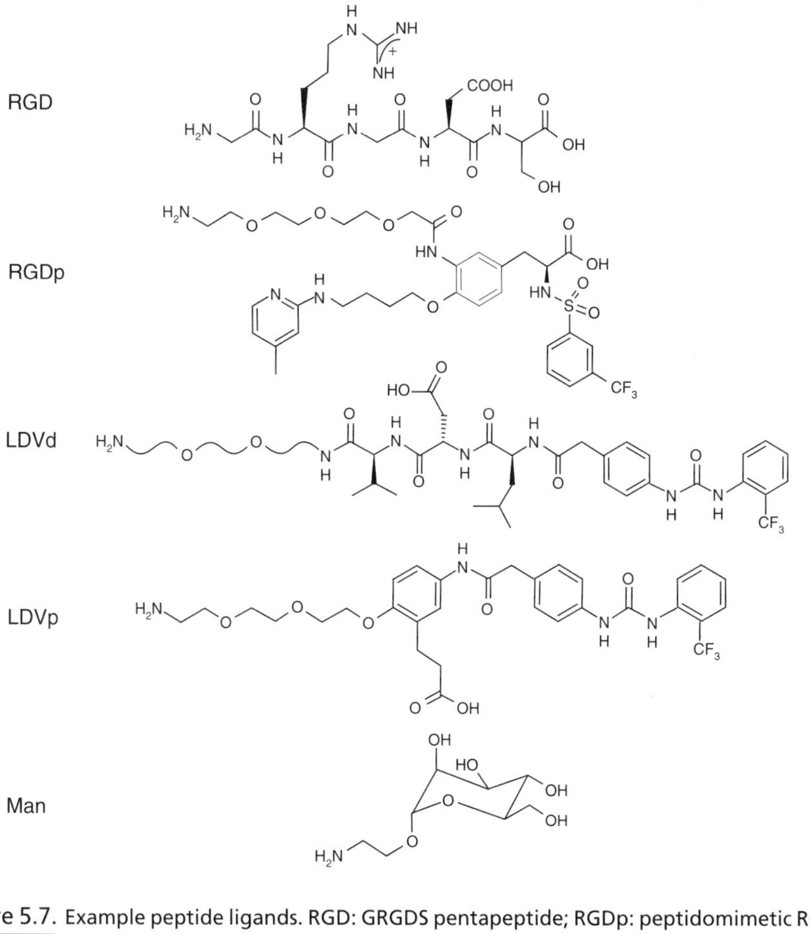

Figure 5.7. Example peptide ligands. RGD: GRGDS pentapeptide; RGDp: peptidomimetic RGD; LDVd: tripeptide; LDVp: peptidomimetic LDV; Man: a derivative of mannose. Reprinted from the European Journal of Pharmaceutics and Biopharmaceutics [152], Copyright (2009), with permission from Elsevier.

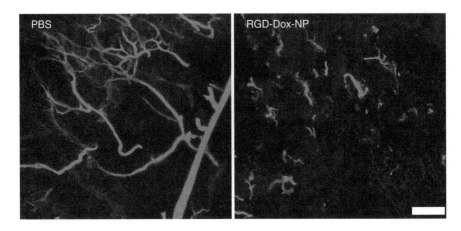

Figure 5.8. Exposure of tumor vasculature to PBS versus RGD-coated DOX-loaded nanoparticles. Reprinted from the National Academy of Sciences [153]. Copyright (2008) National
Academy of Sciences, U.S.A.

elsewhere [129]. By simply grafting integrin-binding peptides to PNPs, these PNPs
now have specific targeting for the easily accessible tumor endothelium, which further
reduces the toxic side effects of the drugs relative to passively targeted systems. For
example, RGD-bound PNPs containing anti-angiogenic DOX had a profound impact
upon tumor vasculature relative to a phosphate buffered saline (PBS) control group
(Fig. 5.8) [153]. There are, however, many different integrin-binding receptors and
other targets present on different cell types that have been found through the use of
phage display and other techniques [154, 155].

In an attempt to reduce nonspecific toxicity, multicoated PNP cancer-targeting
strategies have been achieved using a highly branched copolymer of poly[(amine-
ester)-co-(DL-lactide)]/1,2-dipalmitoyl-sn-glycero-3-phosphoethanolamine   (HPAE-
co-PLA/DPPE). Both cyclic RGD peptide (c(RGDfK)) and transferrin glycoprotein
(Tf) were used as targeting molecules to deliver the anti-tumor therapeutic paclitaxel.
As transferrin is involved in the transport of ferric ions throughout the body, transferrin coating can increase nanoparticle uptake by cells [156]. Transferrin receptors have
also been shown to be more highly expressed on tumor cells than on noncancerous
cells [157]. For instance, to improve drug efficacy, paclitaxel-loaded HPAE-co-
PLA/DPPE nanoparticles (PTX-NPs) were surface conjugated with c(RGDfK) and Tf
(PTX-RGD-NPs and PTX-Tf-NPs). In $\alpha v \beta 3$ integrin-overexpressed human umbilical
vein endothelial cells (HUVECs), RGD-PTX-NPs had a 10-fold lower IC_{50} value
as compared to PTX-NPs. PTX-Tf-NPs showed a similar twofold decrease in IC_{50}
in human cervical carcinoma cells [158]. Specific ligand–receptor interaction led
to enhanced internalization of PTX-RGD-NPs and PTX-Tf-NPs, thereby improving
their anti-tumor efficiency. [158].

However, the largest downfall of using integrin-binding peptides is that many
nontargeted cells and tissues express the same integrins at low levels relative to

cancer cells [159], and so the specific targeting can end up attaching to unintended materials. F3 is a ligand that can be used to get around this issue. This ligand binds to cell-surface nucleolin, a protein, which, although not specific to just cancer cells, is mainly expressed as an endothelial protein *in vivo* in actively angiogenic endothelial cells [160].

A critical part of targeting is selectivity. Shahin et al. [148] performed a comparison of c(RGDfK) and p160 for the selective targeting of paclitaxel-loaded polymeric micelles (PTX-Micelles) to cancer versus endothelial cells. While both the p160 and c(RGDfK) ligands facilitated selective association of PTX-Micelles to MDA-MB-435 cancer cells, the p160 ligand was more effective than RGD at internalization of PTX-Micelles. To attach the peptide to the surface of the PEG-PCL micelle, acetal-PEG-PCL micelles were first synthesized via dropwise addition of the polymer dissolved in DMSO to water with stirring. After dialysis to remove the solvent, an aqueous solution of the peptide was added to facilitate reaction with the acetal groups. The desired peptide-modified micelles were obtained following addition of a reducing agent and subsequent purification by dialysis.

5.4.2.2 Aptamer Ligands.
Aptamers are recently identified nucleic acids used in active targeting. An aptamer is a ligand consisting of single- or double-stranded DNA or RNA that specifically folds and attaches to target ligand(s) with great affinity [161–163]. Aptamers can be used similar to other active targeting molecules, but have advantages that they are of relatively low MW, have limited immunogenicity, and have high affinity when folded into their specific structure [78].

Aptamer-modified polymeric nanospheres have recently been used for the treatment of mercury toxicity in a rat model. Briefly, PEG-PLA was nanoprecipitated with an anti-mercury amino acid, selenomethionine, and conjugated covalently with a targeting aptamer. The results showed significantly reduced mercury concentration in the brain and kidney, with only small toxic side effects [164]. Another property of aptamer ligands is their ability to attach to biologically active cells that cross or are attached to the blood–brain barrier, thereby enabling PNP transport across the barrier. Guo [78] synthesized custom DNA aptamer-coated PEG-PLGA nanospheres containing paclitaxel for use in anti-glioma drug delivery. The nanospheres yielded much higher efficacy and enhanced biodistribution to the tumor compared with traditional anti-glioma chemotherapeutic Taxol® delivered without specific targeting. However, aptamers are a very new targeting technology and there is limited data on the pharmacology of aptamer-conjugated nanoparticles.

5.4.2.3 Antibodies.
Depending upon their method of production, antibodies are available in two main styles, namely, monoclonal or polyclonal. Monoclonal antibodies target one, and only one, specific epitope on the surface of an antigen. They are molecularly homologous with only one variable region. Polyclonal antibodies, on the other hand, represent a heterogeneous population of antibodies that, while targeting the same antigen, can recognize a variety of epitope domains on that particular antigen. Further, polyclonal antibodies can contain different clones that recognize the same epitope, but with vastly different affinities. For this reason, monoclonal antibodies are the

preferred choice for PNP targeting, as they express a much more consistent targeting potential, greatly reducing batch-to-batch variability. However, if recombinant poly-clonal antibodies can be produced through the use of gene libraries, perhaps they can be used to target disease-specific antigens [165]. Monoclonal antibodies have another advantage over polyclonal antibodies in that they can be more easily tailor-made by being produced from gene-modified hybridomas in large supply in the laboratory. A possible additional advantage is the single-targeting ability of monoclonal antibod-ies. While recombinant polyclonal antibodies must be carefully designed to target only applicable moieties on desired cells or tissues, monoclonal antibodies can be chosen that select only a single moiety.

Type IV collagen, NG2 (a proteoglycan surface indicator of pericytes), and ED-B (a form of fibronectin) are some of the markers of angiogenic tissue. These are all selectively produced in tumor vessels, and antibodies have been developed to tar-get these sites for use in delivering toxins [160]. A very significant pitfall to all the aforementioned active targeting coatings that target angiogenesis is that angio-genesis also occurs in tissue with wound healing repair occurring. The occurrence of cancer treatment coinciding with inflammation or an injury could cause seri-ous malfunction with the normal wound repair processes and pose a risk to the patient, and so patients would have to be carefully selected for this option to be a viable one.

One concern with monoclonal antibodies, compared to other targeting, is possi-ble immune activation from nonspecific reticuloendothelial system (RES) uptake. In addition, their large size inhibits movement through vasculature and passive transport across endothelium [4, 166]. A potentially more useful method has been demonstrated where a mimetic antibody peptide was used in lieu of the real antibody. The results showed that there was reduced affinity of the mimetic antibody toward the tumor, but the mimetic antibody showed greater tumor inhibition [166].

Another interesting molecule targeting anti-ovarian cancer is folate (vitamin B9). This vitamin is important in rapidly dividing cells, as in the case of cancerous tis-sue. By surface modifying nanoparticles to include a folate-receptor-binding molecule, these nanoparticles can go through endocytosis to enter into the cytoplasm for drug delivery [139, 167]. Folate-receptor-binding molecules include folic acid and a mon-oclonal antibody that binds to the folate receptor [168].

While systemic targeting is predominantly used in PNP cancer therapy appli-cations, antibody-targeted PNPs are also used in gene therapy. Cationic PNPs form electrostatically stable complexes with DNA and are a widely used alternative to viral gene delivery vectors [169]. An advantage of using antibody-targeted nanoparticles in gene therapy is that a 70 nm nanoparticle can hold around 2000 small interfering RNA (siRNA) segments while keeping the contents safe from external exposure, compared to conjugated antibodies without a nanoparticle carrier, which can only hold less than 10 unprotected siRNA strands [140]. Microparticles and other carriers can have a payload of molecules the same as, if not greater than, that of nanoparticles. However, nanoparticles excel in navigating tumor fenestrations and then delivering the drug to the cytoplasm [139], thereby helping bypass multidrug resistance through entering the cell via receptor-mediated endocytosis [132].

5.4.2.4 Target Epitope Selection. Importantly, if active targeting is to be used, selection of the target epitope must be carefully considered. For instance, the target should be present on the luminal surface of exposed cell types. In particular, this often means the vascular endothelium. Further, the epitope should be spatially and temporally available, that is, the epitope should not be downregulated or hidden. For example, adhesion of activated blood cells and accelerated shedding inhibit targeting some constitutive endothelial determinants [170]. On the other hand, determinants exposed on the endothelial cells under pathological conditions (e.g., selectins) have a distinct transient surface expression profile which may permit selective drug delivery to pathologically altered endothelium, but require exact timing of administration to match duration of target availability. Targeting should not cause harmful side effects in the vasculature. Binding of targeted drugs may cause shedding, internalization, or inhibition of endothelial determinants, which may be detrimental. For example, thrombomodulin, a surface protein responsible for thrombosis containment, is abundantly expressed in the pulmonary vasculature, providing high pulmonary targeting specificity [171]. Yet, its inhibition by antibodies may provoke incidences of thrombosis, which prevents clinical potential for drug delivery. Ideally, engaging of the target should provide therapeutic benefits, such as inhibition of pro-inflammatory molecules.

5.5 PNP CHARACTERIZATION

5.5.1 PNP Characteristics

Ultimately, the success of PNPs is not guaranteed if they are not effectively characterized. Surprisingly, most failures of particles during development have been, in part, due to ineffective characterization of the particles. PNPs' shape, surface properties, and morphology can be determined through imaging, such as scanning electron microscopy (SEM), transmission electron microscopy (TEM), or atomic force microscopy (AFM). Size distribution of PNPs can be checked via nanoscale imaging such as SEM or TEM, or can be analyzed by using dynamic light scattering (DLS). Determining the zeta potential of PNPs is useful both to determine the charge properties of a surface coating and to see if the charge is appropriate for biological use systemically. Surface charge of PNPs is important in determining their stability in suspension, their propensity to aggregate in blood flow, their cellular uptake characteristics, and their likelihood to adhere with oppositely charged particles or cellular membranes [5]. Zeta potential of nanoparticles in dispersion can be measured using laser Doppler electrophoresis (LDE). Characterization techniques such as Fourier transform infrared spectroscopy (FTIR), nuclear magnetic resonance (NMR), or X-ray diffraction (XRD) can be used to determine the chemical groups on the PNP surface.

The stability of PNPs, which is an important characteristic, can easily be checked by looking for degradation products over time in stabilizing media or by checking polydispersity over time. Nanoparticles that aggregate once delivered intravenously can be fatal; thus surface modification to reduce that chance is often necessary [172].

Checking the loading characteristics of PNPs can be as straightforward as simply dissolving/swelling the PNP in an organic solvent to extract the encapsulated drug or degrading the PNP via a method that does not inhibit or destroy the active drug. For instance, if the drug does not degrade in the presence of acid, lowering the pH to dissolve acid-hydrolyzed PNPs is a quick method of degradation, and the concentration of drug released in the supernatant can be determined through an analysis technique such as high performance liquid chromatography (HPLC), UV–visible spectroscopy, fluorometry, or mass spectroscopy. Encapsulation efficiency (EE) is a very commonly used parameter to describe the amount of drug actually loaded into the nanoparticles versus the total amount of drug that was added to the solution of PNP synthesis, as described in Eq. 5.1:

$$\frac{\text{Mass drug loaded into PNP}}{\text{Mass drug added to synthesis solution}} = \text{EE} \qquad (5.1)$$

An easy way to determine EE is to keep track of the mass of drug added to the synthesis solution, form the PNPs, and then centrifuge them into a pellet or run a gel permeation. The supernatant can then be used to back-calculate the encapsulated drug, or a release study can be done with the PNPs to determine the amount of drug released.

5.5.2 Biodistribution

Biodistribution can be determined by both invasive and noninvasive methods. Typically, invasive methods involve histology of targeted organs and tissues after set time periods to detect a marker. For instance, if radiolabeled nanoparticles are used, the tissues can be placed in a gamma counter for comparison over time to find the concentration dynamics. Noninvasive methods are promising in that histology is not required. For instance, if targeted radiopaque PNPs are administered *in vivo*, the subject can be X-ray-imaged over a period to establish biodistribution [173]. Radiopaque polymers can be formed through adding salts containing heavy metals, such as iodine, which absorb X-rays.

Molecular imaging utilizes distinct biomarkers in biological systems to perform characterization at the molecular and cellular level. By delivering a signal-providing, or signal-dampening, probe to a targeted area, 2D and 3D imaging can be produced of that area [174]. A similar branch of molecular imaging, namely, radiogenomics, can detect gene expression radiometrically without performing histology [175]. Different signals can be added to PNPs, such as radioisotopes, which produce either positrons or photons for use in positron emission tomography (PET) or single-photon emission computed tomography (SPECT), respectively, or contrast agents for use in nuclear magnetic resonance imaging (MRI) or optical imaging, etc. Each imaging technique has benefits and caveats because of different sensitivities and approaches. There are many good articles discussing this topic [174, 176–178].

A recent method of detecting biodistribution, while at the same time administering therapeutics, is through the use of theranostic nanoparticles (TNPs) [179–181].

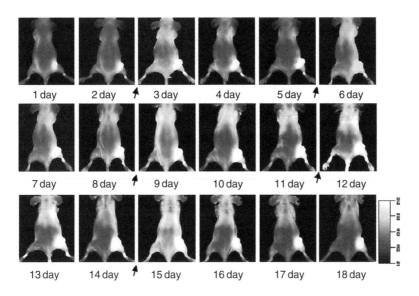

Figure 5.9. Biodistribution of labeled theranostic nanoparticles in a mouse model over 10 days. Reprinted from the Journal of Controlled Release, [181], Copyright (2010), with permission from Elsevier.

TNPs are combinatorial therapeutic nanoparticles that can both deliver drug to combat disease and be used simultaneously as a diagnostic and monitoring tool. As many cancer treatment therapies are for very specific patients, being able to accurately arrive at the treatment necessary is a method to increase the efficacy of the therapy administered [177]. In theory, TNPs can accumulate in diseased tissue that has been passively or actively targeted, and then, by using different imaging techniques available, it is possible to locate and characterize any early stage of disease through use of contrast agents and molecular probes [182].

Figure 5.9 is an example of the combination of theranostics with molecular imaging in a mouse model. Once the tumors reached 7–8 mm, Cy5.5-labeled, paclitaxel-loaded chitosan PNPs were administered intravenously. One can see the increased intensity in the targeted areas and decreased intensity systemically, over time. This shows tumor specificity of the PNPs, as well as the ability of molecular imaging to capture both the concentration of PNPs at the tumor site and the tumor size. Control mice (not shown) had tumors rapidly increasing in size, but mice that received the PNP delivery system showed a constant tumor size up to 15 days and then the tumor size started to decrease [181].

5.5.3 Biocompatibility and Cytotoxicity of PNPs

All systemically injected materials must pass basic safety criteria in order to be approved for use. Owing to the burgeoning area of nanoparticle therapy and the complexity involved, this characterization can be quite extensive and challenging.

However, the principles of determining safety are relatively simple to understand and provide a guiding light to consider as one develops new PNP strategies. At the simplest level, the PNP should be nontoxic, nonimmunogenic, noninflammatory, nonteratogenic, nonthrombogenic, nonbioaccumulating, and stable in blood [130]. As toxicity is easily evaluated in *in vitro* studies and provides a useful indicator of biological toxicity, every PNP should be first evaluated by determining the effect of particles and their degradation products on cellular viability. Cell type selection can be made depending upon the application of interest. Similar to the cellular uptake of PNPs, the cytotoxicity of PNPs can be size- and shape-dependent. Indeed, Kim et al. demonstrated the size-dependent cytotoxicity of polypyrrole nanoparticles (PPy NPs). Human lung fibroblasts and mouse alveolar macrophages were treated with monodispersed PPy NPs of different sizes (20, 40, 60, 80 and 100 nm) [183]. PPy NP cytotoxicity correlated with their size and was in the following order: 60 nm > 20 nm > 40 nm > 80 nm > 100 nm.

Cytotoxicity can be determined by measuring cell viabilities after treating them with different concentrations of PNPs. Before choosing an appropriate cell viability assay, it is necessary to understand what each assay is measuring as an endpoint and how that correlates with cell viability. Assays are available to measure endpoints, such as cell proliferation, number of live cells, number of dead cells, and mechanism of cell death. MTT (3-[4,5-dimethylthiazole-2-yl]-2,5-diphenyl tetrazolium) is a colorimetric assay to measure cell proliferation, wherein the active reductase enzymes in viable cells reduce MTT to a purple-colored formazan product. As a result, formazan formation is directly proportional to the number of viable cells in a culture. However, MTT can also directly react with reducing agents (e.g., polyphenolic antioxidants) to produce formazan crystals. In cases where such reducing agents are involved, MTT or other assays that rely on reductase activity may overestimate cell proliferation [184]. The luminescence-based ATP assay, where luminescence originates from conversion of luciferin to oxyluciferin by a luciferase in presence of ATP, measures luminescence intensity to determine ATP concentration in cells, which is an indicator of cell viability [183]. Live/Dead® assay is a fluorescence-based assay to differentiate live cells from dead cells by simultaneously staining with the green-fluorescing calcein-AM to indicate intracellular esterase activity (marker of live cells) and red-fluorescing ethidium homodimer-1 to indicate loss of plasma membrane integrity (marker of dead cells). Methods of detection for Live/Dead assay include fluorescent spectroscopy, fluorescent imaging, or flow cytometry, and can be used to determine the total number of live and dead cells in a culture. To determine the mechanism of cell death, apoptotic and necrotic cells can be differentiated by detecting phosphatidylserine with fluorescein-5-isothiocyanate (FITC)-bound annexin V and propidium iodide [185]. Furthermore, mitochondrial membrane potential can be measured with flow cytometry to determine if a loss of membrane potential has occurred, a sign of apoptosis in some systems. This can be performed by adding fluorochromes, which reflect the membrane potential via fluorescence. In the case of slow degrading biodegradable PNPs, measuring cytotoxicity of PNPs after short-term exposure (24–72 h) may not be enough, and it is equally important to separately determine the cytotoxicity of water-soluble and insoluble degradation products of PNPs.

While cell viability assays are a good indicator of overall cellular response to a toxin, they do not reveal much about the mechanism of toxicity. Recently, much attention is being given to biomaterial-induced inflammatory response, which is inextricably linked to cellular oxidative stress, where cellular antioxidant defense mechanisms are overwhelmed by excessive generation of reactive oxygen species (ROS) and reactive nitrogen species (RNS) [31]. 2′,7′-Dichlorodihydrofluorescein diacetate (DCFH-DA) is commonly used as a marker of oxidative stress in cells [75]. DCFH-DA, a non-fluorescent form of the dye, is taken up by cells and cleaved to a nonfluorescent DCFH) by active esterases in the cell. DCFH can then react with a variety of ROS and RNS (hydrogen peroxide, peroxynitrite, hydroxyl radical, lipid peroxides, thiol radicals, etc.) to form fluorescent 2′,7′-dichlorofluorescein (DCF). Oxidative stress in the cells can be quantified by measuring the DCF fluorescence. As DCF reacts with a variety of ROS and RNS, it does not provide information about the specific oxidative species involved or about the subcellular compartments (e.g., cytoplasm, plasma membrane) that are at risk of damage by ROS/RNS. Cellular proteins can be measured for their 3-nitrotyrosine (3NT) and protein-bound 4-hydroxy-2-*trans*-nonenal (HNE) content, which are specific markers for protein damage by RNS and lipid peroxidation, respectively [75].

A typical and problematic contaminant in nanoparticle formulations is the endotoxin lipopolysaccharide (LPS). LPS, originating from gram-negative bacteria, is pyrogenic and a major hurdle of nanoparticle formulations in preclinical studies because of its cytotoxicity [186]. Endotoxin levels can be determined via a simple assay, such as the lumilus amebocyte lysate (LAL) assay, which may give a positive result through clot formation, turbidity, or chromogenicity, depending on the test used. The other common method of evaluation for pyrogenic contamination is an *in vivo* rabbit test where qualitative results are measured after injection. Removal of LPS from nanoparticles is very troublesome because of the high surface area to volume ratio of nanoparticles [186], resistance to heat, pH, and inability of removal via sterile filtration; so sterile design and practices may be the most effective method of non-contamination compared to their removal after processing.

5.5.4 Drug Release and Pharmacokinetics

Modeling release characteristics of drugs from PNPs not only gives insight about the release/degradation mechanism in a new PNP formulation, but also helps in choosing PNP design to obtain desired release profiles. As introduced in Chapter 1, Fick's second law of diffusion in spherical coordinates, Eq. 5.2, is a common starting point for modeling drug release from PNPs, and it describes the change in concentration C of drug in a sphere of radius r over time t. D is the diffusivity and a is the constant radius of the sphere. As Fick's second law only describes diffusion, it is not an endpoint equation for PNPs which are degradable or exhibit relaxation effects.

$$\frac{\partial C}{\partial t} = D \left[\frac{\partial^2 C}{\partial r^2} + \frac{2}{r} \frac{\partial C}{\partial r} \right]$$

(5.2)

For one-dimensional diffusion in the radial axis and sink conditions, initial and boundary conditions can be stated as follows:

$$t = 0 \quad 0 < r < a \quad C = C_1$$

$$t = 0 \quad r = 0 \quad \frac{\partial C}{\partial t} = 0$$

$$t > 0 \quad r = a \quad C = C_0$$

where a is the PNP radius, C_1 is the initial concentration in the PNP, and C_0 is the concentration in the surrounding bulk fluid. The series solution to this equation is given by Crank et al. as

$$\frac{M_t}{M_\infty} = 1 - \frac{6}{\pi^2} \sum_{n=1}^{\infty} \frac{1}{n^2} \exp\left[\frac{-Dn^2\pi^2 t}{a^2} \right] \tag{5.3}$$

For short times, Eq. 5.3 can be simplified to

$$\frac{M_t}{M_\infty} = 6\left[\frac{Dt}{\pi a^2} \right]^{\frac{1}{2}} - 3\frac{Dt}{a^2} \tag{5.4}$$

Modeling using non-sink conditions can also be very useful. If the drug delivery is to be in an area where drug may accumulate, such as PNPs meant to be delivered to a tumor site, Fick's second law can be used to derive numerous variations by simply changing the boundary conditions. Historically, the Higuchi equation, originally derived for a slab geometry and simplified in Eq. 5.5, has been the modeling workhorse of diffusive drug delivery [187], showing diffusion following Fick's second law for the first 60% of release. M_t/M_∞ is the mass fraction of the drug released at time t from the total amount contained at $t = 0$, and K is a constant which depends on each system. Over the years, this equation has been the basis for many other equations that take into account other geometries and has been derived from a simple pseudo-steady-state diffusion model. Eq. 5.6, typically called *the power law*, further expands the Higuchi equation into describing the mechanism of drug release by combining diffusive effects with $t^{1/2}$ and relaxation with t^1, as seen in Eq. 5.7. This equation superimposes both relaxation/swelling-based transport and pure Fickian diffusion by allowing alteration of the power n, and again can be used to describe the first 60% of release.

$$\frac{M_t}{M_\infty} = Kt^{1/2} \tag{5.5}$$

$$\frac{M_t}{M_\infty} = Kt^n \tag{5.6}$$

$$\frac{M_t}{M_\infty} = K_1 t^{1/2} + K_2 t \tag{5.7}$$

However, the power values of 0.5 and 1 are useful only for slab geometry, and power values have been derived for systems with other geometries [188]. Concerning spherical geometry, when the exponent n is equal to 0.43, the release mechanism is Fickian diffusion. An exponent between 0.43 and 0.85 is described as transport utilizing both Fickian and case-II swelling, and an exponent of 0.85 is defined as purely case-II relaxation transport. Trivially, a power value of 0 would give no release and 1 would give zero-order release, independent of time.

While the power law is useful for quick characterization, there are some drawbacks in the assumptions made: the particle size distribution must be narrow, sink conditions must always be attained, diffusion must only occur in one direction, edge effects must not exist, the diffusivity of drug must remain constant, the polymer carrier must not dissolve, and the drug must be suspended such that it is much smaller than the thickness of the system [187]. Considering drug delivery applications, sink conditions occur when the drug is released into an area where the limiting condition is the rate of diffusion of the drug from the PNPs, and diffusion of the drug into the surroundings is fast. If the drug is released into an area where local concentration buildup occurs, this model will not fit. If the particle size distribution is tight, setting up an easy experiment with sink conditions is very simple. An example experiment would be to put the PNPs into a dialysis bag, and that bag into a large volume of drug release medium. Then, by calculating the drug release from the particles, the initial and final mass of drug release is known, and parameters K and n can be obtained by fitting the data to a plot.

Nanoparticles can release drugs following several different routes. Possible routes of release include diffusion and degradation of the polymer chains. Diffusion of the drug can occur from the surface, through an expanded polymer matrix, through the wall of a nanocapsule, or through a combination of these processes. Degradation can occur as a result of hydrolysis of bonds, which may increase the mesh size in nanogels or lead to the dissolution of nanospheres, nanocapsules, dendrimers, or micelles.

A common equation used in modeling drug release from nanoparticles is Eq. 5.8.

$$C_{\text{drug}}(t) = Ae^{-\alpha t} + Be^{-\beta t} \tag{5.8}$$

This equation is a biexponential function which describes at time t the concentration of drug in a nanoparticle. A is a diffusion constant, B is a degradation constant, and α and β are rate constants. When it comes to more rigorous modeling, there are a variety of different methods to simulate PNPs, and these methods can be categorized by their end goal. If one is interested in interaction at the molecular level, a macroscale approach will not be as useful as molecular dynamics or Monte Carlo simulations. Molecular dynamics and Monte Carlo simulations rely on molecular interactions, thermodynamics, and kinetics to carry out the simulation. Microscale methods can include Brownian dynamics modeling or dissipative particle dynamics [189]. While molecular dynamics simulations can be more intricate in the modeling of PNPs, there is a large downside in that it usually requires intensive and extensive computation.

Related to drug release, pharmacokinetics, as given in more detail in Chapter 1, can be described through the use of compartmental modeling. Briefly, each compartment describes a biological transport barrier or container, such as the circulatory system, different organs, RES, or cellular barriers. The end goal is to be able to determine concentration at any time in any compartment. The simplest compartmental model is a single-compartment model that describes first-order elimination of a drug following a single bolus injection (Eq. 5.9). For instance, if drug loaded PNPs are injected intravenously and have a single, constant clearance mechanism without any other interaction with any parts of the body, this can be modeled as a single compartment. Solving Eq. 5.9 for the initial condition yields Eq. 5.10, where k_{out} is the elimination rate constant. The constants can be determined through physiologically relevant studies.

$$\frac{dC}{dt} = -k_{out} * C(t) \quad C(0) = C_0 \tag{5.9}$$

$$C(t) = C_0 e^{-k_{out}t} \tag{5.10}$$

Each compartment, in addition to the first, can be organized in the manner necessary to describe the prescribed conditions. Where a single compartment may only utilize simple input and output, a two-compartment model can show equilibrium effects where the drug may be transiently contained. For instance, Fig. 5.10 describes this concept as a block diagram. By utilizing a form of the base Eq. 5.9, the necessary equations can be derived from a mass balance of inputs and outputs, where Q_{in} and Q_{out} represent the volumetric flow rates in and out of the system, V is system volume, and the rate constants are k.

$$V_1 \frac{\partial C_1}{\partial t} = Q_{in} C_0 + k_{21} C_2 V_2 - k_{12} C_1 V_1 - Q_{out} C_1 \tag{5.11}$$

$$V_2 \frac{\partial C_2}{\partial t} = k_{12} C_1 V_1 - k_{21} C_2 V_2 \tag{5.12}$$

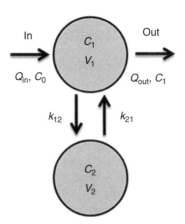

Figure 5.10. Two-compartment model showing equilibrium with a second compartment corresponding to Eq. 5.11 and 5.12.

A simple practical example of Fig. 5.9 is when compartment #1 is the blood space and compartment #2 is tissue space of a particular organ. Blood flows through the organ, and there is local buildup in the tissue space of the organ. This is a simple model, but compartments to represent additional organs or drug depots can be added to increase model accuracy; however, determining appropriate parameters for more complicated models can be challenging.

5.6 MAJOR CLINICAL ACHIEVEMENTS

While there are numerous PNP products in development [143] and several currently in the clinical trial phase [88, 143], there is currently only one PNP approved for use in the US market, Abraxane® for paclitaxel delivery [83]. Interestingly, the story of Abraxane provides an excellent illustration of the advantages to PNP systems. Paclitaxel is a highly hydrophobic anticancer agent that is difficult to deliver in therapeutically relevant doses without some mechanism to increase solubility. Prior to Abraxane, the most common formulation to achieve this was based upon a non-ionic surfactant, Cremophore EL®, and ethanol mix (marketed as Taxol). This mixture is considered to be a predecessor to PNP as, upon injection, Cremophore EL forms a micelle which aides in dispersing and solubilizing paclitaxel [88]. Unfortunately, Cremophore EL has significant side effects, including neuropathy and hypersensitivity. Furthermore, the cremophore micelle has a much higher clearance rate compared to free paclitaxel, which requires more drug to be injected to be effective [88, 190]. In 2005, Abraxis Bioscience (acquired by Celgene in 2010) received approval to market Abraxane in the United States. Abraxane is a 130 nm nanoparticle composed of albumin-bound paclitaxel. Albumin is a long circulating serum protein that is a natural carrier of vitamins and many other different hydrophobic molecules. As such, it was hypothesized that particles composed of albumin would both enhance paclitaxel solubilization and provide improved circulation times. However, it was also found that albumin aides in the transcytosis of the substance it is carrying into endothelial cells by forming caveolae [191]. This effect, in addition to the improved pharmacokinetics with reduced side effects, is a classic example of how PNPs can be designed to improve drug therapy.

Outside the United States, another PNP delivery system has been approved for paclitaxel delivery. Conceptually, a more straightforward approach is to create a micelle system that is less toxic, more stable, and has a longer circulation half-life than Cremophore EL. Genexol-PM® uses a diblock copolymer of poly(ethylene glycol)-*co*-poly(lactic acid) (PEG-PLA), which fulfills many of these requirement, and has already received approval in 2007 for breast cancer treatment in Korea. It is currently being evaluated for use in the United States (Fig. 5.11).

PEG, a hydrophilic nonionic polymer, has excellent anti-adhesive properties, which permits evasion of the MPS, the cell system responsible for the clearance of large particles from circulation. Poly(DL-lactic acid) is a biodegradable hydrophobic polymer. The diblock copolymer of these polymers results in a micelle system that is more stable, and contains a hydrophilic shell that imparts a longer circulation half-life

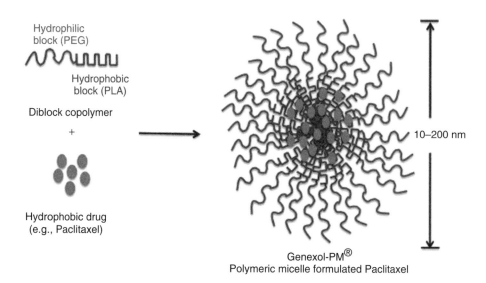

Hydrophilic
block (PEG)

Hydrophobic
block (PLA)

Diblock copolymer

+

Hydrophobic drug
(e.g., Paclitaxel)

10–200 nm

Genexol-PM®
Polymeric micelle formulated Paclitaxel

Figure 5.11. Schematic description of paclitaxel-loaded Genexol-PM®.

compared to other nanoparticle systems. In fact, this longer circulation time resulted in an increase in tumor accumulation due to the EPR effect [88].

5.7 KEY POINTS

- *Importance of PNPs in nanomedicine.* PNPs can increase the effectiveness of a number of functions and properties related to drug delivery. For example, the bioavailability of bioactive molecules and drugs can be enhanced through improved solubility, immunogenic masking, and increased retention time in the systemic circulation. Nanomedicine has profited greatly because of these effects and many exciting applications are arising.

- *Differences in PNP configuration.* While there are several different types of PNPs that can be formed, each configuration has its strengths and weaknesses. Depending on the application required, different configurations may be more or less useful because of their innate properties.

- *Passive targeting.* Targeting of PNPs using passive methods is a common practice and has shown promise toward applications such as anticancer therapies because of a combination of the EPR effect and lowered pH within tumor tissue.

- *Active targeting.* Active targeting can be used in conjunction with passive targeting to enhance therapeutic effects. Adding a targeting molecule to the surface of a nanosphere to select certain cells or tissues can decrease systemic toxicity as a result of less nonspecific binding and higher concentrations of the drug–drug carrier at the target site.

- *Characterization.* Effective PNP characterization involves determination of size, shape, drug loading, and surface charge. This characterization should be made frequently throughout development of a PNP.
- *Biodistribution.* Size, surface charge, surface functionalities, and other properties affect biodistribution of PNPs in the body following administration. Biodistribution and therapy can be combined by using theranostic PNPs which can both sense a target for drug delivery and facilitate visualization of the tissue through noninvasive, molecular imaging techniques.
- *Biocompatibility.* The criteria for biocompatibility require nanoparticle systems be nontoxic, nonimmunogenic, noninflammatory, nonteratogenic, nonthrombogenic, biodegradable, and soluble.

5.8 WORKED EXAMPLE

Floyd Gasleaks is trying to determine what time to take his second, in a series of two, gastrointestinal-medication injections and has asked you for help. The new medication he is using, Vasilyl®, is self-administered intravenously in a bolus injection and consists of drug loaded, actively targeted polymeric nanospheres. Assuming that all the PNPs administered immediately hit their target at once, 90% of the loaded drug remains in the targeted tissue because of endocytosis of the PNPs, while 10% promptly reenters the blood stream as a result of quick diffusive-release effects. $AA = 1$ mg ml^{-1}, $\alpha = 0.1$ s^{-1}, total mass of drug in PNPs $= 100$ mg, systemic volume $= 6$ l, injection volume is 5 ml, $k_{out} = 0.01$ s^{-1}.

1. Determine the time it takes to release the 10% of drug released assuming Eq. 5.8 applies.
2. You know from experience that Floyd should administer another injection when four half-lives of free drug in system have been used up, as that is when the amount of drug locally administered starts to fall below the therapeutic level. If Floyd took his first injection at 8 AM on Monday, determine when Floyd should take his next injection. Use Eq. 5.10.

Solution

1. As drug release is via diffusive effects only, Eq. 5.8 simplifies to

$$C_{drug} = Ae^{-\alpha t}$$

Taking the natural log of both sides and rearranging the equation to explicitly solve for time yields

$$t = \frac{\ln \dfrac{A}{C_{drug}}}{\alpha}$$

10% of drug is 0.1×1 mg $= 0.1$ mg.

Solve for the drug concentration using data given:

$$C_{drug} = \frac{100 \text{ mg}}{6000 \text{ ml}} = 1.7 \times 10^{-2} \text{ mg/ml}$$

Solve for the time:

$$t = \frac{\ln \dfrac{1.0 \text{ mg/ml}}{1.7 \times 10^{-2} \text{ mg/ml}}}{0.1 \dfrac{1}{s}} = 41 \text{ s}$$

2. Four half-lives of the drug is when $100 \text{ mg}/2^4 = 6.25$ mg is remaining. The final concentration would then be $6.25 \text{ mg}/6000 \text{ ml} = 1.0 \times 10^{-3}$ mg/ml. Using Eq. 5.10, take the natural log of both sides and solve explicitly for time; then plug in to solve

$$t = \frac{\ln \dfrac{C_0}{C}}{k_{out}} = \frac{\ln 1.7 \times 10^{-2} \dfrac{\text{mg}}{\text{ml}} / 1.0 \times 10^{-3} \dfrac{\text{mg}}{\text{ml}}}{4 \times 10^{-4} \dfrac{1}{s}} = 42500 \text{ s} = 12 \text{ h}$$

So Floyd should take his next injection at 4 PM on the same day.

5.9 HOMEWORK PROBLEMS

1. State some advantages and disadvantages of using nanospheres, nanocapsules, micelles, and dendrimers.

2. What are the pros and cons of active and passive targeting?

3. State some applications for formulating folate-labeled nanospheres.

4. What is the difference between biodistribution and bioavailability?

5. Following up with the example problem,

   a. Describe where and how the PNPs will travel and ways the drug may be delivered just after IV delivery.

   b. What compartments would you use if you were to design a better compartmental model of the IV drug delivery process?

6. Polymeric nanospheres were added to a solvent to induce drug release, and a total of 5 mg of drug in 1 l of PBS was measured to be released, to a known 60% completion. During synthesis of the same number of nanospheres released, 5 ml of 10 mg ml^{-1} of drug was added. What is the encapsulation efficiency?

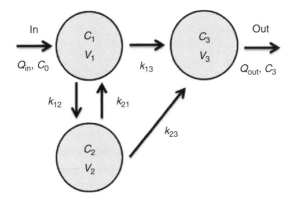

Figure 5.12. Compartment model for homework problem 9A.

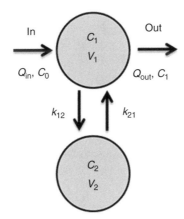

Figure 5.13. Compartment model for homework problem 9B.

7. Determine how much radioactive catalase is to be added to polymeric nanogels during synthesis to produce gamma counts of at least 1000 until release is 95% complete for ^{125}I labeled catalase with initial counts of 200,000 counts per μg and free iodine in solution of 10%. Encapsulation efficiency is 10%, nanogels are 150 nm with a tight distribution, and half-life of ^{125}I is 59.4 days. Assume release can be characterized by Eq. 5.8. $A = 1$ mg ml^{-1}, $\alpha = 1$ h^{-1}, $B = 2$ mg ml^{-1}, $\beta = 0.06$ h^{-1}.

8. Determine constants A, B, α, and β from the following release data of polymeric nanospheres loaded with 1.5 mg drug into 1 ml of PBS. Is release diffusion-based or degradation-based? Use Eq. 5.8.

Time (h)	0.00	0.5	2	12	24	48	72	144	216	288
M_t/M_∞	0.00	0.13	0.30	0.41	0.48	0.59	0.68	0.84	0.92	0.96

9. a. Based upon the compartmental diagram below, write the corresponding set of partial differential equations.

   b. Once again, write the set of equations for the figure below, but this time solve them for C_1 and C_2 assuming that compartment #2 contains a depot of drug and that K_{12} and $C_0 = 0$.

REFERENCES

1. Park JH et al. Polymeric nanomedicine for cancer therapy. Prog Polym Sci 2008; 33(1):113–137.
2. Sahoo SK, Labhasetwar V. Nanotech approaches to delivery and imaging drug. Drug Discov Today 2003;8(24):1112–1120.
3. Vinogradov SV, Bronich TK, Kabanov AV. Nanosized cationic hydrogels for drug delivery: preparation, properties and interactions with cells. Adv Drug Deliv Rev 2002;54(1):135–147.
4. Zhang XX, Eden HS, Chen X. Peptides in cancer nanomedicine: drug carriers, targeting ligands and protease substrates. J Control Release 2011.
5. Kumari A, Yadav SK, Yadav SC. Biodegradable polymeric nanoparticles based drug delivery systems. Colloids Surf, B 2010;75(1):1–18.
6. Dziubla TD, Karim A, Muzykantov VR. Polymer nanocarriers protecting active enzyme cargo against proteolysis. J Control Release 2005;102(2):427–439.
7. Sutton D et al. Functionalized micellar systems for cancer targeted drug delivery. Pharm Res 2007;24(6):1029–1046.
8. Tang R et al. Block copolymer micelles with acid-labile ortho ester side-chains: synthesis, characterization, and enhanced drug delivery to human glioma cells. J Control Release 2011;151(1):18–27.
9. Felber AE, Dufresne MH, Leroux JC. pH-sensitive vesicles, polymeric micelles, and nanospheres prepared with polycarboxylates. Adv Drug Deliv Rev 2012;64(11):979–992.
10. Wadajkar AS et al. Cytotoxic evaluation of N-isopropylacrylamide monomers and temperature-sensitive poly(N-isopropylacrylamide) nanoparticles. J Nanopart Res 2009; 11(6):1375–1382.
11. Urbina MC et al. Investigation of magnetic nanoparticle-polymer composites for multiple-controlled drug delivery. J Phys Chem C 2008;112(30):11102–11108.
12. Chen W et al. Synthesis of PMMA and PMMA/PS nanoparticles by microemulsion polymerization with a new vapor monomer feeding system. Colloids Surf., A 2010;364(1–3):145–150.
13. Monasterolo C et al. Sulfonates-PMMA nanoparticles conjugates: a versatile system for multimodal application. Bioorg Med Chem 2012;20(22):6640–6647.
14. Mohomed K et al. Persistent interactions between hydroxylated nanoballs and atactic poly(2-hydroxyethyl methacrylate) (PHEMA). Chem Commun 2005;26:3277–3279.
15. Oh JK et al. Preparation of nanoparticles of double-hydrophilic PEO-PHEMA block copolymers by AGET ATRP in inverse miniemulsion. J Polym Sci A Polym Chem 2007;45(21):4764–4772.
16. Calvo P et al. Long-circulating PEGylated polycyanoacrylate nanoparticles as new drug carrier for brain delivery. Pharm Res 2001;18(8):1157–1166.

17. Reddy LH, Murthy RR. Influence of polymerization technique and experimental variables on the particle properties and release kinetics of methotrexate from poly(butylcyanoacrylate) nanoparticles. Acta Pharm 2004;54(2):103–118.

18. Huang CY, Chen CM, Lee YD. Synthesis of high loading and encapsulation efficient paclitaxel-loaded poly(n-butyl cyanoacrylate) nanoparticles via miniemulsion. Int J Pharm 2007;338(1–2):267–275.

19. O'Hagan DT, Palin KJ, Davis SS. Poly(butyl-2-cyanoacrylate) particles as adjuvants for oral immunization. Vaccine 1989;7(3):213–216.

20. de Verdiere AC et al. Reversion of multidrug resistance with polyalkylcyanoacrylate nanoparticles: towards a mechanism of action. Br J Cancer 1997;76(2):198–205.

21. Vauthier C et al. Drug delivery to resistant tumors: the potential of poly(alkyl cyanoacrylate) nanoparticles. J Control Release 2003;93(2):151–160.

22. Sadekar S, Ghandehari H. Transepithelial transport and toxicity of PAMAM dendrimers: implications for oral drug delivery. Adv Drug Deliv Rev 2012;64(6):571–588.

23. Mukherjee SP, Davoren M, Byrne HJ. In vitro mammalian cytotoxicological study of PAMAM dendrimers - towards quantitative structure activity relationships. Toxicol In Vitro 2010;24(1):169–177.

24. Liu Y et al. PAMAM dendrimers undergo pH responsive conformational changes without swelling. J Am Chem Soc 2009;131(8):2798–2799.

25. Liu M, Frechet JM. Designing dendrimers for drug delivery. Pharm Sci Technolo Today 1999;2(10):393–401.

26. Srinivas U et al. The Properties of Dendritic Polymers II: Generation Dependence of the Physical Properties of Poly(amidoamine) Dendrimers. ARL-TR-1774 ed. Army Research Laboratory; 1999.

27. Feldstein MM et al. Relation of glass transition temperature to the hydrogen bonding degree and energy in poly(N-vinyl pyrrolidone) blends with hydroxyl-containing plasticizers: 3. Analysis of two glass transition temperatures featured for PVP solutions in liquid poly(ethylene glycol). Polymer 2003;44(6):1819–1834.

28. Bharali DJ et al. Cross-linked polyvinylpyrrolidone nanoparticles: a potential carrier for hydrophilic drugs. J Colloid Interface Sci 2003;258(2):415–423.

29. Lee WC, Chu IM. Preparation and degradation behavior of polyanhydrides nanoparticles. J Biomed Mater Res B Appl Biomater 2008;84B(1):138–146.

30. Pfeifer BA, Burdick JA, Langer R. Formulation and surface modification of poly(ester-anhydride) micro- and nanospheres. Biomaterials 2005;26(2):117–124.

31. Wattamwar PP et al. Synthesis and characterization of poly(antioxidant beta-amino esters) for controlled release of polyphenolic antioxidants. Acta Biomater 2012;8(7):2529–2537.

32. Ko J et al. Tumoral acidic extracellular pH targeting of pH-responsive MPEG-poly (beta-amino ester) block copolymer micelles for cancer therapy. J Control Release 2007;123(2):109–115.

33. Gao GH et al. pH-responsive polymeric micelle based on PEG-poly(beta-amino ester)/(amido amine) as intelligent vehicle for magnetic resonance imaging in detection of cerebral ischemic area. J Control Release 2011;155(1):11–17.

34. Shen Y et al. Degradable poly(beta-amino ester) nanoparticles for cancer cytoplasmic drug delivery. Nanomedicine 2009;5(2):192–201.

35. Min KH et al. Tumoral acidic pH-responsive MPEG-poly(beta-amino ester) polymeric micelles for cancer targeting therapy. J Control Release 2010;144(2):259–266.

36. Beck-Broichsitter M et al. Development of a biodegradable nanoparticle platform for sildenafil: formulation optimization by factorial design analysis combined with application of charge-modified branched polyesters. J Control Release 2012;157(3):469–477.

37. Zheng X et al. Preparation of MPEG-PLA nanoparticle for honokiol delivery in vitro. Int J Pharm 2010;386(1–2):262–267.

38. Gaucher G, Marchessault RH, Leroux JC. Polyester-based micelles and nanoparticles for the parenteral delivery of taxanes. J Control Release 2010;143(1):2–12.

39. Coffin MD, Mcginity JW. Biodegradable pseudolatexes - the chemical-stability of poly(D,L-lactide) and poly (epsilon-caprolactone) nanoparticles in aqueous-media. Pharm Res 1992;9(2):200–205.

40. Lemoine D et al. Stability study of nanoparticles of poly(epsilon-caprolactone), poly(D,L-lactide) and poly(D,L-lactide-co-glycolide). Biomaterials 1996;17(22):2191–2197.

41. Musumeci T et al. PLA/PLGA nanoparticles for sustained release of docetaxel. Int J Pharm 2006;325(1–2):172–179.

42. Mittal G et al. Estradiol loaded PLGA nanoparticles for oral administration: effect of polymer molecular weight and copolymer composition on release behavior in vitro and in vivo. J Control Release 2007;119(1):77–85.

43. Mittal A et al. Cytomodulin-functionalized porous PLGA particulate scaffolds respond better to cell migration, actin production and wound healing in rodent model. J Tissue Eng Regen Med 2012.

44. Fonseca C, Simoes S, Gaspar R. Paclitaxel-loaded PLGA nanoparticles: preparation, physicochemical characterization and in vitro anti-tumoral activity. J Control Release 2002;83(2):273–286.

45. Teixeira M et al. Development and characterization of PLGA nanospheres and nanocapsules containing xanthone and 3-methoxyxanthone. Eur J Pharm Biopharm 2005;59(3):491–500.

46. Hans ML, Lowman AM. Biodegradable nanoparticles for drug delivery and targeting. Curr Opin Solid State Mater Sci 2002;6(4):319–327.

47. Saez A et al. Freeze-drying of polycaprolactone and poly(D,L-lactic-glycolic) nanoparticles induce minor particle size changes affecting the oral pharmacokinetics of loaded drugs. Eur J Pharm Biopharm 2000;50(3):379–387.

48. Barakat NAM et al. Biologically active polycaprolactone/titanium hybrid electrospun nanofibers for hard tissue engineering. Sci Adv Mater 2011;3(5):730–734.

49. Otsuka H, Nagasaki Y, Kataoka K. PEGylated nanoparticles for biological and pharmaceutical applications. Adv Drug Deliv Rev 2003;55(3):403–419.

50. Cheng J et al. Formulation of functionalized PLGA-PEG nanoparticles for in vivo targeted drug delivery. Biomaterials 2007;28(5):869–876.

51. Li YP et al. PEGylated PLGA nanoparticles as protein carriers: synthesis, preparation and biodistribution in rats. J Control Release 2001;71(2):203–211.

52. Ahmed F, Discher DE. Self-porating polymersomes of PEG-PLA and PEG-PCL: hydrolysis-triggered controlled release vesicles. J Control Release 2004;96(1):37–53.

53. Vinogradov S, Batrakova E, Kabanov A. Poly(ethylene glycol)-polyethyleneimine NanoGel (TM) particles: novel drug delivery systems for antisense oligonucleotides. Colloids Surf, B 1999;16(1–4):291–304.

54. Bivas-Benita M et al. PLGA-PEI nanoparticles for gene delivery to pulmonary epithelium. Eur J Pharm Biopharm 2004;58(1):1–6.

55. Lunov O et al. Differential uptake of functionalized polystyrene nanoparticles by human macrophages and a monocytic cell line. Acs Nano 2011;5(3):1657–1669.

56. Paik P, Kar KK. Glass transition temperature of high molecular weight polystyrene: effect of particle size, bulk to micron to nano. NSTI-Nanotech 2006;1.

57. Acharya S, Sahoo SK. PLGA nanoparticles containing various anticancer agents and tumour delivery by EPR effect. Adv Drug Deliv Rev 2011;63(3):170–183.

58. Kean T, Thanou M. Biodegradation, biodistribution and toxicity of chitosan. Adv Drug Deliv Rev 2010;62(1):3–11.

59. Agnihotri SA, Mallikarjuna NN, Aminabhavi TM. Recent advances on chitosan-based micro- and nanoparticles in drug delivery. J Control Release 2004;100(1):5–28.

60. Mundargi RC et al. Nano/micro technologies for delivering macromolecular therapeutics using poly(D,L-lactide-co-glycolide) and its derivatives. J Control Release 2008;125(3):193–209.

61. Panyam J, Labhasetwar V. Biodegradable nanoparticles for drug and gene delivery to cells and tissue. Adv Drug Deliv Rev 2003;55(3):329–347.

62. Vasilakes, A.L., et al., Controlled release of catalase and vancomycin from poly(β-amino ester) hydrogels. Submitted.

63. Anderson DG et al. Structure/property studies of polymeric gene delivery using a library of poly(beta-amino esters). Mol Ther 2005;11(3):426–434.

64. Lu DN et al. Dextran-grafted-PNIPAAm as an artificial chaperone for protein refolding. Biochem Eng J 2006;27(3):336–343.

65. Jiang WW et al. Phagocyte responses to degradable polymers. J Biomed Mater Res A 2007;82A(2):492–497.

66. Fu K et al. Visual evidence of acidic environment within degrading poly(lactic-co-glycolic acid) (PLGA) microspheres. Pharm Res 2000;17(1):100–106.

67. Bat E et al. In vivo behavior of trimethylene carbonate and epsilon-caprolactone-based (co)polymer networks: degradation and tissue response. J Biomed Mater Res A 2010; 95A(3):940–949.

68. Udipi K et al. Modification of inflammatory response to implanted biomedical materials in vivo by surface bound superoxide dismutase mimics. J Biomed Mater Res 2000;51(4):549–560.

69. Fleming C et al. A carbohydrate-antioxidant hybrid polymer reduces oxidative damage in spermatozoa and enhances fertility. Nat Chem Biol 2005;1(5):270–274.

70. Spizzirri UG et al. Synthesis of antioxidant polymers by grafting of gallic acid and catechin on gelatin. Biomacromolecules 2009;10(7):1923–1930.

71. Wang YZ et al. Expansion and osteogenic differentiation of bone marrow-derived mesenchymal stem cells on a vitamin C functionalized polymer. Biomaterials 2006; 27(17):3265–3273.

72. Williams SR et al. Synthesis and characterization of poly(ethylene glycol)-glutathione conjugate self-assembled nanoparticles for antioxidant delivery. Biomacromolecules 2009;10(1):155–161.

73. Whitaker-Brothers K, Uhrich K. Investigation into the erosion mechanism of salicylate-based poly(anhydride-esters). J Biomed Mater Res A 2006;76A(3):470–479.

74. Wattamwar PP et al. Antioxidant activity of degradable polymer poly(trolox ester) to suppress oxidative stress injury in the cells. Adv Funct Mater 2010;20(1):147–154.

75. Wattamwar PP et al. Tuning of the pro-oxidant and antioxidant activity of trolox through the controlled release from biodegradable poly(trolox ester) polymers. J Biomed Mater Res A 2011;99A(2):184–191.

76. Albanese A, Tang PS, Chan WC. The effect of nanoparticle size, shape, and surface chemistry on biological systems. Annu Rev Biomed Eng 2012;14:1–16.

77. Storm G et al. Surface modification of nanoparticles to oppose uptake by the mononuclear phagocyte system. Adv Drug Deliv Rev 1995;17(1):31–48.

78. Guo JW et al. Aptamer-functionalized PEG-PLGA nanoparticles for enhanced anti-glioma drug delivery. Biomaterials 2011;32(31):8010–8020.

79. Veronese FM, Pasut G. PEGylation, successful approach to drug delivery. Drug Discov Today 2005;10(21):1451–1458.

80. Parveen S, Sahoo SK. Long circulating chitosan/PEG blended PLGA nanoparticle for tumor drug delivery. Eur J Pharmacol 2011;670(2–3):372–383.

81. Gref R et al. 'Stealth' corona-core nanoparticles surface modified by polyethylene glycol (PEG): influences of the corona (PEG chain length and surface density) and of the core composition on phagocytic uptake and plasma protein adsorption. Colloids Surf, B 2000;18(3–4):301–313.

82. Bader RA, Silvers AL, Zhang N. Polysialic acid-based micelles for encapsulation of hydrophobic drugs. Biomacromolecules 2011;12(2):314–320.

83. Faraji AH, Wipf P. Nanoparticles in cellular drug delivery. Bioorg Med Chem 2009;17(8):2950–2962.

84. Simone EA, Dziubla TD, Muzykantov VR. Polymeric carriers: role of geometry in drug delivery. Expert Opin Drug Deliv 2008;5(12):1283–1300.

85. Sharma G et al. Polymer particle shape independently influences binding and internalization by macrophages. J Control Release 2010;147(3):408–412.

86. Geng Y et al. Shape effects of filaments versus spherical particles in flow and drug delivery. Nat Nanotechnol 2007;2(4):249–255.

87. Beningo KA, Wang YL. Fc-receptor-mediated phagocytosis is regulated by mechanical properties of the target. J Cell Sci 2002;115(4):849–856.

88. Kim TY et al. Phase I and pharmacokinetic study of Genexol-PM, a cremophor-free, polymeric micelle-formulated paclitaxel, in patients with advanced malignancies. Clin Cancer Res 2004;10(11):3708–3716.

89. Kim SC et al. In vivo evaluation of polymeric micellar paclitaxel formulation: toxicity and efficacy. J Control Release 2001;72(1–3):191–202.

90. Poon Z et al. Highly stable, ligand-clustered "patchy" micelle nanocarriers for systemic tumor targeting. Nanomedicine 2011;7(2):201–209.

91. Nakanishi T et al. Development of the polymer micelle carrier system for doxorubicin. J Control Release 2001;74(1–3):295–302.

92. Matsumura Y et al. Phase I clinical trial and pharmacokinetic evaluation of NK911, a micelle-encapsulated doxorubicin. Br J Cancer 2004;91(10):1775–1781.

93. Photos PJ et al. Polymer vesicles in vivo: correlations with PEG molecular weight. J Control Release 2003;90(3):323–334.

94. Nassar T et al. High plasma levels and effective lymphatic uptake of docetaxel in an orally available nanotransporter formulation. Cancer Res 2011;71(8):3018–3028.

95. Nassar T et al. Novel double coated nanocapsules for intestinal delivery and enhanced oral bioavailability of tacrolimus, a P-gp substrate drug. J Control Release 2009;133(1):77–84.

96. Sheng Y et al. Long-circulating polymeric nanoparticles bearing a combinatorial coating of PEG and water-soluble chitosan. Biomaterials 2009;30(12):2340–2348.

97. Shimoda A et al. Dual crosslinked hydrogel nanoparticles by nanogel bottom-up method for sustained-release delivery. Colloids Surf, B 2012;99:18–44.

98. Hasegawa U et al. Raspberry-like assembly of cross-linked nanogels for protein delivery. J Control Release 2009;140(3):312–317.

99. De Jesus OLP et al. Polyester dendritic systems for drug delivery applications: in vitro and in vivo evaluation. Bioconjug Chem 2002;13(3):453–461.

100. Ihre HR et al. Polyester dendritic systems for drug delivery applications: design, synthesis, and characterization. Bioconjug Chem 2002;13(3):443–452.

101. Gratton SEA et al. Nanofabricated particles for engineered drug therapies: a preliminary biodistribution study of PRINT (TM) nanoparticles. J Control Release 2007;121(1–2): 10–18.

102. Parveen S, Misra R, Sahoo SK. Nanoparticles: a boon to drug delivery, therapeutics, diagnostics and imaging. Nanomedicine 2012;8(2):147–166.

103. Lee JY et al. Intracellular delivery of paclitaxel using oil-free, shell cross-linked HSA - multi-armed PEG nanocapsules. Biomaterials 2011;32(33):8635–8644.

104. Rawat M et al. Nanocarriers: promising vehicle for bioactive drugs. Biol Pharm Bull 2006;29(9):1790–1798.

105. Lai SK, Wang YY, Hanes J. Mucus-penetrating nanoparticles for drug and gene delivery to mucosal tissues. Adv Drug Deliv Rev 2009;61(2):158–171.

106. Beck-Broichsitter M, Merkel OM, Kissel T. Controlled pulmonary drug and gene delivery using polymeric nano-carriers. J Control Release 2012;161(2):214–224.

107. Zhang W et al. The potential of Pluronic polymeric micelles encapsulated with paclitaxel for the treatment of melanoma using subcutaneous and pulmonary metastatic mice models. Biomaterials 2011;32(25):5934–5944.

108. Yoo HS, Lee EA, Park TG. Doxorubicin-conjugated biodegradable polymeric micelles having acid-cleavable linkages. J Control Release 2002;82(1):17–27.

109. Singh R, Lillard JW Jr. Nanoparticle-based targeted drug delivery. Exp Mol Pathol 2009;86(3):215–223.

110. Discher BM et al. Polymersomes: tough vesicles made from diblock copolymers. Science 1999;284(5417):1143–1146.

111. Discher DE, Eisenberg A. Polymer vesicles. Science 2002;297(5583):967–973.

112. Christian DA et al. Polymersome carriers: from self-assembly to siRNA and protein therapeutics. Eur J Pharm Biopharm 2009;71(3):463–474.

113. Ahmed F et al. Biodegradable polymersomes loaded with both paclitaxel and doxorubicin permeate and shrink tumors, inducing apoptosis in proportion to accumulated drug. J Control Release 2006;116(2):150–158.

114. Li SL et al. Self-assembled poly(butadiene)-b-poly(ethylene oxide) polymersomes as paclitaxel carriers. Biotechnol Prog 2007;23(1):278–285.

115. Levine DH et al. Polymersomes: a new multi-functional tool for cancer diagnosis and therapy. Methods 2008;46(1):25–32.

116. Bajpai AK et al. Responsive polymers in controlled drug delivery. Prog Polym Sci 2008;33(11):1088–1118.

117. Morimoto N et al. Hybrid nanogels with physical and chemical cross-linking structures as nanocarriers. Macromol Biosci 2005;5(8):710–716.

118. Shah PP et al. Skin permeating nanogel for the cutaneous co-delivery of two anti-inflammatory drugs. Biomaterials 2012;33(5):1607–1617.

119. Nagahama K, Ouchi T, Ohya Y. Biodegradable nanogels prepared by self-assembly of poly(L-lactide)-grafted dextran: entrapment and release of proteins. Macromol Biosci 2008;8(11):1044–1052.

120. Shidhaye S et al. Nanogel engineered polymeric micelles for drug delivery. Curr Drug Ther 2008;3:209–217.

121. Lee ES et al. A virus-mimetic nanogel vehicle. Angew Chem Int Ed 2008;47(13): 2418–2421.

122. Kopecek J. Polymer chemistry - swell gels. Nature 2002;417(6887):388–391.

123. Kettel MJ et al. Aqueous nanogels modified with cyclodextrin. Polymer 2011; 52(9):1917–1924.

124. Shen W et al. Thermosensitive, biocompatible and antifouling nanogels prepared via aqueous raft dispersion polymerization for targeted drug delivery. J Control Release 2011;152(Suppl 1):e75–e76.

125. Zhang LF, Eisenberg A. Multiple morphologies and characteristics of "crew-cut" micelle-like aggregates of polystyrene-b-poly(acrylic acid) diblock copolymers in aqueous solutions. J Am Chem Soc 1996;118(13):3168–3181.

126. Spataro G et al. Designing dendrimers for ocular drug delivery. Eur J Med Chem 2010;45(1):326–334.

127. Leo E et al. In vitro evaluation of PLA nanoparticles containing a lipophilic rug in water-soluble or insoluble form. Int J Pharm 2004;278(1):133–141.

128. Danhier F et al. Paclitaxel-loaded PEGylated PLGA-based nanoparticles: in vitro and in vivo evaluation. J Control Release 2009;133(1):11–17.

129. Danhier F et al. Targeting of tumor endothelium by RGD-grafted PLGA-nanoparticles loaded with Paclitaxel. J Control Release 2009;140(2):166–173.

130. Ringe K, Walz CM, Sabel BA. Nanoparticle Drug Delivery to the Brain. In: Encyclopedia of Nanoscience and Nanotechnology. American Scientific Publishers; 2004. p 91–104.

131. Gaucher G et al. Block copolymer micelles: preparation, characterization and application in drug delivery. J Control Release 2005;109(1–3):169–188.

132. Xiao L et al. Role of cellular uptake in the reversal of multidrug resistance by PEG-b-PLA polymeric micelles. Biomaterials 2011;32(22):5148–5157.

133. Venkatraman SS et al. Micelle-like nanoparticles of PLA-PEG-PLA triblock copolymer as chemotherapeutic carrier. Int J Pharm 2005;298(1):219–232.

134. Yoo HS, Park TG. Biodegradable polymeric micelles composed of doxorubicin conjugated PLGA-PEG block copolymer. J Control Release 2001;70(1–2):63–70.

135. Nowak AP et al. Rapidly recovering hydrogel scaffolds from self-assembling diblock copolypeptide amphiphiles. Nature 2002;417(6887):424–428.

136. Enlow EM et al. Potent engineered PLGA nanoparticles by virtue of exceptionally high chemotherapeutic loadings. Nano Lett 2011;11(2):808–813.

137. Perry JL et al. PEGylated PRINT nanoparticles: the impact of PEG density on protein binding, macrophage association, biodistribution, and pharmacokinetics. Nano Lett 2012;12(10):5304–5310.

138. Perry JL et al. PRINT: a novel platform toward shape and size specific nanoparticle theranostics. Acc Chem Res 2011;44(10):990–998.

139. Haley B, Frenkel E. Nanoparticles for drug delivery in cancer treatment. Urol Oncol-Semin Ori 2008;26(1):57–64.

140. Davis ME, Chen Z, Shin DM. Nanoparticle therapeutics: an emerging treatment modality for cancer. Nat Rev Drug Discov 2008;7(9):771–782.

141. Lammers T, Hennink WE, Storm G. Tumour-targeted nanomedicines: principles and practice. Br J Cancer 2008;99(3):392–397.

142. Lince F et al. Preparation of polymer nanoparticles loaded with doxorubicin for controlled drug delivery. Chem Eng Res Des 2011;89(11A):2410–2419.

143. Costantino L, Boraschi D. Is there a clinical future for polymeric nanoparticles as brain-targeting drug delivery agents? Drug Discov Today 2012;17(7-8):367–378.

144. Alexis F et al. Factors affecting the clearance and biodistribution of polymeric nanoparticles. Mol Pharm 2008;5(4):505–515.

145. Makhof A, Tozuka Y, Takeuchi H. pH-Sensitive nanospheres for colon-specific drug delivery in experimentally induced colitis rat model. Eur J Pharm Biopharm 2009;72(1):1–8.

146. Ganta S et al. A review of stimuli-responsive nanocarriers for drug and gene delivery. J Control Release 2008;126(3):187–204.

147. Gillies ER, Frechet JMJ. A new approach towards acid sensitive copolymer micelles for drug delivery. Chem Commun 2003;14:1640–1641.

148. Shahin M et al. Decoration of polymeric micelles with cancer-specific peptide ligands for active targeting of paclitaxel. Biomaterials 2011;32(22):5123–5133.

149. Temming K et al. RGD-based strategies for selective delivery of therapeutics and imaging agents to the tumour vasculature. Drug Resist Updat 2005;8(6):381–402.

150. Simnick AJ et al. In vivo tumor targeting by a NGR-decorated micelle of a recombinant diblock copolypeptide. J Control Release 2011;155(2):144–151.

151. Plapied L et al. Fate of polymeric nanocarriers for oral drug delivery. Curr Opin Colloid In 2011;16(3):228–237.

152. Fievez V et al. Targeting nanoparticles to M cells with non-peptidic ligands for oral vaccination. Eur J Pharm Biopharm 2009;73(1):16–24.

153. Murphy EA et al. Nanoparticle-mediated drug delivery to tumor vasculature suppresses metastasis. Proc Natl Acad Sci U S A 2008;105(27):9343–9348.

154. Aina OH et al. From combinatorial chemistry to cancer-targeting peptides. Mol Pharm 2007;4(5):631–651.

155. Petrenko V. Evolution of phage display: from bioactive peptides to bioselective nanomaterials. Expert Opin Drug Deliv 2008;5(8):825–836.

156. Yoon DJ et al. Genetically engineering transferrin to improve its in vitro ability to deliver cytotoxins. J Control Release 2009;133(3):178–184.

157. Byrne JD, Betancourt T, Brannon-Peppas L. Active targeting schemes for nanoparticle systems in cancer therapeutics. Adv Drug Deliv Rev 2008;60(15):1615–1626.

158. Xu Q et al. Anti-tumor activity of paclitaxel through dual-targeting carrier of cyclic RGD and transferrin conjugated hyperbranched copolymer nanoparticles. Biomaterials 2012;33:1627–1639.

159. Wilder RL. Integrin alpha V beta 3 as a target for treatment of rheumatoid arthritis and related rheumatic diseases. Ann Rheum Dis 2002;61:96–99.

160. Ruoslahti E, Bhatia SN, Sailor MJ. Targeting of drugs and nanoparticles to tumors. J Cell Biol 2010;188(6):759–768.

161. Tong R et al. The formulation of aptamer-coated paclitaxel-polylactide nanoconjugates and their targeting to cancer cells. Biomaterials 2010;31(11):3043–3053.

162. Hu X et al. Polymeric nanoparticle-aptamer bioconjugates can diminish the toxicity of mercury in vivo. Toxicol Lett 2012;208(1):69–74.

163. Greenleaf WJ et al. Direct observation of hierarchical folding in single riboswitch aptamers. Science 2008;319(5863):630–633.

164. Hu X et al. Polymeric nanoparticle–aptamer bioconjugates can diminish the toxicity of mercury in vivo. Toxicol Lett 2012;208:67–74.

165. Sharon J, Liebman MA, Williams BR. Recombinant polyclonal antibodies for cancer therapy. J Cell Biochem 2005;96(2):305–313.

166. Qiu XQ et al. Small antibody mimetics comprising two complementarity-determining regions and a framework region for tumor targeting. Nat Biotechnol 2007;25(8):921–929.

167. Garcia-Bennett A, Nees M, Fadeel B. In search of the holy grail: folate-targeted nanoparticles for cancer therapy. Biochem Pharmacol 2011;81(8):976–984.

168. Sudimack J, Lee RJ. Targeted drug delivery via the folate receptor. Adv Drug Deliv Rev 2000;41(2):147–162.

169. Liu G et al. Functional nanoparticles for molecular imaging guided gene delivery. Nano Today 2010;5(6):524–539.

170. Muzykantov VR et al. Endotoxin reduces specific pulmonary uptake of radiolabeled monoclonal antibody to angiotensin-converting enzyme. J Nucl Med 1991;32(3):453–460.

171. Trubetskoy VS et al. Use of N-terminal modified poly(L-lysine)-antibody conjugate as a carrier for targeted gene delivery in mouse lung endothelial cells. Bioconjug Chem 1992;3(4):323–327.

172. Iijima M, Kamiya H. Surface modification for improving the stability of nanoparticles in liquid media. Kona Powder Part J 2009;27:119–129.

173. Galperin A et al. Radiopaque iodinated polymeric nanoparticles for X-ray imaging applications. Biomaterials 2007;28(30):4461–4468.

174. Loudos G, Kagadis GC, Psimadas D. Current status and future perspectives of in vivo small animal imaging using radiolabeled nanoparticles. Eur J Radiol 2011;78(2):287–295.

175. Rutman AM, Kuo MD. Radiogenomics: creating a link between molecular diagnostics and diagnostic imaging. Eur J Radiol 2009;70(2):232–241.

176. Rai P et al. Development and applications of photo-triggered theranostic agents. Adv Drug Deliv Rev 2010;62(11):1094–1124.

177. Xie J, Lee S, Chen XY. Nanoparticle-based theranostic agents. Adv Drug Deliv Rev 2010;62(11):1064–1079.

178. Sakamoto JH et al. Enabling individualized therapy through nanotechnology. Pharmacol Res 2010;62(2):57–89.

179. MacKay JA, Li ZB. Theranostic agents that co-deliver therapeutic and imaging agents? preface. Adv Drug Deliv Rev 2010;62(11):1003–1004.

180. Fang C, Zhang MQ. Nanoparticle-based theragnostics: Integrating diagnostic and therapeutic potentials in nanomedicine. J Control Release 2010;146(1):2–5.

181. Kim K et al. Tumor-homing multifunctional nanoparticles for cancer theragnosis: Simultaneous diagnosis, drug delivery, and therapeutic monitoring. J Control Release 2010;146(2):219–227.

182. Janib SM, Moses AS, MacKay JA. Imaging and drug delivery using theranostic nanoparticles. Adv Drug Deliv Rev 2010;62(11):1052–1063.

183. Kim S et al. Cytotoxicity of, and innate immune response to, size-controlled polypyrrole nanoparticles in mammalian cells. Biomaterials 2011;32(9):2342–2350.

184. Wang PW, Henning SM, Heber D. Limitations of MTT and MTS-based assays for measurement of antiproliferative activity of green tea polyphenols. PLoS One 2010;5(4).

185. Rejinold NS et al. Curcumin-loaded biocompatible thermoresponsive polymeric nanoparticles for cancer drug delivery. J Colloid Interface Sci 2011;360(1):39–51.

186. Dobrovolskaia MA et al. Ambiguities in applying traditional limulus amebocyte lysate tests to quantify endotoxin in nanoparticle formulations. Nanomedicine 2010;5(4):555–562.

187. Siepmann J, Peppas NA. Modeling of drug release from delivery systems based on hydroxypropyl methylcellulose (HPMC). Adv Drug Deliv Rev 2001;48(2–3):139–157.

188. Peppas NA, Sahlin JJ. A simple equation for the description of solute release .3. coupling of diffusion and relaxation. Int J Pharm 1989;57(2):169–172.

189. Zeng QH, Yu AB, Lu GQ. Multiscale modeling and simulation of polymer nanocomposites. Prog Polym Sci 2008;33(2):191–269.

190. Hamaguchi T et al. A phase I and pharmacokinetic study of NK105, a paclitaxel-incorporating micellar nanoparticle formulation. Br J Cancer 2007;97(2):170–176.

191. Hawkins MJ, Soon-Shiong P, Desai N. Protein nanoparticles as drug carriers in clinical medicine. Adv Drug Deliv Rev 2008;60(8):876–885.

6

BLOCK COPOLYMER MICELLES AND VESICLES FOR DRUG DELIVERY

James D. Robertson, Nisa Patikarnmonthon, and
Adrian S. Joseph

Department of Biomedical Science, The University of Sheffield, Sheffield, UK

Giuseppe Battaglia

Department of Chemistry, University College London, London, UK

6.1 INTRODUCTION

Block copolymer amphiphiles self-assemble in aqueous solutions into micelles and vesicles. As drug delivery carriers these vectors offer numerous advantages over their lipid counterparts, including improved stability and reduced permeability. This chapter will review the biological challenges and opportunities associated with block copolymer drug delivery vehicles and outline their successes in the delivery of drugs and nucleic acids *in vitro* and *in vivo*.

Biological barriers serve two important roles in living organisms. They allow compartmentalization of aqueous environments and prevent the entry of toxins and disease-causing pathogens. Drug delivery systems such as block copolymer aggregates can help overcome these biological barriers, which can greatly improve the pharmacokinetics, safety profile, and efficacy of clinical medicines.

Engineering Polymer Systems for Improved Drug Delivery, First Edition.
Edited by Rebecca A. Bader and David A. Putnam.
© 2014 John Wiley & Sons, Inc. Published 2014 by John Wiley & Sons, Inc.

Block copolymer amphiphiles are composed of covalently bound hydrophilic and hydrophobic blocks. Inspired by nature's phospholipids, these block copolymers self-assemble in aqueous solutions to prevent the unfavorable interaction of the hydrophobic block with water. The membrane curvature of copolymer aggregates can be adjusted by altering the packing parameter (p) as defined below:

$$p = \frac{v}{a_o l_c}$$

where v is the volume of the hydrophobic block, l_c is the chain length of the hydrophobic block, and a_o is the optimal surface area of the self-assembled polymer, a parameter controlled by the copolymer hydrophilicity and hydrophobicity. Copolymer aggregates formed with low packing parameters ($\leq 1/3$) have high interface curvatures, which favors the formation of micelles. A packing parameter between 1/3 and 1/2 favors cylindrical micelles and a higher packing parameter ($\geq 1/2$) results in low curvatures favoring the formation of hollow vesicular structures referred to as polymersomes (Fig. 6.1) [1].

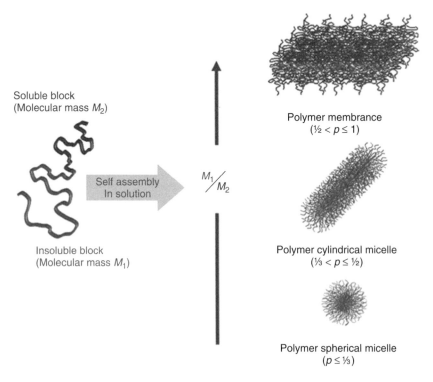

Soluble block
(Molecular mass M_2)

Self assembly
In solution

M_1 / M_2

Insoluble block
(Molecular mass M_1)

Polymer membrance
($\frac{1}{2} < p \leq 1$)

Polymer cylindrical micelle
($\frac{1}{3} < p \leq \frac{1}{2}$)

Polymer spherical micelle
($p \leq \frac{1}{3}$)

Figure 6.1. The self-assembly of micelles, cylindrical micelles or polymersomes in aqueous solutions is dependent on the membrane curvature which can be calculated from the packing factor p. Reprinted from Reference 1, Copyright (2008), with permission from Elsevier.

Block copolymer micelles range from around 5–100 nm in diameter. In aqueous solutions the hydrophilic block forms the outer shell of the aggregate and the inner core contains the hydrophobic portion of the copolymer, which can encapsulate poorly soluble lipophilic drugs. In comparison, polymersomes have a larger range of sizes from around 40 nm to hundreds of micrometers. Polymersomes are also able to encapsulate lipophilic molecules in their hydrophobic membrane, but in addition, can encapsulate hydrophilic molecules within their core.

These drug delivery vectors can be finely tuned by altering the combination of polymers and their molecular weight. In comparison to liposomes they offer thicker more robust membranes, with greater elasticity and mechanical stability. The high mechanical stability of block copolymer aggregates is in part a result of the entropically favorable chain entanglement and interdigitation of the hydrophobic blocks [2]. In 1999, Discher et al. [3] measured the aspiration force required for membrane rupture of liposomes and Polyethylene oxide-poly(butadiene) (PEO-PBD) polymersomes. They found that the polymersome membrane was 10 times more robust and 10 times less permeable to water than the liposome membrane.

The design of intelligent copolymers that respond to specific stimuli has attracted large interest in recent years. By responding to intracellular environments such as lowered pH or redox potential, copolymer aggregates can promote endosomal escape and cargo release. In the extracellular environment, temperature and pH-sensitive polymers can also respond to subtle changes in local tissues, such as tumors.

In order to improve tissue specificity, targeting moieties such as antibodies, growth factors, vitamins, sugars, and peptides can be attached to the copolymer membrane corona, allowing specific binding to functional groups that are exclusive or overexpressed in the target tissue. For instance, as tumors overexpress $\alpha_v\beta_5$ and $\alpha_v\beta_3$ integrins, polymersomes have been functionalized with the arginine-glycine-aspartic acid (RGD) peptide to preferentially target polymersomes to tumor cells [4].

For a copolymer to be successful as a drug carrier in the clinic, they must overcome a number of challenging hurdles. First and foremost, the copolymer aggregates must be biocompatible and nonimmunogenic. Poly(ethylene oxide) (PEO), commonly known as Poly(ethylene glycol) (PEG), is the most common hydrophilic block used in block copolymers because of its minimal toxicity and resistance to protein absorption and adhesion. Other factors in the design of drug delivery systems, such as intracellular delivery, release mechanisms and biodegradability, must also be considered. This chapter will focus on block copolymer micelles and polymersomes, the properties of which make them desirable drug carriers and successful in delivering drug and gene therapies in preclinical disease models.

6.2   DRUG ENCAPSULATION AND RELEASE

For a block copolymer drug delivery vehicle to be effective in the clinic, the efficiency of drug encapsulation and the kinetics of drug release are the key. The ability to retain cargo is necessary in applications that require long circulation times, while controlled

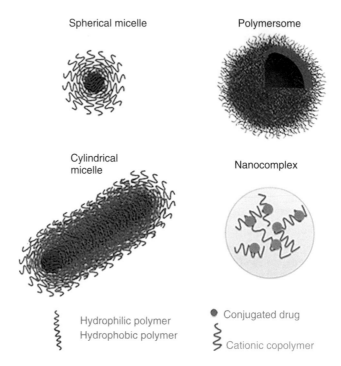

Figure 6.2. Types of block copolymer drug delivery vehicles including a spherical micelle, a polymersome, a cylindrical micelle and a nanocomplex.

leakiness can be advantageous in applications that demand slow extracellular release of the drug.

There are many factors that affect the encapsulation efficiency of block copolymers, ranging from the payload size, hydrophobicity, and method of encapsulation to the type and length of polymer chains. Polymersomes are unique in that both hydrophobic and hydrophilic molecules can be encapsulated and the volume of the core will influence the amount of hydrophilic drug that can be encapsulated.

A number of different block copolymer drug delivery vehicles have been explored [5], some examples of which are shown in Fig. 6.2.

There are several methods described in the literature used for the formation of block copolymer micelles and vesicles and encapsulation of cargo. Some of the methods are outlined in Table 6.1.

6.3 BIOAVAILABILITY AND BIODISTRIBUTION

The main advantages of polymersomes and micelles over other drug carriers are their high stability, high loading capacity and the ability to offer a controlled release, enhancing the bioavailability and biodistribution of the encapsulated drug.

TABLE 6.1. Methods of Block Copolymer Nanoparticle Formation and Drug Encapsulation

Methods	Description	Applications
Solvent evaporation and film rehydration	An aqueous solution of drug is mixed with a polymer film, prepared by solvent evaporation	Mainly used for the encapsulation of hydrophobic molecules [6, 7]
Solvent switch	The block copolymer is dissolved in a solvent compatible with both blocks, another solvent is added (normally water) for which the hydrophobic block is insoluble. This leads to the self-assembly of the block copolymer	This is one of the most common techniques for the formation of block copolymer nanoparticles and is used for the encapsulation of a range of biomolecules. Subsequent removal of solvents by dialysis is necessary for use in biological applications
Condensation	A method whereby encapsulation of cargo is achieved by exploiting electrostatic interactions between the polymer and its cargo	Most commonly used for the encapsulation of nucleic acids such as DNA or siRNA [8]
Water/oil/water double emulsions	Double emulsions are prepared consisting of water droplets surrounded by organic solvent. The block copolymer is dissolved in the solvent and self-assembles on the interface of the double emulsions	This method can be used to prepare monodisperse polymersomes with good encapsulation efficiencies [9] but the technique can be limited to low volumes
Stimuli responsiveness	Certain stimuli-responsive block copolymers can assemble or disassemble in aqueous solutions upon exposure to specific triggers such as pH, temperature, and light.	Block copolymers containing a polybasic hydrophobic block self-assemble into aggregates when the pH is raised above their pKa [10].
Drug conjugation	Molecules can be conjugated directly to the block copolymer during polymer synthesis. This technique can offer high encapsulation efficiencies, but may require a release mechanism for the drug to become functional after delivery	Examples of molecules encapsulated by this method include: anticancer drugs [11, 12], antisense oligonucleotides [13], siRNA [14, 15] and fluorophores [16, 17]
Electroporation	Recently preformed vesicles have been loaded with cargo using electroporation. This is advantageous as it is quick and reproducible but requires vesicles to be made before hand by another method [18]	This method can be used to encapsulate hydrophilic molecules such as dyes, proteins, and nucleic acids [18]

An improved bioavailability minimizes the dosing frequency of the drug, while improving the biodistribution helps to reduce off target side effects. To achieve optimum nanoparticle bioavailability, one must understand and be able to predict and control the fate of these nanoparticles *in vivo*. Nanoparticle fate is controlled by several factors including: the route of administration, particle size, zeta potential, and the type and combination of copolymers.

The route of administration can greatly affect a drug's pharmacokinetics and pharmacodynamics. The most common administration route of nanocarriers *in vivo* is by intravenous injection. This is an easily accessible and reproducible route of administration, making dosage highly tunable and precise. Nanocarriers injected into the blood are immediately exposed to opsonins and phagocytic cells such as monocytes. These cells are very effective in clearing foreign substances from blood; therefore, "stealth" nanocarriers have been designed to minimize phagocytic uptake. Other routes of administration explored include topical, oral, and intratissue injections into the desired organ (e.g., intratumor or intracranial). Injecting nanocarriers directly into organs may help bypass blood clearance by the reticuloendothelial system (RES), the liver and other obstacles such as the blood–brain barrier. One study showed that even direct intratumor injection of two types of polymersomes into mice resulted in a significant accumulation of the copolymers in the liver and spleen [19]. In addition, intratumor injection is not always feasible in cases where tumors have spread and when situated in sensitive areas such as the brain.

Size is probably the most extensively studied parameter affecting nanocarrier clearance *in vivo*. Size directly affects the clearance of nanocarriers by the RES and can also influence their extravasation into other organs. The liver filters blood through sinusoid capillaries and specialized macrophages called Kupffer's cells. The sinusoid capillaries remove particles above around 150 nm, whereas, smaller nanoparticles are often rapidly sequestered by Kupffer's cells. Particles with a diameter of 120–200 nm have proven most effective in escaping liver filtration. In this sense, polymersomes have an advantage over micelles, as they often range between 100 and 400 nm in diameter, whereas micelles are usually smaller than 50 nm. Another organ that avidly up-takes nanocarriers from the blood is the spleen. Interestingly, size is not the only factor dictating mechanical filtration through the spleen. In fact, particles larger than the filtration cutoff (200 nm) can pass through the filter if they are flexible enough. This is an important mechanism in distinguishing between young, healthy erythrocytes and nonfunctional ones that lose their flexibility. Some solid tumors and inflamed tissues have capillary fenestrations in the micrometer scale, allowing nanocarriers to move through. This will be discussed in more detail later. Nanocarriers also interact with plasma proteins in a process known as opsonization. This will facilitate their recognition by leukocytes and increase their size.

The shape of a nanoparticle can also affect its biodistribution. For instance, some cylindrical micelles have long circulation times *in vivo*. In one study, it was shown that the circulation time of cylindrical micelles improved with increasing length, up to a maximum circulation time of 1 week, which is almost an order of magnitude higher than the circulation times recorded for spherical nanoparticles [20]. This may be attributed to fewer high curvature regions on the particles, preventing uptake by phagocytosis [21].

Mitragotri's research group investigated the uptake of geometrically anisotropic polystyrene microparticles by alveolar macrophages [22]. They found that the rate of phagocytosis was highly dependent on the shape of the particle at the point of contact. For instance, polystyrene particles in the shape of elliptical disks were phagocytosed within 6 min if the phagocyte attached along the major axis of the particle but were not phagocytosed even after 2h, if the macrophage attached along the minor axis of the particle.

The zeta potential is another parameter affecting nanoparticle biodistribution. The superficial charge correlates with the rate of opsonization. This means that charged particles tend to clear faster than neutral ones because they are quickly opsonized and cleared by phagocytes. This phenomenon has been widely studied in liposomes and has only recently been investigated in polymersomes and micelles. In one study, Christian et al. [23] observed that, *in vivo*, charged polymersomes were taken up almost solely by the liver, whereas neutral polymersomes were sequestered by both liver and the spleen. In another study, Xiao and coworkers tested seven different micelle formulations of a PEO–cholic acid-based copolymer, each formulation having a similar size of around 22 nm, but with zeta potentials ranging from -27 mV to $+37$ mV. They found that, in comparison with highly charged micelles, the neutral micelles are taken up more readily by tumors and less by the liver, spleen, and lungs [24].

The type and combination of polymers used can also affect the bioavailability of nanocarriers. While the hydrophobic block regulates the mechanical properties of the membrane, it is the hydrophilic block that is responsible for the interactions of nanoparticles with the external environment. A desirable hydrophilic polymer has minimal adsorption to plasma proteins, giving the block copolymer "stealth" properties. As mentioned earlier, the most studied hydrophilic polymer is PEG. Its high hydrophilicity and neutral nature provide an efficient shield against phagocytes and opsonization. The choice of hydrophobic block should balance the requirement for mechanical stability (e.g., cross-linking will improve drug retention) and high flexibility, which can minimize spleen uptake. The hydrophilic block can also dictate the rate of internalization. Our group compared polymersomes of the same hydrophobic block poly(2-(diisopropylamino)ethyl methacrylate) (PDPA) but with different hydrophilic blocks, PEO or poly(2-(methacryloyloxy)ethyl phosphorylcholine) (PMPC). After intratumor injection of the two types of polymersomes, those formed from PMPC–PDPA were internalized by tumor cells more effectively than PEO–PDPA polymersomes; this is in agreement with the reported rapid internalization of PMPC-based polymersomes [19]. PMPC–PDPA was also found to a greater extent in other organs such as the liver and spleen.

To improve the pharmacokinetics and pharmacodynamics of nanocarriers, a number of strategies can be adopted. One approach is to inject the nanoparticles with a large dose of placebo carriers, or with gadolinium chloride to induce transient apoptosis of hepatic and splenic macrophages [25]. Despite being effective, these approaches are not advisable in the clinic because of their cost and increased risk of side effects. Another approach is to imitate nature, such as the way healthy red blood cells and some pathogens escape macrophages. Disher and coworkers recently attempted to mimic the surface charge of red blood cells to prolong the half-life of polymersomes in the blood [23]. Other efforts have been made to modify the surface of polymersomes with markers of "self," for instance decoration of polymersomes with CD47 reduces phagocytic clearance [26].

It is interesting to note that even the longest circulating spherical nanoparticles of optimum size and composition have half-lives no greater than a few hours in mice. It has been suggested that this may be a result of the loss of the protecting hydrophilic layer. This is reasonable for PEG-coated liposomes, but is unlikely to happen to PEG-based polymersomes and micelles which have a uniform brush of PEG. Another explanation may be the *in vivo* degradation of the polymersome membrane in those composed of biodegradable polymers. Finally, even PEG is subject to opsonization, albeit to a lesser extent than most materials. Opsonization will result in polymersome recognition and sequestration by phagocytic cells.

A key question that needs to be addressed is the fate of block copolymers after they are cleared. Examples of polymers already approved by US Food and Drug Administration (FDA) for human drug delivery include the hydrophilic polymer PEG and the hydrophobic biodegradable polymer polylactide PLA. Many of the polymers used in block copolymers have been developed in the past 20 years. This means that, although acute toxicity studies can be performed, there is no data on long-term exposure.

It should be noted that, although there are ways to prolong the half-life of nanocarriers *in vivo* and to avoid RES clearance, in some cases these pharmacodynamics have been exploited to target nanocarriers to the liver, spleen or circulating phagocytes.

6.4   STIMULI RESPONSIVENESS

Stimuli-responsive polymers undergo conformational changes when exposed to specific environments. Common examples of these stimuli include temperature, light, ultrasound, hydrolysis, pH, magnetism, and oxidative and reductive environments. Intelligent block copolymer drug delivery carriers with stimuli-responsive blocks have been developed to allow the copolymer aggregates to respond to specific biological intracellular or extracellular environments.

6.4.1   Temperature

Temperature sensitivity is an attractive feature for a drug vector, as subtle temperature changes are common in disease states. Two types of temperature-sensitive polymers exist. A polymer with a lower critical solution temperature (LCST) becomes insoluble when the temperature is brought below the LCST. Polymers with a higher critical solution temperature (HCST) become insoluble when the temperature is raised above their HCST. This has been exploited in block copolymer aggregates as a method of drug release; once the temperature-sensitive block copolymer becomes insoluble, the aggregate disassembles releasing its cargo.

The most studied thermosensitive polymer is poly(*N*-iso-propylacrylamide) (PNI-PAM), which has a lower critical solution temperature of about 32 °C. Both micelle and polymersome aggregates of the copolymer PEO-*b*-PNIPAM have been reported [27–29]. One group showed that the block copolymer PEO-*b*-PNIPAM could form polymersomes, which were stable at body temperature. The authors showed successful coencapsulation of the hydrophilic chemotherapy drug doxorubicin and the hydropho-bic dye PKH 26. Lowering the temperature below 32 °C resulted in rapid disassembly of the polymersomes and release of their encapsulates [29]. Therapeutically this may provide an excellent tumor-targeting vector when paired with cryotherapy: a treatment where a cryroprobe is implanted to cool tumor tissues.

It is well known that a number of ailments result in local hyperthermia. For instance inflammation caused by tissue damage or infection leads to the release of vasodilators such as histamine, and this increases the blood flow to the area leading to a rise in temperature. Similarly the increased metabolism and blood flow of tumor tissue results in a local rise in temperature of 2–5 °C above body temperature. By responding to these minor changes in temperature, a thermosensitive drug delivery carrier could release its payload specifically at the site of disease. So far, few block copolymer micelles or polymersomes with HCSTs have been reported, although, there is grow-ing interest in block copolymer systems containing poly(2-oxazoline)s which have an HCST in water–ethanol mixtures. For instance, one group showed that the copolymer poly(2-phenyl-2-oxazoline)-*co*-poly(2-methyl-2-oxazoline) (PMeOx-*co*-PPhOx) self-assembled into micelles in water–ethanol mixtures and became insoluble once the temperature was raised above its HCST. The HCST could be tuned by altering the mole percent of the hydrophobic block [30].

6.4.2 Hydrolysis

PLA and poly(caprolactone) (PCL) are susceptible to hydrolytic biodegradation under physiological conditions. When conjugated with PEG as block copolymers they are capable of forming stable polymersomes [31, 32]. The Discher group blended PEG–PLA with inert PEG–polybutadine (PEG–PBD) as a method of extending the biodegradation time *in vivo* [33]. In addition, hydrolysis of these polyesters is more rapid at low pH, which could be exploited to encourage preferential cargo release in acidic environments such as tumor tissue or endolysosomal compartments.

Polyester hydrolysis is greatest at the chain end. As a result, hydrolysis gradually lowers the chain length of the hydrophobic block and thus increases the packing parameter. Eventually, the polymersome membrane becomes unstable and transforms into mixed micellar assemblies resulting in a release of hydrophillic cargo [33].

6.4.3 pH

pH-responsive polymers are one of the most studied stimuli-responsive polymers for drug delivery vehicles. pH-sensitive polymers contain a chemical group with an ion-ization state that is dependent upon the pH. For instance when the pH is raised above its pKa, a polyacid (e.g., poly(acrylic acid) (PAA)) becomes deprotonated, acquiring a negative charge. A polybase (e.g., poly2-vinylpyridine (P2VP)) becomes protonated when the pH is brought below its pKa, giving the polymer a net positive charge [34].

In hydrophobic blocks such as P2VP, pH-dependant protonation results in an increased interaction with water. For this reason, block copolymer aggregates made from pH-sensitive polybase blocks disassemble once the pH is brought below their pKa. As mentioned previously, disassembly in acidic environments allows intracellular cargo release in endolysosomal compartments. One advantage of polybasic block copolymers is that disassembly is rapid and can occur over seconds to minutes, in comparison to the hours to days required for pH-catalyzed hydrolysis observed in PCL and PLA block copolymer aggregates [35]. In addition, cations are membranolytic and dramatically increase the osmotic potential inside these compartments, providing a mechanism of endolysosomal escape for encapsulates into the cell cytosol.

Our research group works primarily on block copolymer polymersomes composed of the biocompatible hydrophilic block (PMPC) and the hydrophobic polybasic block (PDPA). At body temperature, the pKa of PDPA is around 6.4. A pKa just below physiological pH is desirable as it promotes intracellular escape in the early endosome before lysosomal fusion. This avoids the highly oxidative and acidic conditions of lysosomes which can damage the encapsulates and cause cellular toxicity when their contents are released into the cytosol (see Fig. 6.3) [36].

6.4.4   Oxidation

Triblock copolymers formed from a hydrophobic polymer joined to two of the same hydrophillic polymers are referred to as ABA triblock copolymers. Hubbell and coworkers have designed ABA triblock oxidative-responsive polymersomes using the oxidation-sensitive polymer polypropylene sulfide (PPS) and PEG (PEG–PPS–PEG)

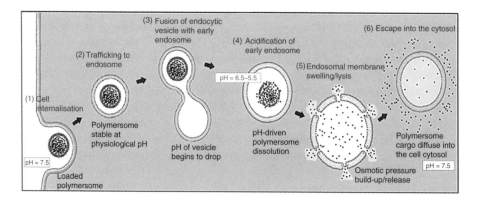

Figure 6.3. The mechanism of pH-sensitive polymersome mediated cytosolic delivery. Polymersomes are internalized by endocytosis and trafficked to an early endosome. A pH drop during endosomal fusion results in polymersome disassembly, temporary endosomal lysis and cargo release. Figure reproduced from Reference 10.

[37]. This may be a useful tool for targeting extracellular oxidative environments such as inflamed and tumor tissues *in vivo*. The hydrophobic block polypropylene is readily oxidized into hydrophilic poly(propylene sulfoxide) and poly(propylene sulfone), resulting in an increase in packing parameter and disintegration of the polymersome into micellular structures. Using cryogenic transmission electron microscopy (cryo-TEM), they showed that exposure to 10-vol% H_2O_2 for as little as 1 minute resulted in a change in morphology from spherical vesicles to long, worm-like micelles.

6.4.5 Reduction

Hydrophilic and hydrophobic blocks connected by a disulfide link are stable in the mildly oxidative extracellular environment. Once internalized, reductive molecules inside the early endosomes such as the amino acid cysteine, break disulfide bonds through the thiol–disulfide exchange. In block copolymer micelles and polymersomes, this results in a sudden disassembly into their hydrophilic and hydrophobic homopolymers.

Reduction-sensitive diblock polymersomes composed of PEG–SS–PPS successfully encapsulated and delivered calcein into mouse macrophages. Analysis using confocal microscopy revealed intracellular fluorescence consistent with endosomal release, after just 10 min of incubation [38].

6.4.6 External Stimuli

Magnetic nanoparticles encapsulated within block copolymer polymersomes and micelles have applications in imaging and drug delivery. Recently, Hu et al. [39] encapsulated commercially available superparamagnetic iron oxide (SPIO) nanoparticles within poly(caprolatone)-*b*-poly(glycerol monomethacylate) (PCL-*b*-PGMA) micelles. These nanoparticles coencapsulated the hydrophobic anticancer drug paclitaxel and were used as a multifunctional tool for combined magnetic resonance imaging (MRI) imaging and drug delivery *in vivo*. Similarly, Sanson et al. [40] coencapsulated doxorubicin with hydrophobically modified γ-Fe_2O_3 magnetic nanoparticles within poly(trimethylene carbonate)-*b*-poly(L-glutamic acid)(PTMC-*b*-PGA) polymersomes, which acted as an effective contrast agent and could be externally guided using a small magnet.

Light- and ultrasound-sensitive block copolymers are an attractive method of promoting site-specific, noninvasive drug delivery. Most photosensitive polymers are responsive to UV light, which has restricted biomedical applications because of toxicity and limited tissue penetration. Zhao and coworkers have developed a block copolymer system containing *O*-nitrobenzyl (ONB) which, in addition to UV sensitivity, could also be cleaved by two-photon near-infrared (700–1000 nm) irradiation [41]. These longer wavelengths of light are more attractive, as they have superior tissue penetration and are less toxic to cells. Ultrasound has also been successfully used as a noninvasive trigger of block copolymer disassembly. Most commonly, these systems are based upon block copolymer micelles of PEG–poly(propylene oxide)–PEG (PEG–PPO–PEG), known commercially as pluronics, which reversibly disassemble upon exposure to ultrasound pulses [42].

6.4.7 Dual Responsive Systems

Recently, block copolymers responsive to multiple stimuli have become fashionable. For instance, dual pH and reduction-sensitive micelles [43] and polymersomes [44] have been employed to maximize the responsiveness of these nanocarriers to the reductive and acidic environments of endosomes and tumors. These systems allow drug release upon exposure to either reductive or acidic environments. On the other hand, one group has designed dual pH reductive block copolymer micelles that release their cargo only upon exposure to both of these environments [45]. This provides an additional safety mechanism to prevent drug release extracellularly and reduce off-target side effects.

Other examples of dual responsive systems include pH- and temperature-responsive micelles [46], light- and redox-responsive micelles [47], and multiresponsive micelles sensitive to pH, reduction, and temperature [48]. Design of these complex smart systems may enable fine-tuning of the location, speed, and efficiency of drug release.

6.5 THE IMMUNE SYSTEM

In drug delivery, the immune system is both a target and an obstacle. The human immune system has evolved a vast array of machinery that makes it capable of recognizing and eliminating almost any synthetic or natural foreign body while maintaining tolerance to "self" antigens. For this reason, many block copolymer vectors that have shown potency *in vitro* are rapidly cleared *in vivo*, providing motivation towards the design of "stealth" nanoparticles that can circumvent these defense mechanisms. In contrast, the immune system has also been targeted for the treatment of inflammatory diseases and for the delivery of antigens for vaccination.

6.5.1 Immunotherapy

Upregulated proinflammatory mediators such as bradykinin and nitric oxide in tumors and inflamed tissues increase the permeability of local blood vessels [49]. This produces vessel fenestrations that promote the extravasation of leukocytes and plasma into the tissue, resulting in local oedema. These vessel fenestrations can also be large enough for nanoparticles to escape the blood stream and accumulate in the inflamed tissue; this phenomenon was first described in 1986, and is known as enhanced permeation and retention (EPR) effect (for a review, see Reference 49). Ishihara et al. [50] showed that micelles encapsulating Cy7-dodecylamine accumulated within the inflamed joints of mice with adjuvant arthritis (see Fig. 6.4). Subsequently, the glucocorticoid betamethasone was encapsulated within these micelles and injected intravenously. A single injection resulted in a 35% decrease in paw inflammation after one day, which was maintained for 9 days. This response was superior to an injection of free betamethasone even with a dose three times greater.

The EPR effect has also been exploited as a method of increasing the specificity of immunosuppressants. Cyclosporine A (CsA) has been used for a number of decades

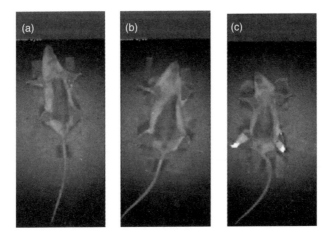

Figure 6.4. Accumulation of Cy7-dodecylamine labeled nanoparticles in the inflamed joints of mice after intravenous injection of micelles or controls. Images were taken using optix *in vivo* fluorescence imaging. (a) An image of a mouse injected with the control Cy7. (b) Nonstealth PLA homopolymer nanoparticles encapsulating Cy7, and (c) stealth micelles encapsulating Cy7, which show the greatest accumulation in the joints. Figure taken from Ishihara et al. with permission Reference 50.

to treat inflammatory disorders such as graft versus host disease and autoimmune diseases. Although CsA has high efficacy, it has a number of clinical drawbacks including poor solubility, low permeability, and some serious long-term side effects such as nephrotoxicity. One group has explored the potential of PEG-*b*-PCL micelles as a CsA drug carrier [51]. *In vivo*, CsA loaded micelles gave immunosuppressive potency comparable to that of the commercial formulation of CsA but were also beneficial in that they gave controlled release of the drug and reduced the accumulation of CsA in the kidneys.

A more radical approach to targeting inflamed tissue was that by Hammer et al. [52] who functionalized Neutravidin coated PEG–PBD polymersomes with biotinylated adhesive molecules sLex and *anti*-ICAM-1; this produced polymersomes with adhesive properties similar to those of leukocytes. They showed that these polymersomes could roll and adhere to ligand-coated surfaces over a range of shear stresses, including physiological shear rates typical in inflammation. These polymersomes may provide a unique mechanism for the specific delivery of antiinflammatory compounds to sites of inflammation.

Another field of immunology that has developed an interest in block copolymer nanocarrier delivery is vaccination. In particular delivery of a DNA sequence encoding an antigen is an attractive approach. When compared to the delivery of a protein antigen, DNA offers lower cost, higher stability, and a greater speed of production. While neutral pluronic micelles cannot encapsulate plasmid DNA, they can act as an adjuvant and facilitate the uptake and nuclear transport of DNA when codelivered [53].

(a)   (b)

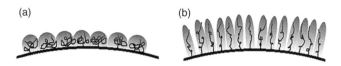

Figure 6.5. A PEGylated surface in the (a) mushroom and (b) the brush configurations.

With the addition of the cationic surfactant benzalkonium chloride (BAK), pluronic can bind to plasmid DNA through electrostatic interactions and enhance the delivery into antigen-presenting cells [54].

6.5.2 Avoiding the Immune System

In most cases, the immune system is seen as an obstacle in drug delivery. Upon administration, foreign materials are opsonized by complement proteins and antibodies, which leads to rapid clearance by circulating phagocytes such as monocytes. In this respect, PEG is considered an attractive hydrophilic block for its resistance to protein adhesion. As the density of the PEG block increases, it becomes more spread and aligned, changing from a mushroom to a brush configuration, and this produces a steric hydrophilic barrier reducing the accessibility of proteins to the particle (see Fig. 6.5). However, even PEGylated nanoparticles are not completely resistant to opsonization, indeed, *anti*-PEG IgM antibodies are found in patients injected with PEGylated liposomes. PEGylated liposomes have higher circulation times than liposomes, but these circulation times are reduced in subsequent doses. This process is referred to as the accelerated blood clearance (ABC) phenomenon [55]. It is worth noting that the ABC phenomenon is considerably lower in PEGylated liposomes than in nonPEGylated ones [56]

The rate of clearance and the extent of complement activation are also strongly dependent on the nanoparticle size, density, and the molecular confirmation. Recently, Hamad et al. [57] explored the effect of pluronic architecture on complement activation. They found that alteration of the PEG coating from a mushroom to brush configuration switched complement activation from the classical to the lectin complement pathway. They also found that properdin, which is synthesized and released by circulating phagocytes, could bind to PEGylated particles in a transitional mushroom–brush confirmation and potentiate the alternative complement pathway.

PEGylated nanoparticles can themselves activate the complement cascade through the alternative pathway, which reacts with hydroxyl groups. Indeed, the numerous hydroxyl groups on the surface of PEGylated nanoparticles have been exploited as a method of activating the complement system in the design of a vaccine [58]. By converting the hydroxyl groups to methoxyl groups alternative complement activation can be reduced [58]. Most PEG copolymers are now based on methoxy-PEG.

As well as opsonizing targets for clearance, the complement system can also trigger inflammatory reactions and anaphylaxis. For instance, a number of acute hypersensitivity reactions have been reported for the FDA-approved Doxil, an anticancer formulation of doxorubicin encapsulated within PEGylated liposomes [59].

Bacteria and parasites have evolved mechanisms of overcoming complement activation. For instance, some bacterial proteins have been found to bind Factor H, a regulatory protein that prevents complement from binding to "self" antigens. It has been suggested that modifying nanoparticles with peptides that bind factor H may provide a mechanism of avoiding complement activation [60].

In comparison to those of PEG, the biocompatibility and immunogenicity of other hydrophilic blocks have been relatively unexplored. Examples of other hydrophilic polymers with proposed steric hindrance include P2VP, poly(2-oxazoline)s, and PMPC. Phosphorylcholine polymers, such as PMPC, stemmed from an observation that the phospholipids composing the inner membrane of erythrocytes were thrombolytic, while the phosphatidylcholine and sphingomyelin that dominated the outer membrane were nonthrombolytic [61]. Later it was shown that the nonthrombolytic nature of the outer leaflet was attributed to phosphorylcholine, the head group of phosphatidylcholine and sphingomyelin [62].

Although the mechanism by which phosphorylcholine-based polymers prevent protein adhesion is not completely understood, a great deal of research has demonstrated that they are very resistant to interactions with blood proteins such as fibrinogen, albumin and immunoglobulins (reviewed in [63]). The highly hydrophilic zwitterionic head group associates with a large amount of water, which allows proteins to bind transiently without undergoing any conformational changes [64]. In addition, MPC has a strong affinity for plasma phospholipid, which builds up on the MPC surface [65]. Resistance to protein adhesion is most likely the result of a combination of these mechanisms.

MPC polymers are now used clinically as nonthrombogenic coatings to coronary stents and contact lenses. The ability of MPC to resist absorption to plasma proteins, including complement component c5a [66], coupled with the extensive *in vitro* cell viability testing on PMPC–PDPA polymersomes [67], suggests that PMPC may provide a suitable alternative hydrophilic block to PEG.

6.6 GENE THERAPY

Transcription of DNA to RNA and translation of RNA to protein are essential processes for all living organisms. Alteration of a single nucleotide in a genome can markedly alter the function of the protein produced. While simple mutations such as these allow species to adapt to changing environments and evolve into more complex organisms, they can also lead to protein malfunction and disease. Many diseases are now known to have a genetic origin and thus the ability to manipulate protein production at the genetic level is highly desirable.

Gene therapy is the treatment of a genetic disorder by the manipulation of protein synthesis. Delivery of whole genes could provide the most effective treatment, but long nucleotides are more easily degraded. Moreover, even if DNA could be efficiently delivered inside the cell cytoplasm, it is still restricted by the nuclear membrane. Genes can be silenced using antisense oligonucleotides (ODNs) or RNA interference (RNAi), which can be more effective because of their small size, lower risk of degradation and the ease of manipulation. Additionally, ODNs and RNAi function in the cytoplasm and so are not limited by the nuclear membrane. Currently, the greatest limiting factor in gene therapy is finding a vector to efficiently deliver these tools into the cells of interest without toxicity or activation of the immune system.

To date, the most successful vectors in gene therapy are viruses, which can offer high transfection efficiency and target specificity. However, even after disease-causing sequences are removed, viruses can still provoke a strong immune response, which can lead to hypersensitivity reactions and fast clearance after repeated doses. Other methods of nucleic acid delivery include physiological techniques such as electroporation [68, 69], sonoporation [70–72], and microneedles [73, 74], such techniques are generally limited to research purposes and can be advantageous in their simplicity, but limitations include the inability to protect nucleic acids from enzymatic degradation, lack of target specificity, and likelihood of cell damage.

Liposomes are another vector that have had some success in gene therapy. Liposomes were discovered more than 50 years ago by Bangham [75], and they are biocompatible and biodegradable vesicles formed from natural lipids. However, their use *in vivo* is limited by low blood circulation times due to their rapid degradation. Block copolymers offer advantages over other vectors because of their potential to be modified for specific requirements.

Figure 6.6 illustrates some examples of the numerous polymeric vectors available for gene therapy [76]. The most commonly used structures are cationic micelles [77] and polyplexes [78].

6.6.1 Polyplexes

Several attempts have been made to design polymers that bind or complex with nucleic acids. Most often this has been achieved by designing polymers with a positive charge that aggregate to form a polyplex. Nucleic acids are negatively charged, which allows cationic polymers to bind and form strong electrostatic interactions. As well as binding to and protecting nucleic acids from degradation, a cationic charge also facilitates endocytosis due to the negative charge of cellular membranes.

The Mallapragada group demonstrated that pH-sensitive pentablock copolymers of poly(diethylaminoethylmethacrylate) (PDEAEM), PEO and PPO could successfully encapsulate and deliver plasmid DNA encoding the luciferase enzyme *in vitro* [78]. They showed that these polyplexes protected the plasmids from enzymatic degradation and showed high transfection efficiencies

Polyplexes can offer high encapsulation efficiencies of nucleic acids but one major disadvantage of using cationic polymers *in vivo* is that the positive charge promotes binding to negatively charged serum proteins such as albumin; this leads to aggregation of the protein–polymer complex and a reduction in cellular delivery. Similarly, opsonins bind readily to the cationic polymers, which results in rapid clearance by phagocytes.

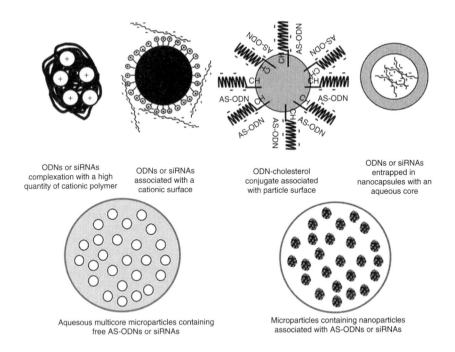

| ODNs or siRNAs complexation with a high quantity of cationic polymer | ODNs or siRNAs associated with a cationic surface | ODN-cholesterol conjugate associated with particle surface | ODNs or siRNAs entrapped in nanocapsules with an aqueous core |

| Aquesous multicore microparticles containing free AS-ODNs or siRNAs | Microparticles containing nanoparticles associated with AS-ODNs or siRNAs |

Figure 6.6. Examples of nano- and micro-technologies used in the delivery of antisense oligonucleotides and siRNA. ODN, oligonucleotides; AS–ODN, antisense oligonucleotides; siRNA, and small interfering RNA. Image taken from Reference 76 with permission.

6.6.2 Micelles

Polyplex micelles formed with PEG can help limit the interaction of nanoparticles with serum proteins. The Kataoka group investigated the antitumor efficacy of pH-sensitive pDNA/micelles from PEG–poly(N-[N-(2-aminoethyl)-2-aminoethyl]aspartamide) (PEG–PAsp(DET)) encoding an antiangiogenic protein [77]. These micelles achieved high *in vitro* gene transfer efficiency and were effective *in vivo* in preventing tumor growth. In another example, polyelectrolyte micelles formed from a complex of polyethylenimine (PEI) and vascular endothelial growth factor (VEGF) siRNA conjugated to PEG. These micelles were introduced into a prostate carcinoma cell line resulting in up to 96% silencing of VEGF expression [79].

Noncationic pluronic micelles cannot encapsulate or bind DNA but when delivered in combination with other cationic or viral vectors can significantly increase gene expression. This is believed to be a result of activation of cellular stress pathways such as NF-κB and upregulation of promoters containing stress response elements [53]. Pluronic is also used to stabilize cationic polyplex dispersions and can enhance DNA uptake and expression through optimization of particle size [80].

6.6.3　Polymersomes

Polymersomes can encapsulate and protect nucleic acids in their core. In comparison to charged carriers they can also offer reduced cytotoxicity and resistance to opsonisation. Kim et al. [81] showed that incubation of A459 cancer cells with PEG–PLA polymersomes encapsulating lamin A/C encoding siRNA gave a 40% knockdown, which is equivalent to the knockdown by the commercially available system Lipofectamine 2000. Similarly our group have shown that PMPC–PDPA polymersomes can efficiently deliver plasmid DNA encoding the green fluorescent protein into Chinese hamster ovary (CHO) and human dermal fibroblast (HDF) cells. In comparison to common protocols using Lipofectamine and calcium phosphate, the polymersomes showed lower cytotoxicity and higher transfection efficiencies [82].

6.7　CANCER THERAPY

Cancer therapy is the most studied application in polymersome drug delivery. Around 50% of potential drugs do not enter clinical trials because of poor bioavailability, poor water solubility, or severe side effects. Encapsulating drugs within nanocarriers can improve bioavailability by accumulating poorly water-soluble drugs in water compatible carriers. Furthermore, nanocarriers isolate the drug from the body until release. This minimizes side effects and protects the drug from degradation. For nanocarriers to deliver cargo selectively to a tumor, they need a long enough blood half-life to reach the tumor. For a more selective delivery of cargo, solid tumors can be targeted either actively or passively, as discussed below.

6.7.1　Passive Targeting

Solid tumor development is dependent on adequate nutrient supply. In most tumors this requirement is satisfied by a rapidly growing network of blood vessels, a process known as angiogenesis. Tumor angiogenesis is characterized by the formation of a chaotic vessel network, rapidly changing, with vessel fenestrations in the micrometer scale. In contrast, healthy tissues have fenestrations of up to 150 nm (hepatic sinusoid). This means that polymersomes tend to selectively extravasate into tumor tissue, whereas, small nanoparticles such as micelles also extravasate into other organs. Furthermore, tumors often exhibit low lymphatic drainage, meaning extracellular liquid is retained in the tissues for longer; as mentioned previously this process is known as the EPR effect (see Fig. 6.7) [83].

Intratumor pressure is greater than intracapillary pressure and is highest at the center of the tumor. His limits the accumulation of nanocarriers to simple diffusion based on concentration gradients. An example of passive targeting to tumors was reported by Discher and coworkers [84, 85]. They showed that an intravenous injection of doxorubicin and paclitaxel loaded polymersomes accumulated in the tumor and effectively shrank it *in vivo*. This has also been supported *in vitro* by another group [86]. Passive targeting can also be achieved by local administration, that is, intratumor delivery of polymersomes. Such an approach was adopted by Murdoch and coworkers [19].

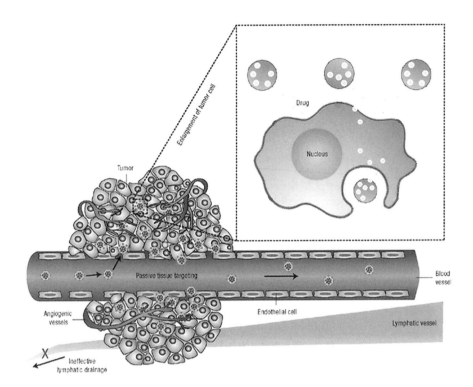

Figure 6.7. The enhanced retention and permeability (EPR) effect. The diagram shows nanoparticles extravasating from the blood stream into tumor tissue where they accumulate and deliver anticancer drugs to cancer cells. Reprinted by permission from Macmillan Publishers Ltd, *Nat Nanotechnol*, Reference 83, Copyright (2007).

6.7.2 Active Targeting

Targeting moieties can be attached to copolymers by conjugation to preformed nanoparticles or by conjugating the moieties to the copolymers before the assembly process. The functionalization chemistries have been recently reviewed in [87, 88].

Active targeting is achieved when a specific marker is overexpressed by the tissue or cells of interest and a moiety is conjugated to the nanoparticle that binds specifically to that marker. This approach increases the proportion of drug delivered to the desired site and can decrease the side effects *in vivo*, resulting in an overall improved therapeutic efficacy. Furthermore, it has been postulated that active targeting using carriers may reduce multidrug resistance (MDR) in some cases [89, 90]. Active targeting has been consistently proven *in vitro*, but currently there are no approved formulations in the clinic. This may be due to the fact that decorating nanoparticles with high molecular weight macromolecules can expose them to faster recognition and clearance by phagocytes.

Because of their unique biochemical characteristics, tumors have a number of up-regulated markers that can be targeted. In one study, the PRb peptide was functionalised onto PEO–PBD polymersomes targeting the $\alpha5\beta1$ receptor; a marker overexpressed by prostate tumor cells [91]. Encapsulated TNFα was delivered into the tumor *in vitro* and the rate of polymersome internalization was found to be dependent on the surface density of the PRb peptide. This resulted in an improved therapeutic efficacy in comparison to free TNFα or untargeted polymersomes. A different approach was taken by the Lecommandoux group, who prepared polymersomes of poly(γ-benzyl l-glutamate)-*block*-hyaluronan (PBLG23-*b*-HYA10). These polymersomes are targeted to CD44, which is overexpressed by some tumor cells [92]. In this study, they showed that these targeted polymersomes encapsulating doxorubicin were more effective in controlling tumor growth than free doxorubicin *in vivo*. In addition, the polymersomes also significantly improved the half-life of doxorubicin in the blood. Finally, as mentioned previously, tumors can also be targeted using stimuli-sensitive polymers such as those responsive to temperature, pH, magnetism or ultrasound.

6.8 CONCLUSIONS

The biological applications of block copolymer micelles and polymersomes are vast and the popularity of these tools has been steadily rising since their discovery. However, despite the extensive literature of successful *in vitro* drug delivery, many systems have failed *in vivo* because of the multiple obstacles that a drug vector faces.

While block copolymer micelles are mainly limited to the delivery of hydrophobic molecules, polymersomes can encapsulate a diverse array of molecules ranging from small chemicals and nucleic acids to large proteins and lipids. In particular, the ability to deliver these molecules intracellularly without inducing cytotoxicity is an exciting prospect, exposing the internal cell machinery as a new target for drug design and gene therapy.

Tissue specific targeting is another attractive quality of block copolymer vehicles. In the case of inflammation and cancer, passive targeting via the EPR effect promotes site-specific accumulation of the drug. Active targeting via decorating moieties can allow preferential drug delivery to almost any tissue in the body. Together these tools expose the possibility of delivering drugs with new targets, superior clinical efficacy and reduced side effects.

6.9 KEY POINTS

- Block copolymer amphiphiles are composed of covalently bound hydrophilic and hydrophobic blocks
- The curvature of a block copolymer aggregate is dependent upon its packing parameter, which dictates the structures formed by self-assembly.
- The bioavailability and biodistribution of a nanoparticle is dependent on many things including the chemistry, shape, size, zeta potential, and route of administration.

- Stimuli-responsive polymers have been engineered to react to specific environments in order to release their cargo at a desired location in the body.
- The immune system can cause rapid clearance of nanoparticles, which lowers the efficiency of the drug delivery.
- Stealth particles, such as PEGylated nanoparticles, can reduce clearance by the immune system by reducing the binding to plasma proteins and opsonins.
- Nanoparticles can be designed to target tumors passively, through the EPR effect, or actively by attaching targeting moieties to the outside of the nanoparticle.

6.10 HOMEWORK PROBLEMS

1. A block copolymer has been synthesized with the following properties:
2. Optimal area per molecule, $a_0 = 0.6$ nm^2; hydrophobic block length $l_c = 2$ nm; hydrophobic molecular volume $v = 0.6$ nm^3
   - Which structure(s) would you expect to form?
   - What could you change to promote the formation of other structures?
3. A drug company would like to manufacture a vector with long circulation times to provide a controlled release of their drug. Discuss the properties of a block copolymer vector that are likely to influence its circulation time.
4. Describe the advantages and disadvantages of the different vectors for gene therapy.
5. What should be considered when designing a block copolymer for the intracellular delivery of sensitive molecules such as nucleic acids?
6. Describe the EPR effect and explain how it can be advantageous in nanoparticle drug delivery.

REFERENCES

1. Smart T et al. Block copolymer nanostructures. Nano Today 2008;3(3–4):38–46.
2. Battaglia G, Ryan AJ. Bilayers and interdigitation in block copolymer vesicles. J Am Chem Soc 2005;127(24):8757–8764.
3. Discher BM et al. Polymersomes: tough vesicles made from diblock copolymers. Science 1999;284(5417):1143–1146.
4. Wang Y et al. RGD-modified polymeric micelles as potential carriers for targeted delivery to integrin-overexpressing tumor vasculature and tumor cells. J Drug Target 2009;17(6):459–467.
5. Bei D, Meng J, Youan BB. Engineering nanomedicines for improved melanoma therapy: progress and promises. Nanomedicine 2010;5(9):1385–1399.
6. Battaglia G, Ryan AJ. The evolution of vesicles from bulk lamellar gels. Nat Mater 2005;4(11):869–876.

7. Lavasanifar A et al. Block copolymer micelles for the encapsulation and delivery of amphotericin B. Pharm Res 2002;19(4):418–422.

8. Dai W et al. The pH-induced thermosensitive poly (NIPAAm-co-AAc-co-HEMA)-g-PCL micelles used as a drug carrier. J Mater Sci Mater Med 2010;21(6):1881–1890.

9. Lorenceau E et al. Generation of polymerosomes from double-emulsions. Langmuir 2005;21(20):9183–9186.

10. Massignani M et al. Enhanced fluorescence imaging of live cells by effective cytosolic delivery of probes. PLos One 2010;5(5).

11. Yokoyama M et al. Preparation of micelle-forming polymer-drug conjugates. Bioconjug Chem 1992;3(4):295–301.

12. Sakai-Kato K et al. Evaluation of intracellular trafficking and clearance from HeLa cells of doxorubicin-bound block copolymers. Int J Pharm 2012;423(2):401–409.

13. Jeong JH, Kim SW, Park TG. A new antisense oligonucleotide delivery system based on self-assembled ODN-PEG hybrid conjugate micelles. J Control Release 2003;93(2): 183–191.

14. Takemoto H et al. Polyion complex stability and gene silencing efficiency with a siRNA-grafted polymer delivery system. Biomaterials 2010;31(31):8097–8105.

15. Lee SH et al. Self-assembled siRNA-PLGA conjugate micelles for gene silencing. J Control Release 2011;152(1):152–158.

16. Ghoroghchian PP et al. Broad spectral domain fluorescence wavelength modulation of visible and near-infrared emissive polymersomes. J Am Chem Soc 2005;127(44):15388–15390.

17. Lomas H et al. Non-cytotoxic polymer vesicles for rapid and efficient intracellular delivery. Faraday Discuss 2008;139:143–159 discussion 213–28, 419–20.

18. Wang L et al. Encapsulation of biomacromolecules within polymersomes by electroporation. Angew Chem Int Ed 2012;51(44):11122–11125.

19. Murdoch C et al. Internalization and biodistribution of polymersomes into oral squamous cell carcinoma cells in vitro and in vivo. Nanomedicine (Lond) 2010;5(7):1025–1036.

20. Geng Y et al. Shape effects of filaments versus spherical particles in flow and drug delivery. Nat Nanotechnol 2007;2(4):249–255.

21. Champion JA, Mitragotri S. Shape induced inhibition of phagocytosis of polymer particles. Pharm Res 2009;26(1):244–249.

22. Champion JA, Mitragotri S. Role of target geometry in phagocytosis. Proc Natl Acad Sci U S A 2006;103(13):4930–4934.

23. Christian DA et al. Polymer vesicles with a red cell-like surface charge: microvascular imaging and in vivo tracking with near-infrared fluorescence. Macromol Rapid Commun 2010;31(2):135–141.

24. Xiao K et al. The effect of surface charge on in vivo biodistribution of PEG-oligocholic acid based micellar nanoparticles. Biomaterials 2011;32(13):3435–3446.

25. Moghimi SM, Hunter AC, Murray JC. Long-circulating and target-specific nanoparticles: theory to practice. Pharmacol Rev 2001;53(2):283–318.

26. Tsai RK, Rodriguez PL, Discher DE. Self inhibition of phagocytosis: the affinity of 'marker of self' CD47 for SIRPalpha dictates potency of inhibition but only at low expression levels. Blood Cells Mol Dis 2010;45(1):67–74.

27. Zhang WQ et al. Thermoresponsive micellization of poly(ethylene glycol)-b-poly(N-isopropylacrylamide) in water. Macromolecules 2005;38(13):5743–5747.

28. Motokawa R et al. Thermosensitive diblock copolymer of poly(N-isopropylacrylamide) and poly(ethylene glycol) in water: polymer preparation and solution behavior. Macromolecules 2005;38(13):5748–5760.

29. Qin S et al. Temperature-controlled assembly and release from polymer vesicles of poly(ethylene oxide)-block-poly(N-isopropylacrylamide). Adv Mater 2006;18(21):2905.

30. Hoogenboom R et al. Tuning solution polymer properties by binary water-ethanol solvent mixtures. Soft Matter 2008;4(1):103–107.

31. Meng FH et al. Biodegradable polymersomes. Macromolecules 2003;36(9):3004–3006.

32. Ghoroghchian PP et al. Bioresorbable vesicles formed through spontaneous self-assembly of amphiphilic poly(ethylene oxide)-block-polycaprolactone. Macromolecules 2006;39(5):1673–1675.

33. Ahmed F, Discher DE. Self-porating polymersomes of PEG-PLA and PEG-PCL: hydrolysis-triggered controlled release vesicles. J Control Release 2004;96(1):37–53.

34. Borchert U et al. pH-induced release from P2VP-PEO block copolymer vesicles. Langmuir 2006;22(13):5843–5847.

35. Ahmed F, Discher DE. Self-porating polymersomes of PEG, ÄìPLA and PEG, ÄìPCL: hydrolysis-triggered controlled release vesicles. J Control Release 2004;96(1):37–53.

36. Lomas H et al. Non-cytotoxic polymer vesicles for rapid and efficient intracellular delivery. Faraday Discuss 2008;139:143–159.

37. Napoli A et al. Oxidation-responsive polymeric vesicles. Nat Mater 2004;3(3):183–189.

38. Cerritelli S, Velluto D, Hubbell JA. PEG-SS-PPS: reduction-sensitive disulfide block copolymer vesicles for intracellular drug delivery. Biomacromolecules 2007;8(6):1966–1972.

39. Hu J et al. Drug-loaded and superparamagnetic iron oxide nanoparticle surface embedded amphiphilic block copolymer micelles for integrated chemotherapeutic drug delivery and MR imaging. Langmuir 2011;28(4):2073–2082.

40. Sanson C et al. Doxorubicin loaded magnetic polymersomes: theranostic nanocarriers for MR imaging and magneto-chemotherapy. ACS Nano 2011;5(2):1122–1140.

41. Jiang JQ et al. Toward photocontrolled release using light-dissociable block copolymer micelles. Macromolecules 2006;39(13):4633–4640.

42. Oerlemans C et al. Polymeric micelles in anticancer therapy: targeting, Imaging and Triggered Release. Pharm Res 2010;27(12):2569–2589.

43. Chen J et al. pH and reduction dual-sensitive copolymeric micelles for intracellular doxorubicin delivery. Biomacromolecules 2011;12(10):3601–3611.

44. Zhang J et al. pH and reduction dual-bioresponsive polymersomes for efficient intracellular protein delivery. Langmuir 2011;28(4):2056–2065.

45. Wei C, Guo J, Wang C. Dual stimuli-responsive polymeric micelles exhibiting "AND" logic gate for controlled release of adriamycin. Macromol Rapid Commun 2011;32(5):451–455.

46. Xiong Z et al. Dual-stimuli responsive behaviors of diblock polyampholyte PDMAEMA-b-PAA in aqueous solution. J Colloid Interface Sci 2011;356(2):557–565.

47. Han D, Tong X, Zhao Y. Block copolymer micelles with a dual-stimuli-responsive core for fast or slow degradation. Langmuir 2012;28(5):2327–2331.

48. Klaikherd A, Nagamani C, Thayumanavan S. Multi-stimuli sensitive amphiphilic block copolymer assemblies. J Am Chem Soc 2009;131(13):4830–4838.

49. Fang J, Nakamura H, Maeda H. The EPR effect: unique features of tumor blood vessels for drug delivery, factors involved, and limitations and augmentation of the effect. Adv Drug Deliv Rev 2011;63(3):136–151.

50. Ishihara T et al. Treatment of experimental arthritis with stealth-type polymeric nanoparticles encapsulating betamethasone phosphate. J Pharmacol Exp Ther 2009;329(2):412–417.

51. Hamdy S et al. The immunosuppressive activity of polymeric micellar formulation of cyclosporine a: in vitro and in vivo studies. AAPS J 2011;13(2):159–168.

52. Hammer DA et al. Leuko-polymersomes. Faraday Discuss 2008;139:129–141.

53. Sriadibhatla S et al. Transcriptional activation of gene expression by pluronic block copolymers in stably and transiently transfected cells. Mol Ther 2006;13(4):804–813.

54. Hartikka J et al. Physical characterization and in vivo evaluation of poloxamer-based DNA vaccine formulations. J Gene Med 2008;10(7):770–782.

55. Dufort S, Sancey L, Coll JL. Physico-chemical parameters that govern nanoparticles fate also dictate rules for their molecular evolution. Adv Drug Deliv Rev 2011;64(2):179–189.

56. Ishida T et al. Effect of the physicochemical properties of initially injected liposomes on the clearance of subsequently injected PEGylated liposomes in mice. J Control Release 2004;95(3):403–412.

57. Hamad I et al. Distinct polymer architecture mediates switching of complement activation pathways at the nanosphere-serum interface: implications for stealth nanoparticle engineering. ACS Nano 2010;4(11):6629–6638.

58. Reddy ST et al. Exploiting lymphatic transport and complement activation in nanoparticle vaccines. Nat Biotechnol 2007;25(10):1159–1164.

59. Chanan-Khan A et al. Complement activation following first exposure to pegylated liposomal doxorubicin (Doxil): possible role in hypersensitivity reactions. Ann Oncol 2003;14(9):1430–1437.

60. Sim RB, Wallis R. SURFACE PROPERTIES Immune attack on nanoparticles. Nat Nanotechnol 2011;6(2):80–81.

61. Zwaal RFA, Comfurius P, Vandeenen LLM. Membrane asymmetry and blood-coagulation. Nature 1977;268(5618):358–360.

62. Hayward JA, Chapman D. Biomembrane surfaces as models for polymer design - the potential for hemocompatibility. Biomaterials 1984;5(3):135–142.

63. Lewis AL. Phosphorylcholine-based polymers and their use in the prevention of biofouling. Colloids Surf B Biointerfaces 2000;18(3–4):261–275.

64. Ishihara K et al. Why do phospholipid polymers reduce protein adsorption? J Biomed Mater Res 1998;39(2):323–330.

65. Ueda T et al. Preparation of 2-methacryloyloxyethyl phosphorylcholine copolymers with alkyl methacrylates and their blood compatibility. Polym J 1992;24(11):1259–1269.

66. Ishihara K et al. Protein adsorption from human plasma is reduced on phospholipid polymers. J Biomed Mater Res 1991;25(11):1397–1407.

67. Massignani M et al. Controlling cellular uptake by surface chemistry, size, and surface topology at the nanoscale. Small 2009;5(21):2424–2432.

68. Murakami T, Sunada Y. Plasmid DNA gene therapy by electroporation: principles and recent advances. Curr Gene Ther 2011;11(6):100.

69. Potter H, Heller R. Transfection by electroporation. Curr Protoc Cell Biol 2011 edited by Bonifacino JS et al. Chapter 20: Unit20.5.1–20.5.6.

70. Zolochevska O et al. Sonoporation delivery of interleukin-27 gene therapy efficiently reduces prostate tumor cell growth in vivo. Hum Gene Ther 2011;22(12):1537–1550.

71. Rodamporn S et al. HeLa cell transfection using a novel sonoporation system. IEEE Trans Biomed Eng 2011;58(4):927–934.

72. Paula DM et al. Therapeutic ultrasound promotes plasmid DNA uptake by clathrin-mediated endocytosis. J Gene Med 2011;13(7–8):392–401.

73. Coulman SA et al. Minimally invasive cutaneous delivery of macromolecules and plasmid DNA via microneedles. Curr Drug Deliv 2006;3(1):65–75.

74. Pearton M et al. Gene delivery to the epidermal cells of human skin explants using micro-fabricated microneedles and hydrogel formulations. Pharm Res 2008;25(2):407–416.

75. Bangham AD, Horne RW. Negative staining of phospholipids and their structural modification by surface-active agents as observed in the electron microscope. J Mol Biol 1964;8:660–668.

76. Fattal E, Barratt G. Nanotechnologies and controlled release systems for the delivery of antisense oligonucleotides and small interfering RNA. Br J Pharmacol 2009;157(2):179–194.

77. Oba M et al. Polyplex micelles prepared from omega-cholesteryl PEG-polycation block copolymers for systemic gene delivery. Biomaterials 2011;32(2):652–663.

78. Agarwal A, Unfer R, Mallapragada SK. Novel cationic pentablock copolymers as non-viral vectors for gene therapy. J Control Release 2005;103(1):245–258.

79. Kim SH et al. PEG conjugated VEGF siRNA for anti-angiogenic gene therapy. J Control Release 2006;116(2):123–129.

80. Gebhart CL et al. Design and formulation of polyplexes based on pluronic-polyethyleneimine conjugates for gene transfer. Bioconjug Chem 2002;13(5):937–944.

81. Kim Y et al. Polymersome delivery of siRNA and antisense oligonucleotides. J Control Release 2009;134(2):132–140.

82. Lomas H et al. Biomimetic pH sensitive polymersomes for efficient DNA encapsulation and delivery. Adv Mater 2007;19(23):4238–4243.

83. Peer D et al. Nanocarriers as an emerging platform for cancer therapy. Nat Nanotechnol 2007;2(12):751–760.

84. Ahmed F et al. Biodegradable polymersomes loaded with both paclitaxel and doxorubicin permeate and shrink tumors, inducing apoptosis in proportion to accumulated drug. J Control Release 2006;116(2):150–158.

85. Ahmed F et al. Shrinkage of a rapidly growing tumor by drug-loaded polymersomes: pH-triggered release through copolymer degradation. Mol Pharm 2006;3(3):340–350.

86. Wang H et al. Enhanced anti-tumor efficacy by co-delivery of doxorubicin and paclitaxel with amphiphilic methoxy PEG-PLGA copolymer nanoparticles. Biomaterials 2011;32(32):8281–8290.

87. Stefan E et al. Functionalization of block copolymer vesicle surfaces. Polymers 2011; 3:252.

88. Meng F, Zhong Z, Feijen J. Stimuli-responsive polymersomes for programmed drug delivery. Biomacromolecules 2009;10(2):197–209.

89. Kobayashi T et al. Effect of transferrin receptor-targeted liposomal doxorubicin in P-glycoprotein-mediated drug resistant tumor cells. Int J Pharm 2007;329(1–2):94–102.

90. Goren D et al. Nuclear delivery of doxorubicin via folate-targeted liposomes with bypass of multidrug-resistance efflux pump. Clin Cancer Res 2000;6(5):1949–1957.

91. Done D et al. PR b-targeted delivery of tumor necrosis factor-a by polymersomes for the treatment of prostate cancer. Soft Matter 2009;5:2011.

92. Upadhyay KK et al. The in vivo behavior and antitumor activity of doxorubicin-loaded poly(Œ≥−benzyl 1-glutamate)-block-hyaluronan polymersomes in Ehrlich ascites tumor-bearing BalB/c mice. Nanomedicine 2012;8(1):71−80.

PART III

IMPLANTABLE POLYMERIC DRUG DELIVERY SYSTEMS

7

IMPLANTABLE DRUG DELIVERY SYSTEMS

Luis Solorio, Angela Carlson,
Haoyan Zhou, and Agata A. Exner

*Department of Radiology, Case Western Reserve University,
Cleveland, OH, USA*

7.1 INTRODUCTION

Delivery of therapeutics to their intended site of action is a complex process filled with numerous barriers. As described in the previous sections, polymeric platforms currently under development for intravenous (IV) delivery help achieve therapeutic drug levels at the target site by protecting agents in micro or nano-constructs. These constructs, in turn, can be manipulated by numerous techniques to be target specific, capable of stimulus-triggered release, detected by various imaging modalities and used for concurrent diagnosis and therapy. Despite the most sophisticated modifications, all of these systems are nonetheless susceptible to the unrelenting transport issues associated with IV administration. Particularly when the therapy objective is site specific, IV administration results in systemic distribution and then refocusing of the delivery to the target site. While this strategy has numerous benefits, in some instances an alternative approach, that at the outset concentrates the therapeutic at the local site, can be of considerable advantage.

Engineering Polymer Systems for Improved Drug Delivery, First Edition.
Edited by Rebecca A. Bader and David A. Putnam.
© 2014 John Wiley & Sons, Inc. Published 2014 by John Wiley & Sons, Inc.

Implantable polymeric systems provide a platform for site-specific therapeutic delivery. In stark contrast to IV delivery, implantable systems are designed to be loaded with a high concentration of the therapeutic agent and implanted at a site only once to deliver a specified level of drug over an extended period of time. The fundamental concept underlying this approach is referred to by many as "controlled drug release." In essence, the implantable formulations, constructed of either degradable or nondegradable polymers, are able to modulate, through a wide range of parameters, the rate of released drug(s) for a period of hours, weeks, or months. Why is this of interest? The primary reason is patient compliance. This may seem like a simplistic goal, but at the core, a therapeutic agent needs to be administered at regular increments in order to keep its plasma concentration within the therapeutic window. If administration is frequent (as often is the case with labile proteins, for example) and requires multiple injections, patient compliance will undoubtedly decrease. Hence, the idea of loading an implant with a drug, placing it into a site and removing the patient from the equation, should improve the overall effectiveness of any number of agents. Such implants have been utilized clinically for decades providing long-term delivery of contraceptives, hormones, and other therapeutic agents.

In addition to improving patient compliance, implantable delivery systems have also been investigated as a means of local drug administration with the primary goal of maximizing drug concentrations in the immediate vicinity of the implants, while reducing systemic drug exposure to minimize unwanted side effects associated with the drug. This is of particular interest in administration of agents with an extremely narrow therapeutic window. The main applications of such devices have been in the treatment of solid tumors with potent anticancer agents, drug eluting stents for reduction of restenosis, and delivery of antibiotics for treatment of periodontal disease.

In this chapter, we discuss the application of polymeric implants in delivery of therapeutics. The following sections outline the role of both nondegradable and degradable implants in systemic and local drug delivery. We expound on the concepts behind controlled release and discuss specific examples of each system that are already utilized in the clinic. We first discuss the application of nonbiodegradable polymers such as silicone and poly(ethylene-vinyl acetate) copolymers in surgically implantable devices. We examine the differences between reservoir devices, where the drug is entrapped within a polymer membrane, and matrix devices, where the drug is distributed throughout the polymer network, and introduce the mathematical models describing drug release profiles from these implants. We also examine specific properties of implants affecting release rate (eg., membrane porosity, pore/mesh size of polymer network, affinity of drug to polymer), and the advantages and disadvantages of this approach. The second part of this chapter discusses implants formulated with biodegradable polymers. We review the formulation techniques, polymer degradation mechanisms, and how these impact implant performance and drug release, and additional factors influencing drug release. Two types of formulations, namely, implantable and injectable, are discussed along with pertinent concepts and case studies. Finally we discuss the relevant challenges associated with these types of implants and provide an overview of the future cutting-edge research directions currently underway in this exciting field.

7.2   NONDEGRADABLE POLYMERIC IMPLANTS

Early attempts at the temporal control of drug administration included tablet coatings that slowly dissolve, suspensions (solid insoluble drugs in a liquid vehicle), as well as emulsions (immiscible liquids combined to form a liquid drug in a liquid vehicle) [1]. Not until the 1960s did the concept of using nondegradable implants for sustained release of therapeutic agents become popular [1–3]. Nondegradable polymers were used because they are relatively inert and biocompatible while offering a simple means of controlling the release via diffusion through a semipermeable matrix [2, 3]. Judah Folkman first proposed that silicone capsules could be used as a drug carrier for a zero order release system due to the constant non-degrading matrix composition and fixed geometry [4]. Silicone has many advantages, for use as a drug eluting polymer depot, in that it is relatively inert, flexible, easily modified, and provides almost constant, linear release of the loaded drug. Modifications can be achieved by adjusting the degree of cross-linking which allows researchers to create tunable periods of controlled long-term drug release [5]. Silicone has been used in several commercially available contraceptive implants such as Norplant® (Leiras, Helsinki, Finland) and Jadelle® (Schering Oy, Berlin, Germany) [2]. Additionally, silicone has been used to deliver antibacterial drugs such as metronidazole and invermectin [6, 7] as well as chemotherapeutic drugs such as carmustine [8, 9].

Another nondegradable polymer commonly used for controlled release applications is poly(ethylene-*co*-vinyl acetate) or EVAc. EVAc is typically used as a drug eluting matrix and can deliver a range of therapeutics from proteins to low molecular weight (Mw) drugs [10, 11]. Clinically, this system has been employed to deliver the drug pilocarpine in order to treat glaucoma (Ocusert®, Johnson and Johnson—formerly Alza Corp.) [12]. EVAc is also used in contraception applications, delivering the hormone etonogestrel from an implantable rod commercially known as IMPLANON® (Organon, Oss Netherlands) [2]. While polydimethylsiloxane (PDMS) and EVAc are two of the most widely used nondegradable polymers in the field of drug delivery, several other polymer systems have been developed over the years. Polyvinyl alcohol (PVA) mixed with ethyl vinyl acetate (EVA) is utilized in Vitrasert (Bausch and Lomb, Rochester, NY), a commercial implant that delivers genciclovir into the eye to control cytomegalovirus retinitis common in AIDS patients [13]. Polyurethane is utilized not only as a covering for silicone breast implants but has also been used as an antibacterial coating for implants [14, 15].

7.2.1   Reservoir Versus Matrix Drug Delivery Systems

As introduced briefly in Chapter 1, most implantable controlled delivery systems can be classified into one of two structure categories: reservoir or matrix systems. Reservoir systems are defined as formulations in which the polymer is used to form a hollow membrane casing that encapsulates a drug reservoir (Fig. 7.1) [5, 16, 17]. In a reservoir system a drug does not need to be dissolved to be loaded into the implant, just encased within the device. One drawback for these release vehicles is that the sole driving force of release is diffusion, and as such the larger the drug is, the slower the

(a)

Drug filled
core

Polymer
membrane

(b)

Drug
distributed
throughout
polymer
matrix

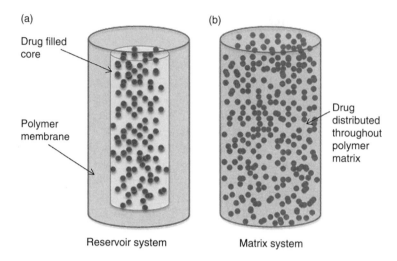

Reservoir system   Matrix system

Figure 7.1. Schematic representation of a reservoir system (a) and matrix system (b).

release rate will be. Additionally, if the membrane of the implant is ruptured, a bolus release of drug may occur, which could be fatal for the patient [5, 18]. A common example of a reservoir system is the Norplant silicone contraceptive implant. Release from a reservoir system is driven by diffusion through a number of barriers. First the drug must travel through the polymer membrane, then through the tissue surrounding the implant and finally into the blood stream. Release from a reservoir system can be modeled using Fick's first law (Eq. 7.1) [19]:

$$J = -D_{\text{d:p}}\frac{dc}{dx} \qquad (7.1)$$

where J is the flux of the drug, $D_{\text{d:p}}$ is the diffusion coefficient of drug through the polymer and dc/dx is the concentration gradient of the drug through the membrane [19]. This equation assumes that diffusion is one-dimensional, the diffusion coefficient is constant and the concentration gradient of drug through the membrane is relatively constant which is plausible only if there is a constant high concentration of drug at the membrane's inner edge [19]. To describe how diffusion changes the drug concentration over time, Fick's first law can be combined with a mass balance equation to derive Fick's second law (Eq. 7.2) [5].

$$\frac{\partial c}{\partial t} = D_{\text{d:p}}\frac{\partial^2 c_{\text{p}}}{\partial x^2} \qquad (7.2)$$

where $D_{\text{d:p}}$ is the diffusion coefficient of drug through the polymer, c_{p} is the concentration of the drug in the matrix, t is time, and x represents the spatial coordinate system of the drug within the matrix. This equation assumes that the drug diffuses into an infinite sink condition, that the implant is a flat plane, and that there is no convection, generation, or consumption of drug within the reservoir. With these assumptions,

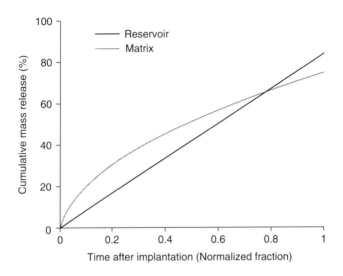

Figure 7.2. Comparison of the release profile from a matrix and reservoir implant.

release from a reservoir system is relatively linear (zero-order) as modeled in Fig. 7.2 [8, 20, 21]. Fick's second law can be modified to describe a spherical or cylindrical implant by changing the coordinate system of the equation.

A matrix based device can be described as a system in which the drug is distributed homogenously (in an ideal scenario) throughout the polymer [5]. This type of drug delivery system is often utilized when the desired drug release rate cannot be controlled sufficiently by use of a biocompatible polymer membrane [22]. The typical release profile from a matrix based implantable device follows first-order kinetics if the matrix is assumed to not swell or degrade [23, 24]. First there is an initial burst release of drug, followed by a slower release until equilibrium is reached (Fig. 7.2). One of the biggest advantages of matrix systems relative to reservoir systems is that there is no hazard of a bolus release of the drug, unless the entire system is damaged. However, one drawback of the release kinetics observed with matrix systems is that the release rate decreases over time [16, 22]. While zero-order release is ideal in many applications, for certain drugs such as leuprolide acetate (which is used to treat prostate cancer), a zero-order release profile would not be adequate. For an effective treatment, this therapy requires a high initial dose of drug followed by a lower maintenance dose [25]. Thus, the first-order release observed in a matrix delivery system can be beneficial.

Park et al. [23] derived an approximate equation to model release at the early stages of a planar non-swelling matrix implant from Fick's second law (Eq. 7.3):

$$\frac{M_t}{M_\infty} \cong 4\left(\frac{D_{d:p}t}{L^2\pi}\right)^2 \tag{7.3}$$

where M_t is the amount of drug inside the matrix over time, M_∞ is the total amount of drug in the matrix initially (and it is assumed that M_t/M_∞ is less than 60%), $D_{d:p}$ is the diffusion coefficient of drug through the polymer, t is time, and L is the length of the implant through which the drug must diffuse [23, 26]. This equation assumes that there is no change in the dimensions or degradation of the implant during the time of release [26]. Further modification of Fick's second law from Equation 7.3 can approximate release from a nonswelling matrix at the end of the release period ($0.4 \leq M_t/M_\infty \leq 1$) (Eq. 7.4) [27].

$$\frac{M_t}{M_\infty} \cong 1 - \left(\frac{8}{\pi^2}\right)\exp\left[\frac{\left(-\pi^2 D_{d:p}t\right)}{L^2}\right] \tag{7.4}$$

There are advantages and disadvantages to both the reservoir and matrix implant designs. Ultimately, the desired release profile will dictate which design can be used.

7.2.2 Factors Affecting Release from Nonbiodegradable Polymer Implants

Unlike the preformed degradable or *in situ* forming implants discussed later in this chapter, nondegradable implants have a fixed geometry and will not degrade or erode once placed within the body. Therefore, the number of factors affecting the release of the preloaded drug from these implants can be reduced to factors that alter the concentration of drug outside of the implant (which are discussed in detail later in this chapter) and factors that affect the diffusivity of the drug through the matrix such as (i) the size of the pore in the polymer membrane or matrix, (ii) the degree of pore connectivity and tortuosity within the matrix, (iii) the distribution of drug throughout the implant, and (iv) and the affinity of the drug for the polymer [8, 28].

The release from a nondegradable reservoir polymer implant system is primarily dependent on the size of the polymer's pores with respect to the size of the drug that will diffuse through them. Studies have shown that a macroporous polymer ($0.1-1$ μm) has pores much larger than the loaded drug, and will therefore have greater release over time. Microporous polymers ($5-20$ nm) release less drug because the pore size is often only slightly larger than the drug molecule, which reduces mass transport [24]. If the drug is larger than the pores, the drug will not diffuse out through the interconnected porous network (which have high diffusivity coefficients), but instead the drug must diffuse through the polymer rich domains (which has diffusivity coefficients that are orders of magnitude smaller) [18, 24, 29].

All reservoir and matrix implants can be considered to be a collection of interconnected pores and the degree of interconnectivity of these pores plays a large role in the release of drug from the preloaded matrix implant. If there are several pathways for the drug to diffuse through, a larger concentration of drug can be released over time from the implant (Fig. 7.3). Additionally, the tortuosity of the pores can play a role in altering drug release. Tortuosity is a measure of how twisted and curved the porous network is [30]. Much like traveling cross country, it is always better to

(a)   (b)

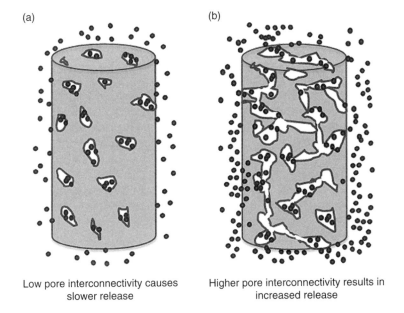

Low pore interconnectivity causes   Higher pore interconnectivity results in
slower release   increased release

Figure 7.3. (a, b) Schematic showing the effect of increased pore interconnectivity on drug release.

fly direct. The more tortuous the path, the longer it takes for the drug to reach its destination outside of the implant [10, 30].

The fraction of drug that is dissolved at any time during the implant lifetime also plays a role in release. In both reservoir and matrix systems there is a direct relationship between drug solubility in the surrounding interstitial fluid of the implantation environment and drug concentration in a dry implant. The higher the drug solubility the faster the release as only dissolved drug is available for diffusion [8, 20, 31, 32]. Distribution of drug throughout the implant matrix can also be a factor in the release profile with homogenous distribution at a low loading density contributing to lower immediate burst release [8, 19, 24].

Another factor that can affect the release of drug from a nondegradable implant is the affinity between the drug and the polymer. The degree of drug hydrophobicity with respect to the polymer will determine whether hydrophobic interactions will counteract or further facilitate the diffusional movement. A hydrophilic drug encapsulated within a hydrophobic polymer will diffuse out rapidly while a hydrophobic drug within a hydrophobic polymer will diffuse out more slowly because of its lack of affinity with the physiological hydrophilic environment surrounding the implant [5]. Drugs may also interact and bind with functional groups on the polymers which will decrease the overall release from the implant. One of the assumptions of purely diffusional release is that the drug is free to move randomly throughout the system and if the drug interacts and binds with polymer functional groups, that free random movement is limited resulting in overall slower release [1, 24]. Release from nondegradable implants can be modified by choosing a polymer with the appropriate properties in order to tailor the release profile to fit the desired application.

7.2.3 Clinical Example and Summary

One of the first and most commercially successful controlled release devices was Norplant, a female contraceptive implant developed in the 1970s [2, 33]. Norplant was successful because it was more effective in preventing pregnancy for a longer duration than any other contraceptive available at the time. The platform was composed of six flexible, silicone cylinders that released a synthetic hormone called levonorgestrel for effective contraception for up to 5 years [33, 34]. Norplant was a reservoir drug delivery system with a very slow, constant release rate; the capsules release 50 µg of levonorgestrel per day for the first 400 days after implantation, followed by a relatively steady release of 30 µg/day for the next 3000 days (or ~8.5 years) [33]. Norplant was typically implanted in a fan-like configuration in the subderma of the patient's upper arm in a minimally invasive outpatient procedure. The first clinical trials for Norplant began in 1980 and within a few years, it was approved by more than 50 countries [34, 35]. By 1992, Norplant was used by over 600,000 women in the United States alone [34, 35]. Post implantation, trials encompassing thousands of women over a ten year period were conducted in which the safety, efficacy, and release from Norplant were scrutinized. Low percentages of women receiving Norplant complained of headaches and weight gain because of the continued use of the hormone. Other more serious complaints such as hair loss, hypertension, uterine fibroids, and breast cancer were reported in less than 1% of the thousands of women surveyed [36, 37]. The most frequent complication seen with Norplant was the difficulty with which the implants were removed. Owing to the long implantation period, fibrous tissue occasionally formed in the area of the implants, making removal difficult. The removal procedures could also be painful and result in incomplete removal because of implant fracture and/or scarring in the area. In extreme cases, sonography was used to determine the exact location of the remaining rod [38]. The difficulty of implant removal seen with the Norplant rods is a common drawback of nondegradable implants.

While synthetic, nondegradable implants are still in use today, a large majority of the research and upcoming clinical applications revolve around the use of biodegradable polymers. This transition is a result of increased control over the release profile, as well as a reduction in possible complications and the number of required procedures, as removal is no longer necessary [1, 8, 11].

7.3 BIODEGRADABLE POLYMERIC IMPLANTS

Biodegradable polymeric implants provide a useful means of controlled drug release without the need for the surgical removal of the implants after their expiration. While degradation results in more complicated implant design, these systems can provide additional, more flexible avenues by which dissolution of drug can be modulated. In this section, we describe the process of drug release from preformed polymer implants and *in situ* forming systems along with the factors that influence implant performance. The mechanisms of polymer degradation and erosion and the factors that influence or alter both processes are discussed. We are also review factors that affect implant-host interactions with the most common biodegradable polymers found in Food and Drug Administration (FDA) approved devices, and provide an overview of clinical applications using these polymers.

7.3.1 Degradation and Erosion

While a specific polymer cannot be approved by the FDA, there are five polymers commonly found in FDA approved devices that have demonstrated an appropriate host tissue response for their designated applications (Fig. 7.4). The polyetherester polydioxanone has been approved for use as suture clips and bone pins marketed as OrthoSorb [17]. The slow degrading semicrystalline poly(caprolactone) has been used for the controlled release of contraceptives and as a suture formerly marketed as Capronor and monocryl [17, 39]. Poly(PCPP-SA anhydride) has been used in the field of drug delivery in order to treat residual tumor cells after surgical resection and are marketed as the Gliadel Wafer® [5, 17, 40]. Finally, poly(glycolic acid) (PGA), poly(lactic acid) (PLA), and their copolymer (PLGA) have been used as degradable sutures, bone pins, and drug delivery vehicles marketed as the Leupron depot, Atrigel, Eligard, Atridox, Dexon, and Vicryl [17, 25, 41–45].

Biodegradable implants lose mass over time as a function of polymer degradation and erosion. Polymer degradation refers to the process by which the repeating structural units of the polymer chain are cleaved resulting in a reduction in Mw (Fig. 7.5). This can be facilitated by a number of factors [5, 46, 47]. For example,

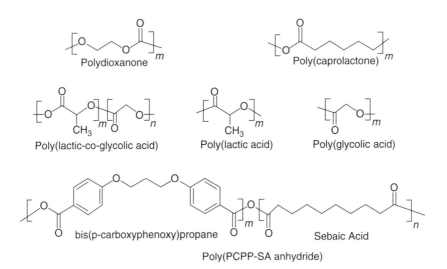

Figure 7.4. Chemical structures of the polymers commonly used in FDA approved devices.

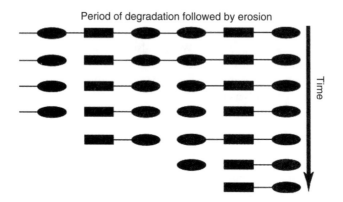

Figure 7.5. Schematic of the degradation and erosion process, where the ellipses and squares represent the subunits of the polymer backbone, and the lines represent the degradable bonds. The top row is the nondegraded polymer. The loss of the lines represents the degradation process while the loss of subunits over time represents erosion after degradation has occurred.

enzymes can catalyze the polymer degradation process which is sometimes referred to as biodegradation. Polymer degradation can also be initiated by external factors such as the presence of UV light, mechanical perturbation, as well as γ-radiation, which is used to sterilize the polymers for clinical applications [46]. For drug delivery purposes, the most common method of degradation occurs through hydrolysis (occurring in both polyesters and polyanhydrides), which is the cleavage of the polymer backbone because of the interactions of the polymer with water [46–48].

After the polymer begins to degrade, the loss of the oligomers and monomers to the surrounding environment facilitates a reduction of polymer mass, and is known as erosion [5, 17, 46, 47, 49]. When erosion is enhanced by physiological processes, it is referred to as bioerosion [5]. As erosion is simply the loss of mass over time, it does not always require degradative processes in order to occur. In the case of a matrix containing water-soluble components, erosion can occur simply through dissolution of the matrix [5], such as a cookie crumbling in milk or a bar of soap reducing in size with use. Erosion is a process that can occur solely on the surface of the implant through a process known as surface erosion (which is the case in the soap example), or throughout the bulk of the polymer, which is then referred to as bulk erosion, as in the cookie example (Fig. 7.6). The primary factor that determines whether the polymer will be surface eroding or bulk eroding is the reaction kinetics of degradation. If the rate of polymer degradation is faster than the rate of water diffusion into the polymer, then the polymer will be surface eroding. If the rate of water diffusion is faster than the reaction kinetics, then the polymer will be bulk eroding [50].

It is the presence of hydrolysable bonds in the polymer backbone that allows for tunable degradation and erosion profiles; therefore, the choice of chemical bond is a critical factor in controlling the rate of degradation and the method by which the polymer will erode. The three most common chemical bonds found in controlled

Bulk eroding implant

Surface eroding implant

Time

Figure 7.6. Schematic illustrating the difference between bulk and surface erosion.

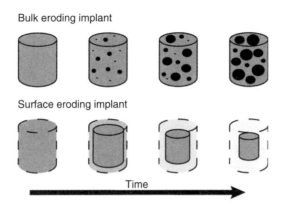

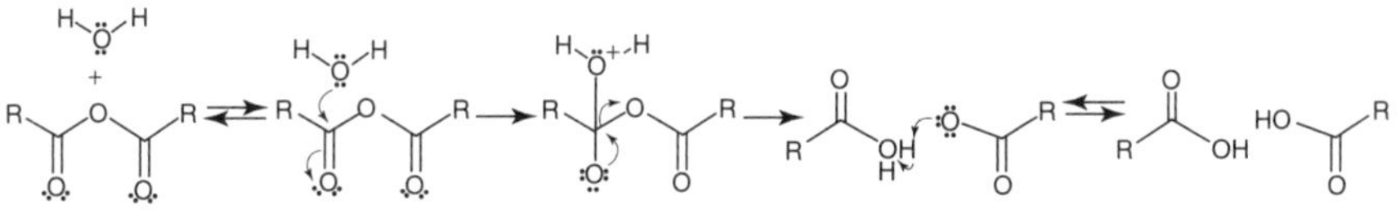

Figure 7.7. Anhydride reaction with water; arrows represent the movement of electrons.

release devices listed in order of reactivity are: anhydrides, esters, and amides [46, 51]. While both esters and amides require either acidic or basic conditions in order for hydrolysis to occur, the reactivity of anhydrides is high enough that hydrolysis occurs under neutral conditions, only requiring the presence of moisture in the air to initiate degradation [51, 52]. The reaction begins when the oxygen of water acts as a nucleophile, and attacks one of the anhydride carbonyls, which leads to the elimination of one carboxylic acid and the formation of a second (Fig. 7.7).

As esters are less reactive than anhydrides, an acidic or alkaline environment is needed for their hydrolysis. When the hydrolysis is acid-catalyzed, the reaction is a reversible process, requiring the presence of excess water or removal of degradation by-product [51, 52]. The two stage reaction begins when a free hydrogen cation associates with the carbonyl, which allows water to act as a nucleophile, forming a tetrahedral intermediate that facilitates the alcohol to act as a leaving group (Fig. 7.8) [52]. When the reaction occurs in an alkaline environment, free hydroxyl anions act as a nuclophile. The nucleophilic attack leads to the formation of a tetrahedral intermediate causing the elimination of an alcohol. Like acid-catalyzed hydrolysis, this reaction leads to the formation of a carboxylic acid and an alcohol, but it is not an equilibrium reaction and will continue until the polymer has completely degraded. The hydrolysis of amides is similar to esters and can occur in either alkaline or acidic environments. However, because the bond is less reactive than an ester linkage, stronger conditions are required in order for hydrolysis to occur [51, 52]. Both ester

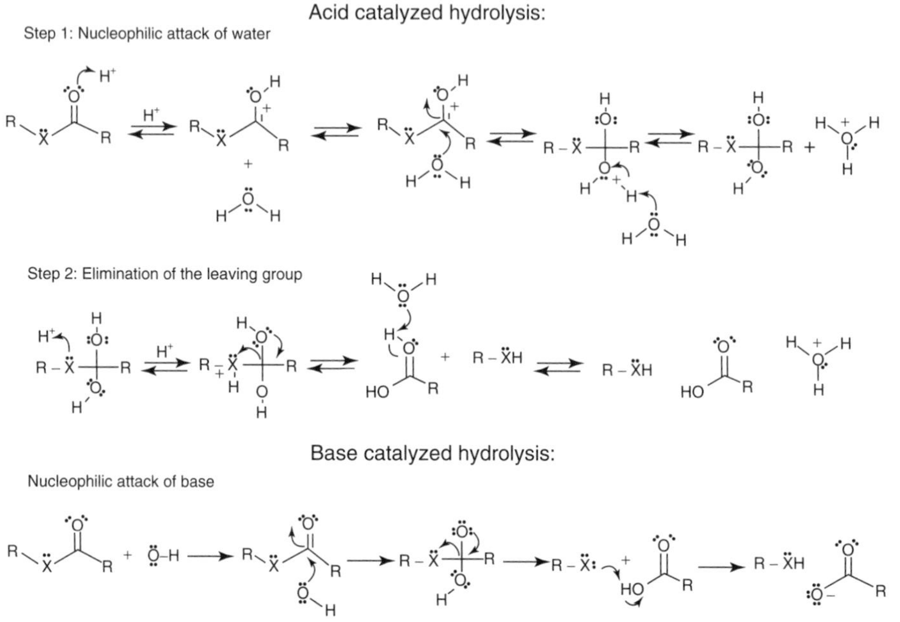

Acid catalyzed hydrolysis:

Step 1: Nucleophilic attack of water

Step 2: Elimination of the leaving group

Base catalyzed hydrolysis:

Nucleophilic attack of base

Figure 7.8. (a) Hydrolysis of an ester in an acidic and alkaline medium resulting in the formation of an alcohol and carboxylic acid, arrows represent the movement of electrons. (b) Hydrolysis of an amide in an acidic medium resulting in the formation of an alcohol and amine, arrows represent the movement of electrons.

hydrolysis and amide hydrolysis leads to the formation of a carboxylic acid, but unlike ester hydrolysis the eliminated group from amide hydrolysis is an amine (Fig. 7.8).

While the chemical bond used to form the polymer backbone is an important factor in controlling the rate of polymer degradation, the groups adjacent to the reactive bond can also be important factors. For example, the methyl group found on PLA, leads to a slower degradation rate than what is observed in PGA because of the presence of the hydrophobic moiety, which sterically hinders the nucleophilic attack of water [46, 53, 54]. As the erosion profile of a polymer is sensitive to both the rate of degradation as well as the rate of water uptake, parameters that decrease the influx of water can be used to alter the erosion profile of the implant. Therefore, the polymer hydrophobicity is an important parameter in controlling whether the polymer will be a surface or bulk eroding polymer.

Crystallinity is a measure of the polymer ability to form a structured array, which occurs as a result of the chain regularity, and is typically reported as a percentage of crystallinity [55]. Owing to the close packing inherent in crystalline domains, the free volume for diffusion is lower in the crystalline regions, which can decrease diffusion coefficients by several orders of magnitude and play a role in altering the rate of polymer degradation [48, 56]. Owing to the random nature of polymers, there will always be amorphous domains such that a polymer can never be purely crystalline [17]. Crystalline domains can be present initially, or can form as a result of oligomer formation caused by polymer degradation, leading to latent crystallization [46, 56, 57].

In addition to polymer crystallinity, the glass transition temperature (T_g) has been shown to play a role in altering the free volume available for diffusion. The T_g is the temperature at which the polymer transitions from a glassy state into a rubbery state. When a polymer is above the glass transition temperature, the free volume is higher, which results in an increased diffusivity [56]. Even the physical dimensions of the polymer can be used to transition a system from bulk eroding to surface eroding [50]. For systems that have low water absorption and rapid degradation kinetics, the implants would have to be extremely small in order to behave as a bulk eroding system. For example a poly(anhydride) disk would need to be smaller than 75 μm thick in order to behave as a bulk eroding system [50]. Conversely, polymer disks that rapidly absorb water with slow degradation kinetics would have to be significantly thicker to behave as a surface eroding system. A poly(α-hydroxy-ester) would need to be at least 7.4 cm thick to surface erode, while a poly(amide) which is even less reactive would need to be at least 13.4 m thick [50].

7.3.2 Biocompatibility

With the insertion of any material into the body, understanding how the host and implant will interact is imperative. Biocompatibility describes the ability of an implanted material to maintain performance without initiating a negative host response [17, 58, 59]. Biocompatibility is often evaluated based on the inflammatory and healing responses of the body to a particular implant [58]. The tissue response continuum, as explained by Anderson et al. [58] organizes the host response to implantation into a sequence of events characterized by the cell types which are present. Phase I, or the acute and chronic inflammatory phase occurs over the course of the first two weeks, and is initiated by the implantation or direct injection of the device. During phase I, neutrophils, monocytes, and lymphocytes will be present with monocytes becoming the dominant cell type within days of implantation. Phase II is characterized by an excess of monocytes and macrophages, leading to the development of a fibrous capsule around the implant. The duration of the second phase is determined by the rate of polymer degradation, and can take as little as 50 days or more than 400 days [58, 60–63]. Phase III is dominated by the degradation of polymer and an increase of fibrous tissue filling the void left behind by the eroding polymer [58]. Histological evaluation of the tissue response has proven useful in categorizing the effect of introducing an implant to the local environment.

One major concern when using a degradable device is the toxicity of the degradation by-products. In the case of PLA, PGA, and their copolymer PLGA, the polymer was designed to degrade into natural metabolites. The hydrolytic degradation of these polyesters results in the formation of lactic and/or glycolic acid, based on the original polymer used [59, 64, 65]. In healthy tissues with high clearance, these intermediates are metabolized by the body into carbon dioxide and water and show no adverse effects on introduction of the material to the body [66]. However, in situations where the clearance is low, which may occur as a result of a diseased state or be a function of injection site with low metabolism and overall clearance, the effect of elevated levels of acidic by-products must be considered. Therefore, the clearance rate of these compounds is an important parameter in implant design.

Other factors to consider when evaluating biocompatibility of a device are additives such as fillers, plasticizers, stabilizers, and excipients. Additives are typically used to modify an implant's properties and to reduce manufacturing costs [67]. For example, fillers and plasticizers are typically used to alter the mechanical properties of the implants and even used to change the outer membrane behavior of some pills [67–75]. The plasticizer di(2-ethylhexyl)phthalate (DEHP) has been used to soften the poly(vinyl chloride) polymer used to make blood storage bags since 1955 [73, 74]. Plasticizers typically increase the flexibility of the plastic by disrupting the crystallinity of the polymer, and increasing the free volume of the material, which lowers the glass transition temperature of the material [76]. Fillers such as carbon black and silica have been used to reinforce the mechanical properties of polymeric devices. The interaction of fillers with the polymer matrix is complex, and reinforcement is not a result of a single interaction [67]. One way in which the fillers can reinforce polymers is by forming a network (when the filler concentration is above the percolation threshold) within a material that provides additional mechanical support [70, 71, 77], and second by interacting with the polymer which alters the chain mobility of the polymer [70, 72, 77]. Other common additives such as stabilizers are used to protect the degradable units within a polymer backbone. Common examples of stabilizers include antioxidants such as vitamin E which has been used to reduce oxidative stress that degrades the amorphous domains in poly(etherurethanes), which are commonly used in medical devices [78]. Excipients are additives which are used to improve drug solubility and biodistribution, but are completely inert in the host, such as cyclodextran [79, 80]. These ring shaped molecules have two distinct domains, a hydrophobic interior and a hydrophilic exterior [79]. When put in contact with poorly soluble drugs (such as doxorubicin), the drug interacts with the interior domain, and the hydrophilic exterior interacts with the aqueous environment leading to improved drug solubility [79].

Some additives not only alter implant behavior, but also have desirable therapeutic properties. For example, the use of a triblock copolymer Pluronic® has been shown to reduce the diffusivity of drug from polymer implants, but these additives have also been shown to inhibit a cell's ability to recover from heat, sensitizing the cell to elevated temperatures [81–85]. Therefore, the effect of additives used must be carefully evaluated to insure that the additive does not induce a negative effect.

7.3.3 Implantable Systems

Drug eluting depots provide a unique way in which plasma concentrations of the delivered therapeutic can be maintained within a narrow window as well as providing a means for achieving elevated local concentrations of drug while limiting systemic involvement [82, 86]. In addition to improving patient compliance, controlling drug release via implantable systems can reduce systemic side effects and patient discomfort [9, 25, 82, 87, 88]. Pre-formed polymer implants have a defined geometric structure, which leads to predictable and reproducible release and degradation profiles for extended periods of time. The therapeutic agent can be trapped homogenously within the encapsulating matrix or formed as a composite for more complex release profiles [82]. While both degradable and nondegradable implants are dependent on the properties of the encapsulating polymer matrix, as the implants degrade over time there is no need for surgical removal [5, 9, 82, 87, 88].

Fabrication of preformed polymer implants can be achieved using a number of techniques including: compression molding, melt casting, solvent casting, and extrusion [9, 81, 86]. Implants fabricated using compression molding are made by first mixing the polymer and drug in a piston shaped mold, then applying elevated pressure at $5-10\,°C$ above T_g to create disk or rod shaped implants [86, 89, 90]. The low fabrication temperature is beneficial for maintaining activity of reactive drugs, since the drug may not be homogenously distributed, there can be a large variability in drug release [86]. Implants formed using melt molding require that the polymer is elevated above T_m, resulting in a viscous solution in which the drug can be homogenously mixed and subsequently solidified in a mold of the desired geometry [86]. The fabricated implant has a reproducible release profile, but the elevated temperature can result in a loss of therapeutic activity if the drug is sensitive to temperature, especially when proteins are used as therapeutics [86]. Solvent casting is performed by dissolving the polymer in a volatile solvent, with drug if the drug is soluble. If the drug is nonsoluble then the powdered drug is homogenously distributed into the polymer solution. The solution can then be added to a mold of the desired geometry and maintained at a lowered temperature so that the solvent will evaporate off slowly [86]. Solvent casting provides a technique with which to fabricate implants loaded with heat sensitive drugs, but this technique has a number of disadvantages. The phase inversion dynamics intrinsic to solvent evaporation can lead to a porous microstructure, resulting in implants with poor mechanical properties, as well as have the potential to deactivate the therapeutic agent [86]. Additionally, because of the amount of time required for the solvent to evaporate, the suspended drug may not stay homogenously distributed in the matrix [86].

Dual release can be achieved through processes known as dip coating, where the preformed implants are dipped into a polymer solution containing a water soluble component such as NaCl or poly(ethylene oxide) and drug in order to form a thin outer membrane [82, 88, 89]. Once implanted into the tissue, the aqueous environment leads to the dissolution of the soluble component and an initial burst release from the porous outer membrane [82, 89]. Ultimately it is the properties of the drug and the desired application that will dictate the fabrication technique used to make the implant.

Drug release is not only affected by the geometry of the implant; the rate of dissolution can be affected by factors such as the ratio of polymer relative to other components in the implant, how the drug is loaded into the implant, the crystallinity of the polymer, the crystallinity of the drug, as well as implant microstructure [16, 46, 49, 56, 57, 86, 91–94].

Percolation theory provides an ideal means by which the effect of drug loading can be evaluated on implant behavior. In percolation theory the matrix is envisioned as a lattice of interconnected points, and the introduction of drug removes a point from the lattice. Initially, the reduction of points in the lattice does not overly disrupt the lattice stability, but as the number of points in the lattice continue to disappear so does the stability of the system. The critical point at which the polymer no longer forms a connected network, is referred to as the percolation threshold [47, 95, 96]. In addition to the percolation threshold, polymer crystallinity can play a role as to where the drug partitions within the system [57, 92]. Typically drug diffuses through the implant pores; therefore, high interconnectivity leads to elevated release.

Similar to nondegradable systems, factors such as the size of the drug diffusing through the polymer network, the affinity of the drug with the polymer, and the tortuosity of the porous network all influence release from the implant [5]. The key difference is that diffusivity of degrading implant systems change as a function of polymer degradation. Simple models of release for bulk eroding systems assume that polymer degradation follows first-order kinetics, leading to an exponential increase in diffusion with respect to time [56].

$$\frac{d[COOH]}{dt} = k[COOH][H_2O][Ester] \tag{7.5}$$

$$D_{eff} = D_0 e^{kt} \tag{7.6}$$

$$\frac{\partial c}{\partial t} = D_{eff} \frac{\partial^2 c_d}{\partial x^2} \tag{7.7}$$

In Eqs. 7.5 and 7.6, [COOH] refers to the concentration of carboxylic acid, $[H_2O]$ refers to the concentration of water, [Ester] refers to the total concentration of degradable esters, k is the first-order degradation kinetic constant of the polymer, D_{eff} is the effective diffusivity as a function of the degradation kinetics, D_0 is the initial diffusivity at time zero before degradation begins, and t is time [56]. The first-order degradation kinetics can be determined from the changes in polymer Mw over time and makes the simplifying assumption that there is a near constant concentration of both the hydrolysable esters and water [48, 97, 98]. The effective diffusivity coefficient can then be used with the general models of diffusion. The result of degradation is an increase in release over time as the polymer diffusivity changes (Fig. 7.9). For surface eroding systems, release of drug is typically proportional to the rate of polymer erosion [86]. For *in vivo* systems, evaluating drug release is more complex because of the presence of cells and microvascularization in the tissue space [9, 89, 99, 100]. Evaluation of release from these systems requires multidimensional analysis of the implant and surrounding tissue, with careful consideration of the boundary conditions between the implant and tissue interface. For this system, the rate of drug distribution within the surrounding tissue involves investigating the diffusion of drug within the

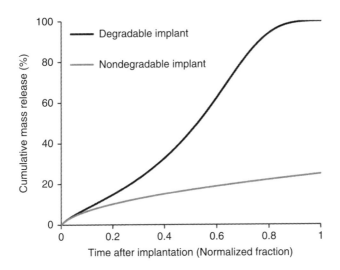

Figure 7.9. Cumulative release over time from a degrading and nondegrading polymer implant.

tissue space from the implant, the elimination of the drug by the vasculature, and the metabolism of the drug by the cells [9, 89, 99, 100].

$$\frac{\partial C}{\partial t} = D\nabla^2 C - v\nabla C - kC \tag{7.8}$$

where k is the rate of drug metabolism, the v accounts for the velocity of the surrounding vasculature, and D is the diffusivity of drug from the implant to the surrounding tissue [9]. A result of diffusion-based local release is that the metabolic activity of the cells and the removal of drug as a function of the microvasculature limits the distribution distance of the drug within the tissue.

7.3.4 Clinical Example of Preformed Polymer Implants

Preformed implants have been successfully implemented as a means for adjuvant therapy, most notably in the form of a surface eroding polyanhydride polymer disk that is inserted directly into the resected tissue space and used to treat malignant gliomas [40, 82, 88, 101–103]. These wafers, commercially known as the Gliadel® wafers (MGI Pharma, Inc., Bloomington, USA) received FDA approval in September of 2006 and are currently the only commercially available solid intratumoral chemotherapeutic device [82, 88, 103]. As these devices were approved by the FDA, they have been used in over 20,000 patients in the United States alone [103].

The wafers are composed of a 20:80 molar ratio of poly(bis[p-carboxyphenoxy]) propane:sebacic acid (PCPP:SA), and loaded with the lipophilic anticancer drug carmustine (1,3-bis(2-chloroethyl)-1-nitrosourea, or BCNU) [103]. The disks slowly erode over the course of 2–3 weeks, with degradation by-products eliminated in the urine or as CO_2 from the lungs [104]. These implants are fabricated to have a 7.25 mm radius and are 1 mm thick loaded with 3.85 wt% drug, and have an average weight of 200 mg [103]. As many as eight wafers can be implanted into the resected tissue space and are used to treat cancer cells that may not have been removed during the surgical procedure. This reduces the risk of recurrence by eliminating residual cancer cells along the tumor periphery. These implant systems have shown modest success in the treatment of malignant gliomas by increasing the chance of survival up to 50%, and increasing the median survival times by 2 months [105].

7.3.5 Injectable Systems

Injectable *in situ* forming implants (ISFIs) are liquid formulations comprised of biodegradable polymers mixed with bioactive therapeutic agents which can be injected into a target tissue. Once in place, the solution forms a solid or semisolid depot from which drugs can be released in a controlled manner. This liquid to solid phase transition takes place in response to a stimulus such as temperature, pH, enzymatic activity, or solvent miscibility. In recent years, ISFIs have garnered increased attention because of their versatility, ease of manufacturing, potential for improved patient compliance, and minimally invasive placement using needles as small as 21-gauge for the implant injection. This is in contrast to preformed implant systems which often require local anesthesia and minimally invasive surgical placement [106]. ISFIs can be divided into five categories based on the mechanism of transition from liquid to solid: (i) thermoplastic pastes, (ii) thermally induced gelling systems, (iii) *in situ* cross-linked systems, (iv) *in situ* solidifying organogels, and (iv) *in situ* precipitating or phase inverting implants [107]. Table 7.1 summarizes each of these categories.

Thermoplastic pastes (or thermopastes) are polymers that can be injected in the molten form and solidify as they cool down to body temperature. These polymers typically have a low melting temperature, ranging from 25 to 65 °C, and have an intrinsic viscosity ranging from 0.05 to 0.8 dl/g (determined and measured at 25 °C) [108]. Common thermopastes include PLA, PGA, PCL, and poly(trimethylene carbonate) [108, 109].

Conversely, thermally induced gelling systems are liquid at room temperature, and form a gel at temperatures above the lower critical solution temperature (LCST). Lower critical phase separation is governed by the balance between hydrophobic and hydrophilic moieties on the polymer chain and is driven by the negative entropy of mixing. The Gibbs free energy change for the mixing of two phases is negative below the LCST and positive above. When temperature increases to the LCST, the hydrogen bonding between polymer and water becomes energetically unfavorable compared to polymer–polymer and water–water interactions. Then an abrupt transition occurs as the hydrated hydrophilic molecule quickly dehydrates and changes to a more hydrophobic structure [110]. A number of polymer modifications can be used to alter the temperature at which this transition occurs [106, 111, 112]. Examples of this system include poly(*N*-isopropyl acrylamide) (poly(NIPAAM)), PEO–PPO–PEO

TABLE 7.1. Summary of *In Situ* Forming Implant (ISFI) Categories

ISFI Category	Formation and System Requirements	Representative Polymers
Thermoplastic pastes	Polymers injected in the molten state and form an implant when cooling down to body temperature Low melting temperature of 25–65 °C and an intrinsic viscosity from 0.05 to 0.8 dl/g, at 25 °C are required [108]	poly(D,L-lactide) poly(glycolide) poly(Ccaprolactone) poly(trimethylene carbonate) [108, 109]
Thermally-induced gels	Temperature is used to control critical phase separation in thermosensitive polymers. Systems are liquid at room temperature, and form a gel at and above the lower critical solution temperature (LCST) [106, 111, 112]	poly(N-isopropyl acrylamide) poly(ethylene oxide) PEO–PPO–PEO triblock copolymers poly(ethylene oxide)-poly(L-lactic acid) PEG–PLGA–PEG [113, 114, 165, 115, 116]
Cross-linked systems	Polymer chains cross-linked to form solid polymers or gels Cross-linking source can be: heat initiation, photon absorption, and ionic mediated reactions [166]	poly(D,L-lactide-*co*-caprolactone) PEG-oligoglycolylacrylates alginate 1,2-bis(palmitoyl) glycero-3-phosphocoline 1,2-bis(myristoyl)-glycero-3-phophocoline [118–121]
In situ solidifying organogels	Amphiphilic organogels are waxy at room temperature and form a cubic liquid crystal phase on injection into aqueous medium Glycerol esters of fatty acid-based systems are most common [122]	Amphiphilic lipids oils such as peanut oil waxes [124–126]
In situ precipitating systems	Implant forms through a process called phase inversion where solvent diffuses into the aqueous environment while water diffuses into polymer system [129, 130] Typically comprising water insoluble polymer dissolved in a water miscible, biocompatible solvent	poly(DL-lactide) poly(DL-lactide-*co*-glycolide) poly(DL-lactide-*co*-Ccaprolactone) Poly(ethylene carbonate) Fluoroalkyl-poly(ethylene glycol) [106, 107, 118, 131]

copolymers (Pluronics®), and PEG–PLA as well as PEG–PLGA–PEG copolymers [113–117].

In situ cross-linked polymer systems form cross-links at the injection site because of heat, photon absorption, or ionic mediated interactions. On initiation of the cross-linking reaction, the solutions can then transition into a solid polymer depot or gel *in situ*. Polymers such as PCL, PEG-oligoglycolylacrylates, alginate, 1,2-bis(palmitoyl)-glycero-3-phosphocoline (DPPC), 1,2-bis(myristoyl)-glycero-3-phophocoline (DMPC) have been used with *in situ* forming cross-link systems [118–121]. For example, a photon initiated biodegradable hydrogel drug delivery system introduced by Hubbell et al. [119] consists of a polymer with at least two free radical-polymerizable regions (PEG-oligoglycolylacrylates), a photosensitive initiator (eosin dye) and a photon source (visible light). The polymer begins to cross-link and form a network after it is exposed to the photoinitiator and light source. The formed networks can be used to deliver drugs at a controlled rate.

In situ solidifying organogels are amphiphilic organogel waxes at room temperature and transition into a cubic liquid crystal phase on injection into aqueous medium [122]. Cubic liquid crystal phases are unique structures formed by amphiphilic molecules which organize into a tortuous array of hydrophilic and hydrophobic domains [123]. This unique structure provides regions for both hydrophilic and hydrophobic drugs to accumulate, and because of the tortuous paths, provide a means of controlling release from these structures [122]. Amphiphilic lipids, oils such as peanut oil, waxes, and glycerol esters of fatty acids are among the most commonly used organogels for drug delivery applications [124–126].

Another class of ISFI uses phase sensitivity to elicit a transition into a solid drug eluting depot, and will be the focus of the remainder of the chapter. Phase sensitive ISFI are comprised of a water insoluble biodegradable polymer dissolved in an organic biocompatible solvent [127, 128]. Drugs can be suspended into this polymer solution with mechanical agitation or dissolved directly into the polymer solution [118, 127]. Counter transport of solvent and water begins the instant the polymer solution is in contact with an aqueous environment. The solvent/nonsolvent exchange results in the precipitation of the polymer, forming an implant once the water concentration becomes sufficiently high to stabilize the tertiary system [129, 130]. The transition into a solid depot is known as phase inversion. These implants have received significant attention as the phase transition only requires contact with an aqueous environment while other ISF categories typically require an external initiator such as heat or light. The phase inversion process is illustrated in Fig. 7.10. Common polymers used in this system are PLGA, PCL, PLA, poly(ethylene carbonate), sucrose acetate isobutyrate, and fluoroalkyl-ended poly(ethylene glycol) [106, 107, 118, 131].

Earlier in this chapter we examined how polymer degradation and erosion affect drug release. ISFI behavior and resulting drug release are also dependent on these processes, however phase inversion can also significantly alter the release profile. Phase inverting systems are typically classified into two categories, fast phase inverting (FPI) implants and slow phase inverting (SPI) implants [91–93, 128, 132]. FPIs require a highly water miscible solvent such as *N*-methyl-2-pyrrolidone (NMP) or dimethyl sulfoxide (DMSO) [91, 132]. The high solvent miscibility results in a rapid rate of phase

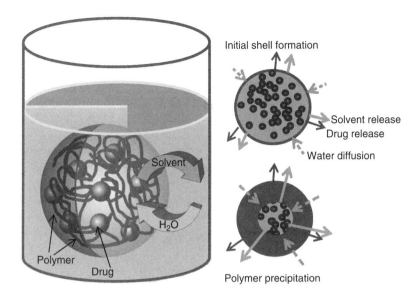

Figure 7.10. Schematic representation of the phase inversion process.

inversion, leading to the formation of a thin, dense shell which acts as a diffusional barrier. Inside the interfacial polymer shell, droplets called polymer-lean domains form, which consist of both solvent and nonsolvent. Owing to the reduced nonsolvent/solvent exchange, polymer-lean domains begin to expand [133]. As a result, the implants develop a vast network of interconnected pores and macrovoids (Fig. 7.11) [134–137]. As a consequence of the resultant morphology, drug release is elevated. Initially, there is a burst release of drug, followed by a diffusion facilitated phase which will begin to plateau as the drug trapped within the interconnected porous network is depleted (Fig. 7.11). Finally, the release rate increases as the polymer degrades and the diffusivity of the drug increases [137, 138].

SPIs require a solvent that has low miscibility in water, such as ethyl benzoate. The low miscibility of the solvent reduces the counter transport responsible for phase inversion, leading to a slow rate of polymer precipitation [91, 93, 128, 136]. The slow rate of solvent exchange leads to the formation of a dense matrix with low diffusivity and negligible pore formation [134, 139]. The absence of the porous network observed with FPI systems, forces drug to diffuse through the viscous polymer. Therefore, a nearly zero-order release can be achieved with this system. These solutions often have a high viscosity (especially when compared with FPIs), which can make injection extremely difficult. Combined solvent systems have also been developed to achieve intermediate release profiles [93, 140–143]. The combination of NMP and triacetin has been shown to reduce the rate of drug release [144], changing the morphology into a less porous structure [93]. Also the addition of water miscible solvents has been shown to decrease the solution viscosity and improve the injectability of SPI systems [142, 145, 146].

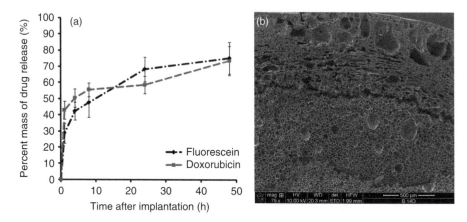

Figure 7.11. (a) Doxorubicin/fluorescein (drug/drug model) release profile showing FPI effects. (b) Morphology of an FPI system as imaged by scanning electron microscope (SEM). Adapted from Reference [137] with kind permission from Springer Science and Business Media.

Additives have also been used to modify the release rate from FPI systems. The surfactant Pluronic® has been used to reduce burst release by decreasing the diffusivity of drug within the porous network [147, 148]. The hydrophobic PPO block of Pluronic is hypothesized to incorporate with the polymer phase, while the hydrophilic PEO block extends into the polymer-lean region. When the concentration of Pluronic is significantly high, the additive fills the interconnected pores and acts as a barrier for diffusion and reduces the burst release [147]. If the Pluronic concentration exceeds the percolation threshold, there will no longer be a sufficient mass of polymer available resulting in an elevated release of drug [148]. Other additives that have been reported to effectively reduce the rate of drug release are heptanoate and glycerol [149]. While the majority of the additives are utilized to reduce burst release, some additives such as polyvinylpyrrolidone (PVP) and aliphatic esters have the opposite effect, which have been shown to increase the drug release [93, 150].

Like the cosolvent system, a combined polymer system can also be used to control drug release profiles and fit the specific delivery requirements [151–155]. Many studies have been done to tune the drug release profile by changing the polymer properties such as the Mw of the polymer and the polymer concentration in the solvent [148, 156–158]. For instance, Lambert and Peck studied changing solvent, polymer Mw, polymer concentration in the system to manipulate the release of FITC-bovine serum albumin from PLGA implants. They found that for high PLGA Mw (75–115 kDa) higher polymer concentration will lead to smaller burst release. For low Mw (10–15 kDa), the initial burst of drug release was eliminated by a much higher concentration of polymer in solution [159]. The results are shown in Fig. 7.12.

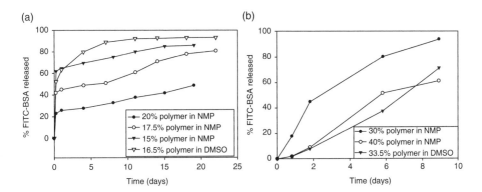

Figure 7.12. (a) FTIC-BSA release from high MW 50:50 system, polymer concentration is between 15–20%. (b) FITC-BSA release from low MW 50:50 system, polymer concentration is between 30–40%. Reprinted from the Journal of Controlled Release, Reference [159], Copyright (1995), with permission from Elsevier.

7.3.6 Clinical Applications of ISF Implants

A number of ISF implant systems have been used in clinical applications. Products such as Eligard® (Sanofi-Aventis Inc., France), Atridox® (Zila Inc, Fort Collins, CO), and Zoladex® (AstraZeneca, UK) all use ISF technology [106]. Eligard is a formulation of leuprolide acetate (a luteinizing hormone-releasing hormone (LHRH) agonist) in the polymer solution Atrigel® (Atrix Laboratories, Fort Collins, CO), which consists of PLGA (PLA:PGA=75:25) dissolved in NMP [94, 127, 160]. Leuprolide acetate can be released for a period of up to 6 months from this system [161], and suppresses plasma testosterone levels which inhibits prostatic tumor growth.

Atridox is another ISFI system that uses Atrigel® to deliver the antibiotic doxycycline for the treatment of periodontal disease for a period of 21 days [106, 162]. As administration is minimally invasive, Atridox requires no anesthesia and can be administered in the dentist's office. The SABER® (Durect Corp., Cupertino, CA) delivery system utilizes a high viscosity polymer, sucrose acetate isobutyrate (SAIB), and a hydrophobic solvent such as benzyl benzoate to provide a depot with low viscosity and slow solvent diffusion for release times ranging from several hours to several weeks. Zoladex® is also a marketed product using this system to treat prostate cancer [106, 162].

7.3.7 Phase Inverting Implants and their Characterization

Most implantable systems are preformed using relatively standardized and reproducible manufacturing processes ensuring consistent shape and size [14]. The reproducible geometry provides them with a more consistent release behavior when compared to injectable systems. However, preformed implants require surgical placement and subsequent surgical removal if the implants are nondegradable, such as silicon elastomers [14]. For injectable phase inverting systems, the preparation is much simpler and the implants are administered with a simple injection. The release of drugs from both preformed systems and ISF systems is dependent on the surrounding physiological environment. Local micro-vasculature, cell metabolism of drugs, and potential interactions between drugs and the extracellular matrix will all reduce the distribution volume of drug in the tissue [9, 89, 99, 100]. Furthermore, owing to the *in situ* forming nature of injectable systems, the implant shape and size are not consistent and highly dependent on mechanical and chemical properties of the local environment. Thus their drug release profiles are more difficult to control [16, 17]. One study by Patel et al. [37] demonstrated that the poor *in vitro* and *in vivo* correlation of ISFIs was, in part, a result of the various physical properties of the surrounding environment.

In order to better understand the behavior of this system *in vivo*, recent research has focused on the development of noninvasive characterization techniques able to quantify longitudinal implant behavior. Ultrasound imaging is a technique recently applied for this purpose by Solorio et al. [157] (Fig. 7.13). In this technique, a transducer linearly emits short bursts of ultrasonic waves into a sample and echoes that reflect from materials of different properties are recorded. The backscattered signal can be characterized as a function of acoustic impedance which is determined by the material density and speed of sound in the material. Therefore, as the polymer system goes through the phase inversion process, the acoustic impedance changes, resulting in the development of an echo signal which can be detected by ultrasound [157]. This technique provides unique properties such as real time visualization of the phase inversion process and can be used to trace shape and composition changes

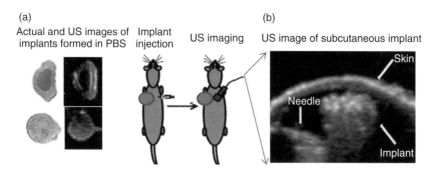

Figure 7.13. ISF implant formation imaged with ultrasound. (a) Images of two different implants formed in PBS along with photos of their cross-section. Dark areas on ultrasound image indicate more water-like core while lighter areas indicate precipitated polymer. (b) Ultrasound image of implant injection subcutaneously; arrows highlight the needle, skin and implant. Adapted from the Journal of Controlled Release, Reference [157], Copyright (2010), with permission from Elsevier.

of the implants over time. The technique is noninvasive, allowing an entire set of *in vivo* time course data to be collected using the same implant, thereby reducing environmental variability and the number of animals used [156].

Two other imaging techniques have been used to characterize injectable implant behavior: dark ground optics and electron paramagnetic resonance (EPR) [138]. Dark ground optics fuses both a dark ground fringe image and a reflected light image. The dark ground image shows the polymer distribution of the reactive index near the diffusion front while the reflected light image shows the solidification of the polymer. The fused image can be used to obtain information such as diffusion coefficients, liquid–liquid phase separation, and gel formation [163]. This method is simple and fast; however, it cannot be used to analyze implants *in vivo* [138].

EPR is based on interactions between electrons and a magnetic field. Electrons are aligned with the magnetic field that has been applied in a resonator, and, at the resonance frequency, unpaired electrons of the sample will be excited [138]. EPR can be used as an *in vivo* characterization technique, but the type and accuracy of the data collected are limited. For instance, the size and shape of the injected implant cannot be determined by EPR alone because EPR is more sensitive to mobility and kinetics of solvent/nonsolvent exchange. The direct biological environment influence of implant formation is also not available from EPR [164]. Furthermore, small Mw paramagnetic spin probes are required during the measurement, introducing another variable that can affect implant performance [157].

7.4   CONCLUSIONS AND FUTURE PERSPECTIVES

Implantable delivery systems are capable of overcoming many issues associated with enteral and IV administration of therapeutic agents. When used as a subcutaneous or intramuscular "storage depot" for extended systemic delivery, they can considerably improve the dosage schedule and can maintain an agent within its therapeutic window without inconveniencing the patient. They can also be used to focus the delivery of an agent at the desired site of action whether it is a solid unresectable tumor, an artery, or the eye. While not without issues, in many cases the strategies have been able to revolutionize the standard of care.

The evolution of implantable systems has been relatively rapid and has occurred with the changing needs of the clinical applications. Like the shift from nondegradable to more patient friendly biodegradable polymers used in their formulation, implants continue to adapt to the unyielding slew of new information, new technology, and new tools available for their design, engineering, and analysis. Continuing discovery and deeper understanding of the implants themselves and the impact of the implantation site on implant behavior *in vivo* has narrowed the criteria needed for engineering reproducible, successful systems.

Outstanding challenges still remain. With all implants, improved control, and on-demand modulation of drug release are of interest to many. Understanding the factors most influential in the poor *in vitro–in vivo* correlations of many implantable systems, and improving implant formulations to overcome these factors are also necessary.

Along the same lines, the development of more sophisticated *in vitro* phantoms that can better mimic the eventual clinical application is also of crucial importance. Such phantoms would permit simple, inexpensive, yet accurate, testing of new implantable formulations, streamlining research, discovery, and translation. Finally, for implants delivering drugs locally, an array of tools that can characterize their performance (implant formation, drug release, polymer degradation) *in vivo* is of great importance for the advancement of the field. Research into all of these aspects is ongoing and producing exciting developments every day. Advancements in implant technology will continue to escalate and increase future academic, industrial, and clinical interest.

7.5   KEY POINTS

- Administration from an implantable drug depot facilitates improved patient compliance over time, especially when dosing is frequent and inconvenient.
- Implantable technology can be used to achieve special and temporal control of drug delivery.
- Biodegradable implants are more patient friendly than nonbiodegradable implants.
- Patient compliance can be further improved by using injectable systems that form biodegradable networks *in vivo*.

7.6   HOMEWORK PROBLEMS

1. Re-create the release of Norplant in graphical format as well try to model the release by using a modification of Fick's first law.
2. What is the difference between erosion and degradation, how can these parameters be used to predict changes in drug release over time?
3. What effect does reaction kinetics have on determining whether a material will behave as a surface eroding or bulk eroding material? What parameters dictate how a material will erode? Predict what effect changes in the surrounding solution pH (i.e., a pH of 13 vs. a pH of 7) may have on degradation kinetics for a poly(α-hydroxy-ester), will it always behave as a bulk eroding polymer regardless of the solution pH?
4. Using the given assumptions for the first-order degradation kinetics, solve the underlying problem and describe how this can be used to determine the rate kinetics. Apply this equation to the general solution and demonstrate the effect that degradation kinetics have on cumulative drug release.
5. What are the benefits of local delivery, and what effect does the metabolic activity of the surrounding tissue have on the spatial distribution of drug released from these implants?
6. What causes the burst release of drug from the ISFIs and what can be done to eliminate this burst release?

REFERENCES

1. Langer R. Implantable controlled release systems. Pharmacol Ther 1983;21(1):35–51.

2. Shastri PV. Toxicology of polymers for implant contraceptives for women. Contraception 2002;65(1):9–13.

3. Pillai O, Panchagnula R. Polymers in drug delivery. Curr Opin Chem Biol 2001; 5(4):447–451.

4. Folkman J, Long DM. The use of silicone rubber as a carrier for prolonged drug therapy. J Surg Res 1964;4:139–142.

5. Saltzman WM. Drug Delivery: Engineering Principles for Drug Therapy. Oxford University Press; 2001. 198 Madison Ave., New York, New York 10016

6. Maeda H, Brandon M, Sano A. Design of controlled-release formulation for ivermectin using silicone. Int J Pharm 2003;261(1–2):9–19.

7. Malcolm RK et al. Controlled release of a model antibacterial drug from a novel self-lubricating silicone biomaterial. J Control Release 2004;97(2):313–320.

8. Dash AK, Cudworth GC. Therapeutic applications of implantable drug delivery systems. J Pharmacol Toxicol Methods 1998;40(1):1–12.

9. Saltzman WM, Fung LK. Polymeric implants for cancer chemotherapy. Adv Drug Deliv Rev 1997;26(2–3):209–230.

10. Hsu TT, Langer R. Polymers for the controlled release of macromolecules: effect of molecular weight of ethylene-vinyl acetate copolymer. J Biomed Mater Res 1985;19(4):445–460.

11. Pillai O, Dhanikula AB, Panchagnula R. Drug delivery: an odyssey of 100 years. Curr Opin Chem Biol 2001;5(4):439–446.

12. Okabe K et al. Intraocular tissue distribution of betamethasone after intrascleral administration using a non-biodegradable sustained drug delivery device. Invest Ophthalmol Vis Sci 2003;44(6):2702–2707.

13. Dhillon B, Kamal A, Leen C. Intravitreal sustained-release ganciclovir implantation to control cytomegalovirus retinitis in AIDS. Int J STD AIDS 1998;9(4):227–230.

14. Basak P et al. Sustained release of antibiotic from polyurethane coated implant materials. J Mater Sci Mater Med 2009;20:213–221.

15. Schierholz JM et al. Controlled release of antibiotics from biomedical polyurethanes: morphological and structural features. Biomaterials 1997;18(12):839–844.

16. Siepmann J, Siepmann F. Modeling of diffusion controlled drug delivery. J Control Release 2012;161(2):351–362.

17. Ratner BD. Biomaterials Science, Second Edition: An Introduction to Materials in Medicine. 2nd ed. Elsevier Academic Press; 2004;24-28 Oval Road, London NW1 7DX, UK.

18. Peppas NA, Gurny R. Relation between the structure of polymers and the controlled release of active ingredients. Pharm Acta Helv 1983;58(1):2–8.

19. Langer R. Polymer-controlled drug-delivery systems. Acc Chem Res 1993;26(10): 537–542.

20. Baker R. Controlled Release of Biologically Active Agents. Vol. 40. New York: John Wiley & Sons, Inc.; 1987.

21. Mantanus J et al. Near infrared and Raman spectroscopy as process analytical technology tools for the manufacturing of silicone-based drug reservoirs. Anal Chim Acta 2011;699(1):96–106.

22. Siegel RA. Pharmacokinetic transfer functions and generalized clearances. J Pharmacokinet Biopharm 1986;14(5):511–521.

23. Ferrero C, Massuelle D, Doelker E. Towards elucidation of the drug release mechanism from compressed hydrophilic matrices made of cellulose ethers. II. Evaluation of a possible swelling-controlled drug release mechanism using dimensionless analysis. J Control Release 2010;141(2):223–233.

24. Grassi M, Grassi G. Mathematical modeling and controlled drug delivery: matrix systems. Curr Drug Deliv 2005;2:97–116.

25. Ravivarapu HB, Moyer KL, Dunn RL. Sustained suppression of pituitary-gonadal axis with an injectable, in situ forming implant of leuprolide acetate. J Pharm Sci 2000; 89(6):732–741.

26. Fu Y, Kao WJ. Drug release kinetics and transport mechanisms of non-degradable and degradable polymeric delivery systems. Expert Opin Drug Deliv 2010;7(4):429–444.

27. Park K, Shalaby W, Park H. Biodegradable Hydrogels for Drug Delivery. Vol. 191. Technomic publishing company; 1993 851 New Holland Ave, Box 3535, Lancaster, PA, 17604.

28. Saltzman WM, Langer R. Transport rates of proteins in porous materials with known microgeometry. Biophys J 1989;55(1):163–171.

29. Ballal G, Zygourakis K. Diffusion in particles with varying cross-section. Chem Eng Sci 1985;40(8):1477–1483.

30. Fournier RL. Basic Transport Phenomenon in Biomedical Engineering. Taylor and Francis; 1999 325 Chestnut St., Philadelphia, PA, 19106.

31. Higuchi T. Rate of release of medicaments from ointment base containing drugs in suspension. J Pharm Sci 1961;50:874–879.

32. Lee PI. Novel-approach to zero-order drug delivery via immobilized nonuniform drug distribution in glassy hydrogels. J Pharm Sci 1984;73(10):1344–1347.

33. Sivin I. International experience with NORPLANT and NORPLANT-2 contraceptives. Stud Fam Plann 1988;19(2):81–94.

34. Sivin I et al. The performance of levonorgestrel rod and Norplant contraceptive implants: a 5 year randomized study. Hum Reprod 1998;13(12):3371–3378.

35. Meirik O, Fraser IS, d'Arcangues C. Implantable contraceptives for women. Hum Reprod Update 2003;9(1):49–59.

36. Mansour D. The benefits and risks of using a levonorgestrel-releasing intrauterine system for contraception. Contraception 2012;85(3):224–234.

37. Pritts EA et al. Angiogenic effects of norplant contraception on endometrial histology and uterine bleeding. J Clin Endocrinol Metab 2005;90(4):2142–2147.

38. Berg WA, Hamper UM. Norplant implants: sonographic identification and localization for removal. AJR Am J Roentgenol 1995;164(2):419–420.

39. de la Puerta B et al. In vitro comparison of mechanical and degradation properties of equivalent absorbable suture materials from two different manufacturers. Vet Surg 2011;40(2):223–227.

40. Attenello FJ et al. Use of Gliadel (BCNU) wafer in the surgical treatment of malignant glioma: a 10-year institutional experience. Ann Surg Oncol 2008;15(10):2887–2893.

41. Dunn RL, Garrett S. The drug delivery and biomaterial attributes of the ATRIGEL technology in the treatment of periodontal disease. Expert Opin Investig Drugs 1998; 7(9):1483–1491.

42. Gad HA, El-Nabarawi MA, El-Hady SSA. Formulation and evaluation of PLA and PLGA in situ implants containing secnidazole and/or doxycycline for treatment of periodontitis. AAPS Pharmscitech 2008;9(3):878–884.

43. Sartor O. Eligard (R) 6: a new form of treatment for prostate cancer. Eur Urol Suppl 2006;5(18):905–910.

44. Paajanen H et al. Randomized clinical trial of tissue glue versus absorbable sutures for mesh fixation in local anaesthetic Lichtenstein hernia repair. Br J Surg 2011;98(9):1245–1251.

45. Sakamoto A et al. An investigation of the fixation materials for cartilage frames in microtia. J Plast Reconstr Aesthet Surg 2012;65(5):584–589.

46. Gopferich A. Mechanisms of polymer degradation and erosion. Biomaterials 1996; 17(2):103–114.

47. Gopferich A. Polymer bulk erosion. Macromolecules 1997;30(9):2598–2604.

48. Alexis F. Factors affecting the degradation and drug-release mechanism of poly(lactic acid) and poly[(lactic acid)-co-(glycolic acid)]. Polym Int 2005;54(1):36–46.

49. Gopferich A, Langer R. Modeling of polymer erosion. Macromolecules 1993;26(16): 4105–4112.

50. von Burkersroda F, Schedl L, Gopferich A. Why degradable polymers undergo surface erosion or bulk erosion. Biomaterials 2002;23(21):4221–4231.

51. Wade LG. Organic Chemistry. Prentice Hall; 2003 Upper Saddle River, NJ 07458.

52. Morrison RT, Boyd RN. Organic Chemistry. 6 ed. Prentice Hall; 1992 Upper Saddle River, NJ 07458.

53. Jager J, Jan BF, Engberts N. Inhibition of water-catalyzed ester hydrolysis in hydrophobic microdomains of poly(methacrilic acid) hypercolis. J Am Chem Soc 1984;106:3331–3334.

54. Seo T et al. Ester hydrolysis by poly(allylamines) having hydrophobic groups: Catalytic activity and substrate specificity. J Macromol Sci Part A 1996;33:1025–1047.

55. Callister WD. Fundamentals of Materials Science and Engineering. Somerset, NJ: John Wiley & Sons, Inc.; 2004.

56. Siepmann J, Gopferich A. Mathematical modeling of bioerodible, polymeric drug delivery systems. Adv Drug Deliv Rev 2001;48(2–3):229–247.

57. Hurrell S, Cameron RE. The effect of initial polymer morphology on the degradation and drug release from polyglycolide. Biomaterials 2002;23(11):2401–2409.

58. Anderson JM, Shive MS. Biodegradation and biocompatibility of PLA and PLGA microspheres. Adv Drug Deliv Rev 1997;28(1):5–24.

59. Williams DF, Mort E. Enzyme-accelerated hydrolysis of polyglycolic acid. J Bioeng 1977;1(3):231–238.

60. Visscher GE et al. Effect of particle size on the in vitro and in vivo degradation rates of poly(DL-lactide-co-glycolide) microcapsules. J Biomed Mater Res 1988;22(8):733–746.

61. Visscher GE, Robison MA, Argentieri GJ. Tissue response to biodegradable injectable microcapsules. J Biomater Appl 1987;2(1):118–131.

62. Visscher GE et al. Biodegradation of and tissue reaction to 50:50 poly(DL-lactide-co-glycolide) microcapsules. J Biomed Mater Res 1985;19(3):349–365.

63. Visscher GE et al. Biodegradation of and tissue reaction to poly(DL-lactide) microcapsules. J Biomed Mater Res 1986;20(5):667–676.

64. Ignatius AA, Claes LE. In vitro biocompatibility of bioresorbable polymers: poly(L, DL-lactide) and poly(L-lactide-co-glycolide). Biomaterials 1996;17(8):831–839.

65. Schakenraad JM et al. Enzymatic activity toward poly(L-lactic acid) implants. J Biomed Mater Res 1990;24(5):529–545.

66. Kulkarni RK et al. Biodegradable poly(lactic acid) polymers. J Biomed Mater Res 1971; 5(3):169–181.

67. Chabert E et al. Filler-filler interactions and viscoelastic behavior of polymer nanocomposites. Mater Sci Eng 2004;381(1–2):320–330.

68. Abdul S, Chandewar AV, Jaiswal SB. A flexible technology for modified-release drugs: multiple-unit pellet system (MUPS). J Control Release 2010;147(1):2–16.

69. Bailly M, Kontopoulou M, El Mabrouk K. Effect of polymer/filler interactions on the structure and rheological properties of ethylene-octene copolymer/nanosilica composites. Polymer 2010;51(23):5506–5515.

70. Fritzsche J, Kluppel M. Structural dynamics and interfacial properties of filler-reinforced elastomers. J Phys Condens Matter 2011;23(3).

71. Koga T et al. Structure factors of dispersible units of carbon black filler in rubbers. Langmuir 2005;21(24):11409–11413.

72. Nunes RCR, Fonseca JLC, Pereira MR. Polymer-filler interactions and mechanical properties of a polyurethane elastomer. Polym Test 2000;19(1):93–103.

73. Sampson J, de Korte D. DEHP-plasticised PVC: relevance to blood services. Transfus Med 2011;21(2):73–83.

74. Shaz BH, Grima K, Hillyer CD. 2-(Diethylhexyl)phthalate in blood bags: is this a public health issue? Transfusion 2011;51(11):2510–2517.

75. Yu JG, Wang N, Ma XF. Fabrication and characterization of poly(lactic acid)/acetyl tributyl citrate/carbon black as conductive polymer composites. Biomacromolecules 2008;9(3):1050–1057.

76. Cadogan DF, Howick CJ. Plasticizers. In: Ullmann's Encyclopedia of Industrial Chemistry. Weinhein: Wiley-VCH; 2000.

77. Wang ZH et al. Novel percolation phenomena and mechanism of strengthening elastomers by nanofillers. Phys Chem Chem Phys 2010;12(12):3014–3030.

78. Schubert MA et al. Vitamin E as an antioxidant for poly(etherurethane urea): in vivo studies. J Biomed Mater Res 1996;32(4):493–504.

79. Stella VJ, He QR. Cyclodextrins. Toxicol Pathol 2008;36(1):30–42.

80. Thompson DO. Cyclodextrins - enabling excipients: their present and future use in pharmaceuticals. Crit Rev Ther Drug Carrier Syst 1997;14(1):1–104.

81. Exner AA et al. Enhancement of carboplatin toxicity by Pluronic block copolymers. J Control Release 2005;106(1–2):188–197.

82. Exner AA, Saidel GM. Drug-eluting polymer implants in cancer therapy. Expert Opin Drug Deliv 2008;5(7):775–788.

83. Krupka TM et al. Effect of intratumoral injection of carboplatin combined with pluronic P85 or L61 on experimental colorectal carcinoma in rats. Exp Biol Med (Maywood) 2007;232(7):950–957.

84. Krupka TM et al. Injectable polymer depot combined with radiofrequency ablation for treatment of experimental carcinoma in rat. Invest Radiol 2006;41(12):890–897.

85. Weinberg BD et al. Combination of sensitizing pretreatment and radiofrequency tumor ablation: evaluation in rat model. Radiology 2008;246(3):796–803.

86. Tamada J, Langer R. The development of polyanhydrides for drug delivery applications. J Biomater Sci Poly Ed 1992;3(4):315–353.

87. Langer R. Polymer implants for drug delivery in the brain. J Control Release 1991; 16(1–2):53–59.

88. Solorio L et al. Advances in image-guided intratumoral drug delivery techniques. Ther Deliv 2010;1(2):307–322.

89. Qian F et al. Combined modeling and experimental approach for the development of dual-release polymer millirods. J Control Release 2002;83(3):427–435.

90. Qian F, Szymanski A, Gao JM. Fabrication and characterization of controlled release poly(D,L-lactide-co-glycolide) millirods. J Biomed Mater Res 2001;55(4):512–522.

91. Brodbeck KJ, DesNoyer JR, McHugh AJ. Phase inversion dynamics of PLGA solutions related to drug delivery. Part II. The role of solution thermodynamics and bath-side mass transfer. J Control Release 1999;62(3):333–344.

92. DesNoyer JR, McHugh AJ. Role of crystallization in the phase inversion dynamics and protein release kinetics of injectable drug delivery systems. J Control Release 2001;70(3):285–294.

93. Graham PD, Brodbeck KJ, McHugh AJ. Phase inversion dynamics of PLGA solutions related to drug delivery. J Control Release 1999;58(2):233–245.

94. Ravivarapu HB, Moyer KL, Dunn RL. Parameters affecting the efficacy of a sustained release polymeric implant of leuprolide. Int J Pharm 2000;194(2):181–191.

95. Caraballo I et al. Percolation theory: application to the study of the release behaviour from inert matrix systems. Int J Pharm 1993;96:175–181.

96. Leuenberger H, Rohera BD, Haas C. Percolation theory - a novel-approach to solid dosage form design. Int J Pharm 1987;38(1–3):109–115.

97. Tsuji H, Mizuno A, Ikada Y. Properties and morphology of poly(L-lactide). III. Effects of initial crystallinity on long-term in vitro hydrolysis of high molecular weight poly(L-lactide) film in phosphate-buffered solution. J Appl Polym Sci 2000;77(7):1452–1464.

98. Wu XS, Wang N. Synthesis, characterization, biodegradation, and drug delivery application of biodegradable lactic/glycolic acid polymers. Part II: biodegradation. J Biomater Sci Poly Ed 2001;12(1):21–34.

99. Weinberg BD et al. Modeling doxorubicin transport to improve intratumoral drug delivery to RF ablated tumors. J Control Release 2007;124(1–2):11–19.

100. Weinberg BD et al. Model simulation and experimental validation of intratumoral chemotherapy using multiple polymer implants. Med Biol Eng Comput 2008; 46(10):1039–1049.

101. Affronti ML et al. Overall survival of newly diagnosed glioblastoma patients Receiving carmustine wafers followed by radiation and concurrent temozolomide plus rotational multiagent chemotherapy. Cancer 2009;115(15):3501–3511.

102. Noel G et al. Retrospective comparison of chemoradiotherapy followed by adjuvant chemotherapy, with or without prior gliadel implantation (Carmustine) after initial surgery in patients with newly diagnosed high-grade gliomas. Int J Radiat Oncol Biol Phys 2012; 82(2):749–755.

103. Panigrahi M, Das PK, Parikh PM. Brain tumor and gliadel wafer treatment. Indian J Cancer 2011;48(1):11–17.

104. Fleming AB, Saltzman WM. Pharmacokinetics of the carmustine implant. Clin Pharmacokinet 2002;41(6):403–419.

105. Westphal M et al. Gliadel (R) wafer in initial surgery for malignant glioma: long-term follow-up of a multicenter controlled trial. Acta Neurochir 2006;148(3):269–275.

106. Packhaeuser CB et al. In situ forming parenteral drug delivery systems: an overview. Eur J Pharm Biopharm 2004;58(2):445–455.

107. Hatefi A, Amsden B. Biodegradable injectable in situ forming drug delivery systems. J Control Release 2002;80(1–3):9–28.

108. Bezwada, RS. Liquid copolymers of epsilon-caprolactone and lactide. US Patent. 1995; p 15.

109. Einmahl S et al. A viscous bioerodible poly(ortho ester) as a new biomaterial for intraocular application. J Biomed Mater Res 2000;50(4):566–573.

110. Stile RA, Burghardt WR, Healy KE. Synthesis and characterization of injectable poly(N-isopropylacrylamide)-based hydrogels that support tissue formation in vitro. Macromolecules 1999;32(22):7370–7379.

111. Hoffman AS. Applications of thermally reversible polymers and hydrogels in therapeutics and diagnostics. J Control Release 1987;6:297–305.

112. Stile RA, Burghardt WR, Healy KE. Synthesis and characterization of injectable poly(N-isopropylacrylamide)-based hydrogels that support tissue formation in vitro. Macromolecules 1999;32(22):7370–7379.

113. Schild HG. Poly(N-isopropylacrylamide): experiment, theory and application. Prog Polym Sci 1992;17:163–249.

114. Alexandridis P, Hatton TA. Poly(ethylene oxide)–poly-(propylene oxide)–poly(ethylene oxide) block copolymer surfactants in aqueous solutions and at interfaces: thermodynamics, structure, dynamics and modeling. Colloid Surf 1995;96:1–46.

115. Jeong B et al. New biodegradable polymers for injectable drug delivery systems. J Control Release 1999;62(1–2):109–114.

116. Jeong B, Bae YH, Kim SW. Drug release from biodegradable injectable thermosensitive hydrogel of PEG-PLGA-PEG triblock copolymers. J Control Release 2000; 63(1–2):155–163.

117. Jeong B, Bae YH, Lee DS, Kim SW. Biodegradable block copolymers as injectable drug delivery systems. Nature 1997;388:860–862.

118. Dunn RL, English JP, Cowsar DR, Vanderbelt DD, Biodegradable in-situ forming implants and methods of producing the same. USA. U.S.A Patent Application Date: 03 Oct 1988 Publication Date: 03 July 1990 Publication number 4938763.

119. Hubbell JA, Pathak CP, Sawhney AS, Desai NP, Hill JL, Photopolymerizable biodegradable hydrogels as tissue contacting materials and controlled release carriers. 1995: USA. U.S.A Patent Application Date: 01 March 1993 Publication Date: 25 Apr 1995 Publication number 5410016.

120. Viegas TX, Reeve LE, Henry RL, Medical uses of in-situ formed gels. USA. U.S.A Patent Application Date: 28 Dec 1993 Publication Date: 24 Dec 1996 Publication number 5587175.

121. Papahadjopoulos D et al. Phase transitions in phospholipid vesicles. Fluorescence polarization and permeability measurements concerning the effect of temperature and cholesterol. Biochim Biophys Acta 1973;311(3):330–348.

122. Engstrom S, Engstrom L. Phase-behavior of the lidocaine-monoolein-water system. Int J Pharm 1992;79(2–3):113–122.

123. Scriven LE. Equilibrium bicontinuous structure. Nature 1976;263(5573):123–125.

124. Ericsson B et al. Cubic phases as delivery systems for peptide drugs. ACS Symp Ser 1991;469:251–265.

125. Gao Z, Shukla AJ, Johnson JR, Crowley WR. Controlled release of contraceptive steroid from biodegradable and injectable gel formulations: in-vitro evaluation. Pharm Res 1995;12(6):857–864.

126. Gao Z, Crowley WR, Shukla AJ, Johnson JR, Reger JF. Controlled release of contraceptive steroids from biodegradable and injectable gel formulations: in-vivo evaluation. Pharm Res 1998;12(6):864–868.

127. Ravivarapu HB, Moyer KL, Dunn RL. Sustained activity and release of leuprolide acetate from an in situ forming polymeric implant. AAPS PharmSciTech 2000;1(1):E1.

128. McHugh AJ. The role of polymer membrane formation in sustained release drug delivery systems. J Control Release 2005;109(1–3):211–221.

129. Smolders CA et al. Microstructure in phase inversion membranes. Formation of macrovoids. J Membr Sci 1992;73:259–275.

130. Tsay CS, McHugh AJ. A technique for rapid measurement of diffusion-coefficients. Ind Eng Chem Res 1992;86(1):449–452.

131. Chandrashekar BL, Zhou M, Jarr EM, Dunn RL, Controlled release liquid delivery compositions with low initial drug burst. 2000: USA. U.S.A. Patent Filed Oct 28, 1998 Date of Patent: Nov. 7, 2000 Patent Number: 6,143,314.

132. Brodbeck KJ, Pushpala S, McHugh AJ. Sustained release of human growth hormone from PLGA solution depots. Pharm Res 1999;16(12):1825–1829.

133. Smolders CA et al. Microstructures in phase-inversion membranes .1. Formation of macrovoids. J Membr Sci 1992;73(2–3):259–275.

134. Smolders CA, Reuvers AJ, Boom RM, Wienk IM. Microstructure in phase inversion membranes. Formation of macrovoids. J Membr Sci 1992;73:259–275.

135. Vogrin N et al. The wet phase separation: the effect of cast solution thickness on the appearance of macrovoids in the membrane forming ternary cellulose acetate/acetone/water system. J Membr Sci 2002;207(1):139–141.

136. Raman C, McHugh AJ. A model for drug release from fast phase inverting injectable solutions. J Control Release 2005;102(1):145–157.

137. Solorio L et al. Effect of cargo properties on in situ forming implant behavior determined by noninvasive ultrasound imaging. Drug Deliv Transl Res 2012;2(1):45–55.

138. Solorio L, Solorio LD, Gleeson S, Exner AA. Phase inverting polymer systems in drug delivery and medicine. In: Ehlers TP, Wilhelm JK, editors. Polymer Phase Behavior. Nova Science Publishers, Inc; 2011. 400 Oser Ave Suite 1600, Hauppauge, NY 11788.

139. Tsay CS, McHugh AJ. A technique for rapid measurement of diffusion-coefficients. Ind Eng Chem Res 1992;86(1):449–452.

140. Chen S, Singh J. Controlled delivery of testosterone from smart polymer solution based systems: in vitro evaluation. Int J Pharm 2005;295(1–2):183–190.

141. Chen S et al. In vivo absorption of steroidal hormones from smart polymer based delivery systems. J Pharm Sci 2010;99(8):3381–3388.

142. Dhawan S, Kapil R, Kapoor DN. Development and evaluation of in situ gel-forming System for sustained delivery of insulin. J Biomater Appl 2011.

143. Singh S, Singh J. Phase-sensitive polymer-based controlled delivery systems of leuprolide acetate: in vitro release, biocompatibility, and in vivo absorption in rabbits. Int J Pharm 2007;328(1):42–48.

144. Liu QF et al. In vitro and in vivo study of thymosin alpha1 biodegradable in situ forming poly(lactide-co-glycolide) implants. Int J Pharm 2010;397(1–2):122–129.

145. Singh S, Singh J. Controlled release of a model protein lysozyme from phase sensitive smart polymer systems. Int J Pharm 2004;271(1–2):189–196.

146. Yapar A, Baykara T. Effects of solvent combinations on drug release from injectable phase sensitive liquid implants. Turk J Pharm Sci 2010;7(1):49–56.

147. DesNoyer JR, McHugh AJ. The effect of Pluronic on the protein release kinetics of an injectable drug delivery system. J Control Release 2003;86(1):15–24.

148. Patel RB et al. Characterization of formulation parameters affecting low molecular weight drug release from in situ forming drug delivery systems. J Biomed Mater Res A 2010;94A(2):476–484.

149. Bakhshi R et al. The effect of additives on naltrexone hydrochloride release and solvent removal rate from an injectable in situ forming PLGA implant. Polym Adv Technol 2006;17(5):354–359.

150. Mashak A et al. The effect of aliphatic esters on the formation and degradation behavior of PLGA-based in situ forming system. Poly Bull 2010. DOI: 10.1007/s00289-010-0386-7.

151. Packhaeuser CB et al. In situ forming parenteral drug delivery systems: an overview. Eur J Pharm Biopharm 2004;58(2):445–455.

152. Royals MA et al. Biocompatibility of a biodegradable in situ forming implant system in rhesus monkeys. J Biomed Mater Res 1999;45(3):231–239.

153. Okumu FW et al. Sustained delivery of human growth hormone from a novel gel system: SABER. Biomaterials 2002;23(22):4353–4358.

154. Tae G, Kornfield JA, Hubbell JA. Sustained release of human growth hormone from in situ forming hydrogels using self-assembly of fluoroalkyl-ended poly(ethylene glycol). Biomaterials 2005;26(25):5259–5266.

155. Ueda H et al. Injectable, in situ forming poly(propylene fumarate)-based ocular drug delivery systems. J Biomed Mater Res A 2007;83A(3):656–666.

156. Patel RB et al. Effect of injection site on in situ implant formation and drug release in vivo. J Control Release 2010;147(3):350–358.

157. Solorio L et al. Noninvasive characterization of in situ forming implants using diagnostic ultrasound. J Control Release 2010;143(2):183–190.

158. Liu H, Venkatraman SS. Effect of polymer type on the dynamics of phase inversion and drug release in injectable in situ gelling systems. J Biomater Sci Polym Ed 2012;23.

159. Lambert WJ, Peck KD. Development of an in situ forming biodegradable poly-lactide-co-glycolide system for the controlled release of proteins. J Control Release 1995;33:189–195.

160. Sartor O. Eligard: leuprolide acetate in a novel sustained-release delivery system. Urology 2003;61(2 Suppl 1):25–31.

161. Schulman C et al. Expert opinion on 6-monthly luteinizing hormone-releasing hormone agonist treatment with the single-sphere depot system for prostate cancer. BJU Int 2007;100(1 Suppl):1–5.

162. Solanki HK, Thakkar JH. Recent advances in implantable drug delivery. Int J Pharm Sci Rev Res 2010;4(3):168–177.

163. Mchugh AJ, Miller DC. The dynamics of diffusion and gel growth during nonsolvent-induced phase inversion of polyethersulfone. J Membr Sci 1995;105(1–2):121–136.

164. Kempe S et al. Non-invasive in vivo evaluation of in situ forming PLGA implants by benchtop magnetic resonance imaging (BT-MRI) and EPR spectroscopy. Eur J Pharm Biopharm 2010;74(1):102–108.

165. Jeong B et al. Biodegradable block copolymers as injectable drug-delivery systems. Nature 1997;388(6645):860–862.

166. D. Annavajjula, K. Yim, S.C Rowe. Drug Delivery System for Recombinant Human Growth Hormone with Photopolymerized Hydrogels. In: 28th International Symposium on Controlled Release of Bioactive Materials; 2001.

8

POLYMERIC DRUG DELIVERY SYSTEMS IN TISSUE ENGINEERING

Matthew Skiles and James Blanchette

Department of Biomedical Engineering, University of South Carolina, Columbia, SC, USA

8.1 INTRODUCTION

Tissue engineering and regenerative medicine are fields that merge developmental biology with material science to achieve the controlled generation of tissue. Whether occurring in a host or *ex vivo*, tissue generation (natural or induced) relies on many common, yet complex underlying processes. These processes involve the dynamic interplay between cellular, structural, and biochemical components of a tissue.

The inspiration for regenerative strategies is often derived from our understanding of natural biological pathways involved in tissue growth and repair. Many of the most important of these pathways are regulated by chemical cues known as growth factors, which rapidly relay information to cells about their local microenvironment and affect cellular behaviors such as survival, migration, proliferation, and differentiation. It is now well understood that the ability to engineer tissues is dependent upon our ability to control and direct cell behavior through regulated application of these factors.

The manner in which growth factors are delivered (temporally and spatially) and the microenvironment in which they interact with cells greatly influence the nature of

Engineering Polymer Systems for Improved Drug Delivery, First Edition.
Edited by Rebecca A. Bader and David A. Putnam.
© 2014 John Wiley & Sons, Inc. Published 2014 by John Wiley & Sons, Inc.

cellular responses. Therefore, approaches for tissue generation have been developed in the fields of tissue engineering and regenerative medicine, which focus on the controlled delivery of growth factors from polymeric systems capable of regulating temporal and spatial release and (sometimes) providing their own beneficial interaction with cells. Such systems take many lessons from natural processes in which materials (the extracellular matrix) and bioactive molecules (growth factors) interact to achieve ideal temporospatial growth factor presentation, stabilization, and activity.

This chapter is concerned with current methods for the delivery of bioactive factors in tissue engineering and regenerative medicine. We will briefly explore the native healing processes that serve as a template for many regenerative therapies and then discuss some of the most common growth factors applied in tissue engineering and regenerative medicine. We will also highlight some important growth factor–matrix interactions to consider when selecting a delivery material. Finally, we will detail material-based and cell-based strategies for growth factor delivery. Because they can offer fine control over release kinetics, exhibit highly modifiable characteristics, and can be engineered to incorporate material–biomolecule interactions, polymers are most commonly used for growth factor delivery applications.

8.2 WOUND HEALING AS A PROTOTYPE FOR ADULT TISSUE GENERATION

Wound healing is the process by which a damaged tissue achieves restored anatomical configuration and function [1]. Healing pathways involve reciprocal interaction between cells, growth factors, and the ECM. The complex and overlapping processes involved in wound healing are responsible for restoring homeostasis, removing debris, repopulating voided space, and re-forming and organizing anatomical structures. These processes, particularly (re)population, organization, and maturation, are also involved in the successful engineering of tissues. Furthermore, it is important to understand that implantation of an engineered tissue or scaffold will often trigger the wound healing response, resulting in a specific microenvironment that can further promote tissue development and integration. Thus, an understanding of the wound healing response can provide insights into how these processes result in the formation of a tissue and how they can be induced and/or modified in order to achieve desirable outcomes in tissue generation.

8.2.1 The Wound

A wound is defined as a disruption of normal anatomical structure and function and can result from internal or external events [1]. In a healthy body, the intrinsic pathways that exist for the ordered and timely repair of a wound can be categorized into four phases which overlap in a continuous event: hemostasis, inflammation, proliferation, and remodeling. Different tissues and different forms of tissue damage will exhibit variations in these processes. For instance, different tissues will express different tissue-specific growth factors; require maturation of different, tissue-specific cell types;

and exhibit production of different tissue-specific extracellular matrix (ECM) proteins. However, in general, these processes as a whole apply to all wound repair. The most common end result of successful progression through wound healing is the restoration of tissue homeostasis through formation of a scar. Dysfunction of one or more of the phases of healing can be associated with wound pathology and a failure to heal. Regenerative medicine supposes that careful modification of wound healing processes can result in superior regenerative healing in which the repaired tissue is almost structurally and functionally identical to the original tissue. Likewise, tissue engineers attempt to stimulate pathways similar to those that occur in wound healing in order to encourage the growth of a functional replacement tissue either *in vitro* or *in vivo*.

It should be noted that wound healing and tissue generation are extremely complicated events and many of the shortcomings of tissue engineering and regenerative medicine result from an incomplete understanding or failure to re-create this intricacy. Tissues are complex, heterogeneous combinations of extracellular materials, cells (of various phenotype), and biochemicals. Optimal regeneration of a given tissue often involves directing growth of the primary tissue (e.g., skin, bone, muscle), as well as many other associated tissues such as blood vessels and nerves. Thus, researchers implement therapeutic techniques.

8.2.2 The Wound Healing Response

Wound healing can occur in any tissue of the body, to various degrees, through a network of common underlying processes. This suggests that there is potential for (re)generation of any bodily tissue. Though a complex, dynamic, and continuous process, healing can be better understood through definition of four phases, each characterized by specific physiological events. These phases are hemostasis, inflammation, proliferation, and remodeling. Associated with each stage are distinct physiological, biological, and mechanical actions and the biochemical cues that regulate them. An understanding of these events and how specific biochemical signals affect and direct the intricate cellular tasks involved in tissue repair is vital to the development of viable regenerative therapeutic approaches. Furthermore, the timing of therapeutic intervention is key, as the local microenvironment will change as healing processes progress. A summary of the phases of wound healing follows [2–7].

8.2.2.1 Hemostasis. In an injury that disrupts vascular integrity, the healing response begins with a series of events designed to stop blood loss and maintain hemostasis. Though restoration of hemostasis is not usually the immediate goal of tissue engineering or regenerative medicine, events associated with tissue damage, vascular disruption, and clotting lead to the formation of a biochemical microenvironment that is highly conducive to the formation of new tissue. Blood platelets contact exposed ECM proteins, notably collagen, in the vessel wall and surrounding tissues and trigger the coagulation cascade. The activated platelets release a number of factors, including platelet-derived growth factor (PDGF), transforming growth factor (TGF)-α/β, fibroblast growth factor (FGF)-2, and epidermal growth factor (EGF), which stimulate activation of other local platelets, as well as immune cells, endothelial cells, and fibroblasts. They also release clotting factors, which results in the deposition of a cross-linked fibrin plug consisting of fibrin, fibronectin, vitronectin, thrombospondin, and incorporated platelets. This network blocks blood loss from the wound, prevents further entry of foreign material and microorganisms, and serves as a provisional matrix for the subsequent stages of healing.

8.2.2.2 Inflammation.
As coagulation and clotting restore hemostasis, the cytokine factors released from local platelets initiate transition of wound healing into the inflammation stage. Permeability of surrounding blood vessels is increased, creating a swollen wound site and facilitating diffusion of dissolved bioactive molecules. PDGF secreted from platelets stimulates the initial chemotaxis of neutrophils into the wound and later that of monocytes, fibroblasts, and smooth muscle cells. Arriving neutrophils destroy and phagocytize bacteria and collect foreign material and cellular and matrix debris. TGF-β and fibrin attract monocytes and stimulate their secretion of additional cytokines, including IL-1, FGF-2, TNF-α, PDGF, and more TGF-β. In the wound, monocytes transform into macrophages that clean debris from the wound (including bacteria-laden neutrophils and nonfunctional host cells) and are essential to the progression of healing.

A rich network of cytokines develops in the wound during this time through secretory contributions from platelets during homeostasis and macrophages during inflammation as well as growth factors liberated by damage to the ECM. Presence of these factors drives repopulation of the wound during the next phase of healing. PDGF induces mitogenesis of fibroblasts and smooth muscle cells, and TGF-β induces their chemotaxis. TGF-β, in particular, is known to regulate a large number of other fibroblast behaviors, including acceleration of collagen synthesis and deposition, which is also assisted by FGF-2. EGF and vascular endothelial growth factor (VEGF) released during hemostasis and inflammation can begin to stimulate chemotaxis of epithelial and vascular endothelial cells, respectively. It is important to note that many of these bioactive molecules develop three-dimensional (3-D) concentration gradients within the local matrix, which contribute to directed effects on local cells.

8.2.2.3 Proliferation.
The proliferative phase of wound healing is marked by decreased presence of macrophages, invasion of the wound site by fibroblasts, and increased wound tissue strength due to the deposition of new matrix. The initial secretion of TGF-β from platelets stimulates increased proliferation of local fibroblasts. With the additional release of TGF-β from macrophages, more fibroblasts are recruited to the wound and begin to proliferate rapidly. During their migration, fibroblasts attach to the fibrin network produced during hemostasis. The goal of the proliferative phase of wound healing is to repopulate the injury with cells and matrix in order to re-establish continuity with the surrounding tissue, increase its strength and stability, and provide a platform for future remodeling. TGF-β triggers a decrease in matrix metalloprotease (MMP) release and stimulates the upregulation of matrix protein production in the fibroblasts, which quickly deposit collagen, fibronectin, and proteogylcans to form a stronger, more stable matrix in the wound tissue.

The recruitment of more specialized cells, including epithelial, endothelial, smooth muscle, and neuronal cells, also proceeds during the proliferation phase. Of particular importance is revascularization of the wound in order to supply nutrients and oxygen to surviving residual cells and to meet the high metabolic demands of migrating and proliferating cells. FGF-2 that has been secreted by macrophages and VEGF that is released from oxygen-deficient cells as a result of reduced local blood delivery stimulate the activity of endothelial cells residing in intact capillaries in the wound periphery. These cells break down the basal lamina of the parent vessel through protease activity, migrate through the extracellular matrix toward the cytokine source, and proliferate and remodel to form microvessels in the wound.

8.2.2.4 Remodeling. The final stage of wound healing is remodeling. Many events activated by stimulatory cytokines reach equilibrium with competing inhibitory cytokine pathways during this time. As the wound regains continuity with the surrounding tissue and becomes more fully occupied by both cellular and sturdy matrix components, fibroblast proliferation and matrix deposition slow. Presence of both macrophages and neutrophils is further reduced. The wound is now stabilized, but often lacks significant mechanical stability. Over time, repeated breakdown and reformation of matrix fibers results in a more organized and aligned matrix with improved mechanical strength. Collagen bundles thicken and become more cross-linked, and residual hyaluronic acid and fibronectin are degraded. The wound is now a mature scar. With extended time, more mature cells of the native tissue type can eventually become present, and additional remodeling can allow the tissue to more closely resemble the prewound tissue, but scar tissue will never truly recapitulate the anatomical and functional properties of the original.

8.2.3 Homeostasis Versus Regeneration in Tissue Repair

While effective, the healing processes in adult tissues are not the gold standard of regenerative therapies. Natural pathways tend to emphasize rapid homeostasis and restoration of mechanical stability rather than exact anatomical and functional replication of the original tissue. New matrix that is formed during the proliferation and remodeling phases of wound healing differs significantly from that of native ECM, with fibers that are disorganized and unaligned. Its material composition differs as well, with collagen III present in a higher percentage than in native matrix (30% vs. 10–20%, respectively) and elastin, which gives native tissue its elasticity, being entirely absent. Furthermore, the cellular component of a healing tissue is less than that of a native tissue and is further reduced over time with remodeling. Together, these characteristics mean that the scar tissue formed through natural wound healing pathways is often inferior to rather than identical to the tissue that previously existed.

Because of this, it is hardly beneficial in tissue engineering or regenerative medicine to merely re-create native regenerative processes. Instead, an understanding of natural pathways allows for their educated modification to achieve superior therapeutic results. In other words, innate regenerative pathways represent a starting point for tissue formation but can be improved through tissue engineering approaches that promote beneficial cell behaviors while repressing undesirable behaviors. This is illustrated by topical wound treatments that attempt to suppress inflammation—reduced inflammation leads to reduced fibroblast recruitment, less collagen deposition, and reduced scar tissue formation. The trade-off is that healing takes more time. Such therapies that at the same time encourage the proliferation and maturation of progenitor cells into tissue-appropriate phenotypes can promote regenerative healing, with the mature cells depositing ECM more typical of the original tissue. Thus a common strategy in tissue engineering is controlling the induction or suppression of innate signaling and response pathways in order to direct cell behaviors to a desirable outcome.

8.3 BIOACTIVE FACTORS IN TISSUE ENGINEERING AND REGENERATIVE MEDICINE

Tissue engineering scaffolds and the bioactive factors associated with them guide cell phenotype. Bioactive molecules can be utilized to control cell adhesion, mobility, migration, survival, proliferation, differentiation, and secretion profiles (Fig. 8.1). However, the presentation of such factors, both spatially and temporally, can have a large impact on their functionality. Thus polymeric carrier/delivery systems which localize bioactive factors to a specific site and regulate their release are also integral

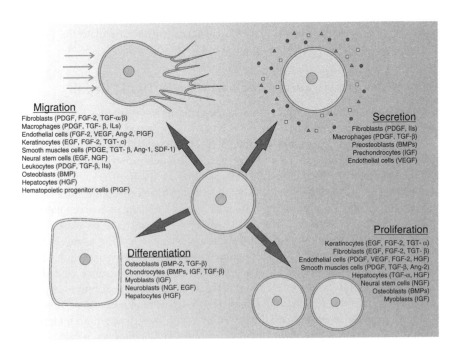

Migration
Fibroblasts (PDGF, FGF-2, TGF-α/β)
Macrophages (PDGF, TGF- β, ILs)
Endothelial cells (FGF-2, VEGF, Ang-2, PIGF)
Keratinocytes (EGF, FGF-2, TGT- o)
Smooth muscles cells (PDGE, TGT- β, Ang-1, SDF-1)
Neural stem cells (EGF, NGF)
Leukocytes (PDGF, TGF-β, Ils)
Osteoblasts (BMP)
Hepatocytes (HGF)
Hematopoietic progenitor cells (PIGF)

Secretion
Fibroblasts (PDGF, Ils)
Macrophages (PDGF, TGF-β)
Preosteoblasts (BMPs)
Prechondrocytes (IGF)
Endothelial cells (VEGF)

Proliferation
Keratinocytes (EGF, FGF-2, TGT- α)
Fibroblasts (EGF, FGF-2, TGT- β)
Endothelial cells (PDGF, VEGF, FGF-2, HGF)
Smooth muscles cells (PDGF, TGF-β, Ang-2)
Hepatocytes (TGF-α, HGF)
Neural stem cells (NGF)
Osteoblasts (BMPs)
Myoblasts (IGF)

Differentiation
Osteoblasts (BMP-2, TGF-β)
Chondrocytes (BMPs, IGF, TGF-β)
Myoblasts (IGF)
Neuroblasts (NGF, EGF)
Hepatocytes (HGF)

Figure 8.1. Bioactive molecules regulate many aspects of cell behavior.

to the successful regulation of cell behavior. We will next discuss the characteristics of common bioactive factors relevant to tissue engineering and regenerative medicine followed by an examination of ways in which they interact with the ECM *in vivo*.

8.3.1   Common Bioactive Proteins in Tissue Engineering

Most bioactive molecules utilized in tissue engineering and regenerative medicine are soluble polypeptide cytokines naturally produced and released by living cells. These factors interact with cells nonenzymatically in small concentrations over relatively short distances to regulate cell functions [8, 9]. Most bioactive factors used in tissue engineering can be classified as growth factors. Compared to other soluble, inter-cellular signaling molecules, it appears that the central role of growth factors is to control the (re)modeling of tissues [9]. Bioactive proteins can promote and/or inhibit cell migration, motility and adhesion, proliferation, differentiation, and secretion to regulate cell behavior. Thus they represent a unique and powerful group of tools available to tissue engineers. Systemically, growth factor half-life is often short, with cell responses to growth factors being concentration dependent. In native tissue regen-eration, the timing of growth factor release is precisely controlled and is triggered by the process of repair [10].

As should be clear from our discussion of wound healing (Section 8.2.2), biochem-ical regulation of pathways can be complex, with a variety of bioactive factors being produced by homogenous or heterogeneous cell populations and individual factors capable of acting on different cell types with different effects. Additionally, multi-ple factors with different availability profiles may act concurrently or in sequence to modulate an effect on cell behavior (Fig. 8.2). For tissue engineering uses, bioactive

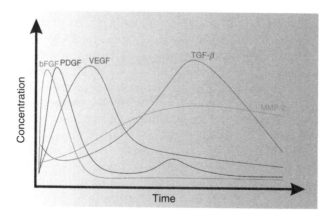

Figure 8.2. In the body, a given biological process will involve the activity of multiple bioactive factors, often in distinct temporal and spatial profiles. Possible profiles of several factors found in the local wound microenvironment during repair are shown here, illustrating the complexity involved in regenerative processes. In tissue engineering, it is desirable to recreate such profiles as closely as possible to achieve favorable tissue regeneration.

proteins can be applied exogenously, for instance, by delivery from a laden polymeric device, or cells can be induced to produce the desired factor themselves by provision of a suitable biomaterial/biochemical environment. It is not the purpose of this chapter to provide a comprehensive list of every known bioactive agent and its activity; in fact, the optimal temporospatial network of factors required for any given biological activity is an active area of research. However, as we increase our understanding of growth factor activities in the body, we become better able to rationally design regenerative therapies. Currently, bioactive proteins (primarily growth factors) are central tools in tissue engineering and regenerative medicine, and we will examine those factors whose use is most relevant, summarizing their important properties and activities. An overview of these bioactive agents is provided in Table 8.1, and the reader is directed to References 10–12 for additional reviews on this topic.

It should be noted that while the above growth factors represent those most commonly and broadly used in tissue engineering and regenerative therapies, other factors exist that have very powerful and specific activities in specific tissues. Such factors may not be employed in all tissue engineering and wound healing strategies, but may be very important to therapies aimed at the regeneration of a specific type of tissue. Consideration of such specific factors as well as those listed below illustrates the importance of signaling molecules in tissue engineering and the need to develop strategies for their controlled administration. Such strategies can take a lesson from the native biochemical–biomaterial interactions that occur between growth factors and the ECM *in vivo*.

8.3.2   Growth Factors Interact with the Extracellular Matrix

In the body, the ECM serves as more than just a structural framework, but dynamically interacts with both cells and biochemicals [117]. As growth factors continue to be better understood, it is becoming apparent that the ECM is a key contributor to the proper activity of most (if not all) growth factors. While unbound bioactive factors can diffuse in the extracellular fluid and are available for immediate cellular interaction, factors that exhibit ECM binding are often present in spatiotemporal gradients, which as a whole impact cellular responses and prolong growth factor activity [118]. In this sense, cooperative action between growth factors and the ECM allow the two to be considered as a single functional unit forming an "information network" that regulates cell activities [119]. When designing a polymeric device for the delivery of growth factors, it is important to consider native growth factor–matrix interactions and understand how they impact growth factor stability, presentation, and activity.

8.3.2.1   *Matrix Sequestration of Growth Factors.*   The ECM is a heterogeneous network made up of several types of components: fibers (e.g., collagen, elastin), polysaccharides (e.g., hyaluronic acid), proteoglycans (e.g., heparin, heparin sulfate), and other proteins (e.g., fibronectin, laminin). Growth factors can be directly bound by matrix proteins, including fiber components, nonfiber components, and

TABLE 8.1. Bioactive Agents Commonly used in Tissue Engineering

Name	Molecular weight (MW), kDa	Stability	Origins	Cellular effects	Comments	References
EGF— (epidermal growth factor)	6.2	Rapidly internalized (1–3 min) and degraded (30–50 min) upon cell binding Quickly cleared from systemic circulation	Macrophages Keratinocytes	Mitogenesis of keratinocytes and fibroblasts Chemotaxis of keratinocytes and neural stem cells Differentiation of neural stem cells	6–12 h of continuous exposure required for mitogenic effect Used in wound healing and skin engineering	13–21
PDGF— (platelet-derived growth factor)	PDGF-AA: 28.5 PDGF-AB: 25.5 PDGF-BB: 24.3	Rapidly cleared from systemic circulation (half-life <2 min)	Platelets Macrophages Endothelial cells Keratinocytes Smooth muscle cells	Chemotaxis of fibroblasts, leukocytes, macrophages, and smooth muscle cells Mitogenesis of fibroblasts, endothelial cells and smooth muscle cells	Cationic 8–10 h of exposure required to induce matrix deposition Involved in matrix remodeling and used in wound healing and vascular engineering Binds to heparin sulfate and to osteonectin	22–30

(continued)

TABLE 8.1. (*Continued*)

Name	Molecular weight (MW), kDa	Stability	Origins	Cellular effects	Comments	References
				Activation of matrix secretion from fibroblasts (upregulation of collagen V, fibronectin, hyaluronan, and MMPs) Activation of growth factor secretion from leukocytes and macrophages		
FGF-2—(fibroblast growth factor-2, or basic fibroblast growth factor)	High MW isoforms: 22 22.5 24 Low MW isoform: 18	Rapidly cleared from systemic circulation (half-life 3 min)	Macrophages Fibroblasts Endothelial cells	Chemotaxis of fibroblasts, keratinocytes, and endothelial cells Mitogenesis of fibroblasts, keratinocytes, endothelial cells Inhibits apoptosis of endothelial cells Strong induction of angiogenesis Induces proteolysis of ECM	Basic Widely used in tissue engineering for vascularization Also used in wound healing Binds to heparin sulfate and to matrix-associated FGF receptors	31–36

Name	MW		Source cells	Functions	Uses/Notes	
TGF-α — (transforming growth factor-α)	5.5		Macrophages Keratinocytes	Chemotaxis of keratinocytes and fibroblasts Mitogenesis of keratinocytes and hepatocytes	Very similar in function to EGF, but more potent with lower intracellular degradation	37–39
TGF-β — (transforming growth factor-β)	25	Rapidly cleared from systemic circulation (half-life <3 min)	Platelets Macrophages Fibroblasts Endothelial cells Keratinocytes Smooth muscle cells	Chemotaxis of fibroblasts, leukocytes, macrophages, and smooth muscle cells Mitogenesis of fibroblasts and smooth muscles cells Mitogenesis and differentiation of preosteoblasts Antiproliferative effect in epithelial cells	Used in wound healing, vascular engineering, and especially engineering of osteochondrogenic tissue Can bind to collagen IV, fibronectin, or microfibers (in latent form) directly in the matrix or to matrix-associated accessory proteins or heparin	40–50

(continued)

TABLE 8.1. (*Continued*)

Name	Molecular weight (MW), kDa	Stability	Origins	Cellular effects	Comments	References
				Activation of growth factor secretion from leukocytes and macrophages Activation of matrix deposition; inhibition of MMPs		
VEGF— (vascular endothelial growth factor, vascular endothelial growth factor-A, vascular permeability factor (VPF)) isoforms: $VEGF_{121,165,189,xxxb}$	46 ($VEGF_{165}$ as representative)	Cleared from systemic circulation within 50 min.	Mesenchymal cells	Enodthelial cell mitogenesis, chemotaxis, survival, and secretion of MMPs Increases vascular permeability Angiogenesis Maintenance of survival of other cell types, including neuronal and hepatic	Dimeric glycoprotein closely related to PDGF $VEGF_{165}$ is the primary isoform with strong activity and heparin binding (50–70% bound to ECM) $VEGF_{189}$ is almost entirely sequestered in the ECM and released by MMPs, heparinase and/or plasmin. Its activity on endothelial cells is dependent upon their source.	51–58

					VEGF$_{121}$ is almost entirely soluble with no ECM binding. VEGF$_{121}$ alone leads to disordered vascular formation. VEGF is widely used in angiogenesis and wound healing for tissue engineering. VEGF$_{xxxb}$ isoforms inhibit angiogenesis	
BMP— (bone morphogenetic protein, growth differentiation factor (VDF)) isoforms: include BMP-2,3,4,5,6,7,9	26-38	Systemic half-life of only several minutes	Mesenchymal cells	Osteoblastic differentiation Mitogenesis and chemotaxis of osteoblasts Chondrogenesis Activation of matrix deposition	Member of the TGF-β super family. Requires continuous residence at site of action. BMP-2 is the key inducer of osteogenesis and is also important in chondrogenesis. Is also involved in neuronal development. It binds to heparin sulfate and to collagen IV.	59–67

(continued)

TABLE 8.1. (*Continued*)

Name	Molecular weight (MW), kDa	Stability	Origins	Cellular effects	Comments	References
					BMP-3 is an antagonist to osteogenesis	
					BMP-4 is important to bone formation from mesoderm, with involvement in bone repair. It also binds to heparin sulfate.	
					BMP-5 is involved in cartilage formation.	
					BMP-6 is involved in maintaining cartilage integrity.	
					BMP-7 is a potent inducer of osteoblast differentiation and is important in renal development and repair. It is bound in a proto form to ECM through fibrillin, and in a cleaved form to heparin sulfate.	

Ang— (angiopoietin) Isoforms: Ang-1, Ang-2	70	Ang-1: Platelets, Mesenchymal cells-notably smooth muscle Ang-2: Endothelial cells	Chemotaxis and survival of endothelial cells Chemotaxis of smooth muscle cells Reduction of vascular permeability (anti-inflammatory) Regulation of adipose tissue growth/regression	BMP-9 promotes chondrogenic differentiation and is involved in hepatic glucose homeostasis Ang-1 is less active in promoting endothelial cell proliferation than VEGF. Coadministration of Ang-1 with VEGF enhances angiogenesis. Ang-1 also promotes blood vessel maturation, reducing vessel permeability. It is down regulated by TGF-β. Ang-1 can be matrix immobilized.	68–76

(continued)

TABLE 8.1. (*Continued*)

Name	Molecular weight (MW), kDa	Stability	Origins	Cellular effects	Comments	References
					Ang-2 acts as an antagonist to Ang-1. In presence of VEGF, it promotes angiogenesis, while in absence of VEGF, vessel regression occurs.	
NGF—(nerve growth factor)	26	Rapidly cleared from systemic circulation (half-life in rats <6min.)	Neurons Peripheral neuronal tissue	Mitogenesis, differentiation, and survival of neural stem cells	Used in neural regeneration and tissue engineering to promote innervation.	77–82
				Growth but not proliferation of mature neural cells	Pretreatment of stem cells with FGF followed by addition of NGF promotes cell proliferation. Then, upon removal of NGF, neural differentiation is observed	
				Neurotrophism		
				Proliferation of B and T-lymphocytes		
				Degranulation of mast cells		
				Growth and proliferation of hematopoietic cells		

HGF— (hepatocyte growth factor)	103	Rapidly cleared from systemic circulation (half-life in rats <4 min.)	Mesenchymal cells	Strong mitogenesis and chemotaxis of hepatocytes Mitogenesis of epithelial and endothelial cells	Involved in liver regeneration and wound healing Suggested to have angiogenic activity and assist in muscle repair Sequential administration of IGF-1 then HGF assist myocardial repair Binds to heparin sulfate, fibronectin, and vitronectin	83–91
IGF— (insulin-like growth factor)	7.5	Half-life of 6 h. following subcutaneous injection [89]	Liver cells Skeletal muscle cells	Induction of cartilage ECM protein secretion and chondrogenic differentiation of mesenchymal stem cells Proliferation and differentiation of myoblasts	Chondrogenic differentiation of MSCs is significantly enhanced with co-application of TGF-β Enhanced cartilage repair with co-application of BMP-7 In concert with growth hormone, IGF moderates muscle development *in vivo*	92–98

(continued)

TABLE 8.1. (Continued)

Name	Molecular weight (MW), kDa	Stability	Origins	Cellular effects	Comments	References
					IGF can bind to ECM through matrix-bound IGF binding protein-5, or can be heparin bound when associated with IGF-binding protein-2	
SDF-1—(stromal-derived factor-1, CXCL-12)	7.8		Stromal cells	Strong migration and homing of mesenchymal stem cells Chemotaxis of lymphocytes	Basic Can enhance wound healing and angiogenesis Augments the effects of a variety of other growth factors Binds to heparin sulfate	99–105
PlGF—(placental growth factor)	46		Various tissues but not kidney or pancreas	Chemotaxis of endothelial cells, and hemotopoietic progenitor cells Increases vascular permeability Chemotaxis and activation of monocytes	Homodimeric glycoprotein member of the VEGF family Augments the effects of VEGF Useful in vascular engineering and wound healing	106–108

IL—(interleukin) Many isoforms: IL-1-35	16–45	Leukocytes Macrophages MSCs Fibroblasts Various cell types for different interleukins	Chemotaxis and activation of leukocytes and macrophages Activation of fibroblasts and keratinocytes Inflammation Collagen deposition in wound healing Immunity Stimulation of angiogenesis	Very numerous with a variety of activities. See References 111, 112	109–116

matrix-integrated growth factor receptors. Examples of growth factors binding directly to structural ECM components are numerous. TGF-β and bone morphogenetic protein (BMP)-2 bind to regions of collagen IV, and TGF-β can also be bound by fibronectin and in latent form by microfibrillar structures. FGFs can bind to a matrix-embedded form of the FGF receptor, and PDGF-AB/BB bind to osteonectin, a basement membrane protein.

However, the most prominent and well-characterized category of ECM–growth factor interaction involves proteoglycan binding. Proteoglycans consist of a protein core attached to at least one glycosaminoglycan (GAG) chain, and many growth factors exhibit a proteoglycan-binding region. In particular, the proteoglycans heparin and heparin sulfate have been shown to exhibit high binding affinity for a large range of growth factors [120], including bFGF, TGF-β, VEGF, hepatocyte growth factor (HGF), platelet-derived growth factor (PDGF), BMPs, insulin-like growth factor (IGF), SDF-1, certain interleukins (ILs), and a form of EGF termed heparin-binding EGF (see Table 8.1). Variations in heparin-binding affinity between different isoforms of growth factors largely determine differences in their *in vivo* solubility and the area of their effective action.

8.3.2.2 *Modulation of Growth Factor Activity by Matrix Binding.* More than just providing storage, ECM binding can modulate growth factor activity in a variety of ways. The function of some bioactive agents is dependent upon matrix association. For instance, binding of bFGF to heparin sulfate imparts stability and prolonged activity to the factor [121–123] and is required for a cellular response to occur [124, 125]. In this case, heparin sulfate stabilizes a bFGF receptor pair and coordinates proper spatial presentation of a bound bFGF pair to facilitate ligation. Likewise, HGF activated by local tissue injury functions when bound to both a cell surface receptor and heparin sulfate, showing increased mitogenic activity in hepatocytes [126, 127]. Latent TGF-β can be activated by binding of the matrix protein thrombospondin [128]. Matrix binding can also promote growth factor activity less directly by localizing an active factor to enhance its regional effect. IL-3 activity can be modulated in this manner through heparin sulfate binding of the functional factor [129].

On the other hand, many bioactive agents become inactive upon matrix binding or are secreted directly into the matrix in an inactive form. In this case, matrix binding negatively regulates the growth factor activity, but simultaneously allows for its regional storage in a readily available form for rapid localized action upon future release. Growth factors sequestered in this way are often protected from clearance and degradation processes that would affect soluble proteins. TGF-β is produced as a latent matrix-associated complex of proteins, allowing it to be present in high concentrations in a tissue without immediate activity. HGF is likewise secreted in a latent, matrix-bound form. Matrix immobilization of such factors allows for the development of standing gradients that contribute to organized and directed cell responses upon growth factor release/activation. Heparin-binding isoforms of VEGF show reduced mitogenic and vascular permeability effects when matrix bound, but like TGF-β, they form immobilized concentration gradients that are vital to directing angiogenic endothelial cell migration upon release from the matrix [130].

8.3.2.3 Release of Matrix-Bound Factors.

For factors that are sequestered by ECM binding, mechanisms of release can provide positive regulation of activity. Liberation of growth factors from the matrix is accomplished primarily through the activity of proteases, including MMPs, thrombin, and plasmin, which can specifically cleave various matrix components to free incorporated growth factors or expose functionally active matrix–growth factor complexes. Cleavage of matrix-bound proteins in the latent TGF-β complex by plasmin results in the release of active TGF-β. Likewise, matrix-bound VEGF and colony stimulating factor-1 (CSF-1) are freed from the matrix by plasmin. PDGF-B is released from the matrix in a functionally active form through the activity of thrombin [131–134]. MMP cleavage of various collagens can also expose regions of active growth factors that were previously inaccessible to cells. Furthermore, heparinases can liberate heparin-binding growth factors from association with heparin sulfate. Some ECM fragments that result from proteolytic cleavage function as signaling molecules themselves. Such fragments can be termed *matrikines*. For instance, MMP-cleaved laminin-5 creates an epitope that binds different integrins than the intact molecule, thus inducing epithelial cell migration [135]. MMP2/9 cleavage of collagen IV creates a fragment that is proangiogenic, while MMP-7 and elastin cleavage of collagen XVIII produces an antiangiogenic fragment [136]. Certain collagen I fragments are known to reduce focal adhesion of smooth muscle cells. Fibronectin fragments can inhibit cell proliferation, induce proteinase gene expression, promote adipocyte differentiation, and induce cell migration [136].

8.3.2.4 Sequestered Growth Factors Form 3-D Standing Gradients in Tissues.

As mentioned, many matrix-bound bioactive factors present a 3-D standing gradient. This activity seems to be a unique property of growth factor signaling. Most growth factors are chemotactic and direct cell migration along these gradients toward regions of high concentration. Migrating cells secrete proteases in order to traverse through the ECM, and in the process liberate growth factors in their direct vicinity, which in turn act on the cell to further regulate behavior. Cells also secrete their own growth factors, altering the biochemical identity of the local ECM and creating new bioactive gradients for future cell signaling. Thus, sequestration of growth factors in the matrix creates a standing "blueprint" for cell activity which is accessed by the cell itself. As compared to cell signaling via *de novo* protein synthesis, the ECM–growth factor unit represents a readily available and rapidly effective means for propagating information about a local microenvironment and directing appropriate cell responses.

Overall, then, the matrix serves as a depot for bioactive agents, allowing for their extended stability, precise localization, rapid activity, and functional regulation. As a unit, the matrix/growth factor network allows for multiple cell signals to be presented in a complex and adaptable spatiotemporal gradient for precise regulation of cell behavior. In order to achieve the degree of control over cell behavior required for generation of quality engineered tissue, growth factor delivery systems must attempt to emulate such reciprocal interaction.

8.4   DELIVERY OF GROWTH FACTORS IN TISSUE ENGINEERING AND REGENERATIVE MEDICINE

Growth factors intended to have a controlled effect on tissue growth in tissue engineering must be made available to the appropriate cells through some manner of delivery. The simplest forms of administration include systemic intravenous delivery and bolus injection. However, the nonlocalized nature of such delivery can contribute to ineffectuality and undesired side effects [11, 13, 138]. It is for this reason that current approaches to growth factor administration employ more specialized delivery systems.

Delivery refers to the process in which drug solutes migrate from the initial position in the polymeric system to the polymer's outer surface and then to the release medium [139, 140]. Release kinetics are affected by properties of the release medium (including pH, temperature, ionic strength, and presence of enzymes), properties of the agent being delivered (including size, charge, solubility, stability, and material interactions), and properties of the delivery matrix (including chemical composition, structure, swelling, and degradation) [140]. For *in vivo* and *in vitro* approaches to tissue engineering, the medium into which an agent is released is either extracellular fluid or culture medium, respectively. Because the medium is specifically formulated to ensure cellular growth and survival, its makeup cannot be readily altered in order to affect delivery. Likewise, the chemical identity and structure of natural bioactive agents are properties that define their biological functions and cannot be greatly altered without affecting their efficacy. Thus the material properties of a delivery matrix remain as the most readily engineered factor for achieving controlled delivery of therapeutic agents in tissue engineering.

Polymers are useful materials for constructing a delivery matrix because of the way in which their assembly can be controlled to provide a large range of chemical and mechanical properties that affect delivery. Growth factor release rate can be easily modified, for example, by varying the identity and molecular weight of component monomers and the cross-linking density of polymer chains. In the following sections we will discuss key considerations for the design of a polymer-based growth factor delivery device as well as different polymers that are commonly employed for the purpose of growth factor delivery in tissue engineering and regenerative medicine.

8.4.1   Considerations for Design of a Growth Factor Delivery Device

The concepts of delivery, as overviewed in Chapters 1 and 2, can be applied to the administration of a wide range of natural and synthetic agents. For each, properties of the specific agent impact decisions for the design of an appropriate delivery construct. As discussed in Section 8.3.1, the commonly applied agents in tissue engineering are protein growth factors. Thus, unique properties of growth factors are important to consider when endeavoring to develop an effective growth factor delivery construct. Compared to many synthetic drugs, growth factors are of high molecular weight, yet highly soluble, readily dissolving in the extracellular fluid. They function in small concentrations, but as proteins they are subject to degradative enzymatic and oxidative processes and thus exhibit short half-lives in solution in most tissues [141, 142]. Also, unlike endocrine agents, such as hormones, growth factors are paracrine or autocrine, functioning over relatively short distances. To this end, direct interaction with the matrix allows for the development of 3-D signaling gradients that both prolong growth factor function and provide an added level of control over cell behavior. Thus, there are several considerations for the development of devices intended to deliver growth factors [10, 11, 143].

- There must be knowledge about the growth factor(s) to be delivered. This includes a decision as to which factor(s) is/are therapeutically appropriate for the given application as well as an understanding of the characteristics and activities of those factors. Some factors are involved in tissue regeneration in general, while others have potent tissue-specific activity. Section 8.3.1 discussed common growth factors used in tissue engineering.

- The mode of factor delivery should encourage some manner of specificity. In other words, delivery should be targeted to the cells of interest, with minimal delivery to nontarget cells or locations. This can be accomplished simply through local delivery from a matrix vehicle in close proximity to the target cells, or through more complex mechanisms that actively present the factor only to the target cells. In terms of specificity, polymeric delivery should provide some advantage over systemic delivery or bolus injection, such as increased factor activity, decreased dose requirement, and/or minimization of systemic side effects.

- The polymeric delivery system must provide a well-controlled profile of growth factor release. Both temporal and spatial dynamics of growth factor presentation impact cell responses, and thus both the timing and amount of factor release must be considered. Material properties and fabrication processes can greatly affect delivery kinetics. Polymer parameters that can be manipulated to affect growth factor release include pore size and mesh density, loading capacity, load distribution, hydrophobicity/-philicity, binding affinity, and degradation or erosion rate. Furthermore, bioresponsive polymers can release incorporated factors in response to changes in pH, temperature, and osmolarity, or by activity of endogenous enzymes. It is generally desirable to recreate the native concentration profile using such tools when possible.

- Growth factor functionality must be maintained throughout the process of device fabrication, storage, and use. Proteins are somewhat susceptible to denaturation outside physiological conditions. Polymer fabrication techniques that require high temperatures, extreme pHs, or harsh solvents can damage growth factor function. Additionally, if a growth factor is bound to the polymer, it must be ensured that its active site is still accessible. In the body, long-term stability and activity of growth factors are often achieved by their sequestration in the ECM which provides them with protection (Section 8.3.2). Polymeric systems that mimic this action will be best able to provide prolonged activity of the factor they are delivering.

8.4.2 Polymers for Growth Factor Delivery

Polymers are composed of repeated monomer subunits that can be homogeneous or heterogeneous. This contributes to their great diversity of properties. The polymers commonly used for growth factor delivery can be classified as naturally derived or synthetic. Natural polymers are those that naturally occur in biological organisms. Synthetic polymers do not exist in nature and are chemically engineered. Hybrid polymers can also be created that incorporate both natural and synthetic components, combining the favorable characteristics of each. Detailed discussions of natural and synthetic polymers can be found elsewhere in this text, but we will briefly identify those polymers commonly used for growth factor delivery, highlighting pros and cons of their use.

8.4.2.1 Natural Polymers. Natural polymers are generally grouped as polysaccharide-based or protein-based. Polysaccharide polymers include hyaluronic acid, alginate, and chitosan (and heparin as a growth factor stabilizer). Protein polymers include materials such as natural collagen, denatured collagen (gelatin), and fibrin. These polymers are usually derived from the matrix material of various animal species. In general, protein-based biopolymers are mechanically stronger than polysaccharide-based biopolymers in their unmodified forms. Most natural polymers are highly water-soluble, allowing for gentle aqueous processing of growth factors and polymer at the same time, which can improve the percentage loading and distribution within a device. Natural polymer delivery matrices can be formed, for instance, through freeze drying, aqueous cross-linking in the presence of divalent cations, or in response to mild temperature changes. A large advantage of using natural polymers in tissue engineering is that they exhibit inherent interactions with growth factors and cells without need for modification. They are also degraded through natural physiological processes into nontoxic components, releasing incorporated factors as well as bioactive matrix fragments (Section 8.3.2).

However, compared to synthetic polymers, natural polymers are somewhat less available and more expensive to isolate. In their native forms, they also exhibit lower mechanical strength than many synthetic polymers with a smaller range of inherent mechanical properties. Also, native natural polymers may be more difficult to modify than synthetic polymers, resulting in somewhat less control over tunability of release. Properties of some common natural polymers used in growth factor delivery are given in Table 8.2. The reader is directed to Reference 144 for an additional review on this topic.

8.4.2.2 Synthetic Polymers. Synthetic polymers have several advantages over natural polymers in growth factor delivery. Because they are not derived from animal sources, they carry less danger of immunogenicity and transfer of disease. They provide a wide range of chemical and mechanical properties, which can be superior to and easier to predict than those exhibited by natural polymers. The greatest benefit of synthetic polymers is their capacity and ease with which they can be modified, functionalized, and configured. This allows for the tailoring of

TABLE 8.2. Natural Polymers Commonly used for Growth Factor Delivery in Tissue Engineering

Polymer	Molecular weight (MW), kDa	Properties	Degradation	Growth factor interactions	Uses	References
Polysaccharides						
Hyaluronic Acid (HA)	5–20	Nonsulfated GAG with MW dependant upon the tissue from which it is isolated ECM component which can associate with other GAGs or collagen	Degrades within 2–4 wk *in vivo*, depending upon degree of cross-linking. Degraded by specific hyaluronidases	Electrostatic	Used in hydrogel and scaffold delivery systems HA derivatives can form thin films	144–147
Alginate	30–270	Unbranched, linear, anionic polysaccharide polymer derived from seaweed Can be prepared with MW from 50 to 100,000 residues (with higher MW holding more water) Release is mainly diffusion driven	Degrades within about 12 wk *in vivo* Not a native human polysaccharide; degraded by nonspecific enzymatic, hydrolytic, and lysozymal processes	Electrostatic	Used to form hydrogel and scaffold delivery systems Hydrogel tensile strength can be improved by addition of gluronic acid Often combined with PLL	144, 148

(continued)

TABLE 8.2. (*Continued*)

Polymer	Molecular weight (MW), kDa	Properties	Degradation	Growth factor interactions	Uses	References
Chitosan	7–200	Cationic amniopolysaccharide fiber derived from chitan, typically produced as a 2000 saccharide monomer unit. Can promote wound healing on its own With collagen, among the mechanically stronger natural polymers	Degrades in the range of 10–84 days *in vivo*, depending upon degree of deacetylation. Not a human-derived; degraded by nonspecific enzymatic, hydrolytic, and lysozymal processes	Electrostatic	Used to form hydrogel and scaffold delivery systems Tensile strength can be enhanced by using long, branched chains	144, 149
Proteins Collagens	~300	Protein helices that can be harvested as an insoluble network, *en masse*, or can be digested to soluble subunits	Degrades within 1–2 wk, *in vivo*, depending upon the degree of cross-linking. Degraded by MMP and specific protease activity.	Specific growth factor affinities (e.g., BMP-2 and TGF-β)	Used in fibril, thin film, hydrogel, and scaffold delivery systems Duration of growth factor release can be increased by increased cross-linking	144, 150

		ECM component which can interact with many growth factors and with cells				
		With chitosan, among the mechanically stronger natural polymers				
Gelatin	5–100	Denatured collagen	Degraded *in vivo* by the same processes as collagen and over the same timeframe	Does not exhibit specific affinity for growth factors due to denaturing.	Used in fibril, thin film, hydrogel, and scaffold delivery systems	144

(continued)

TABLE 8.2. (*Continued*)

Polymer	Molecular weight (MW), kDa	Properties	Degradation	Growth factor interactions	Uses	References
				Can associate with growth factors through electrostatic interactions, its surface charge can be varied through processing.		
Fibrin	180	Fibrous polymer formed from glycoprotein protofibrils. ECM component which can interact with several growth factors as well as cells	Degrades within 7–14 days *in vivo* through the activity of thrombin	Specific growth factor affinities (e.g., bFGF and VEGF)	Used as biological glue/sealant and in thin film and hydrogel delivery systems	144

properties such as cross-linking density, pore size, and degradation rate which affect growth factor release rates. They can also be modified to covalently bind growth factors for various forms of responsive release.

However, fabrication of synthetic polymers can sometimes utilize harsh processes that exclude the integration of growth factors during production because of protein denaturation or deactivation that wound result. In these cases, growth factors must be added following polymer production. Because they are foreign to the body, synthetic polymers can sometimes trigger unwanted immune responses. Likewise, many offer little inherent interaction with growth factors in the absence of modification. Finally, synthetic polymer degradation products can sometimes lead to the formation of nonconducive biological microenvironments, by lowering the local pH for example. Table 8.3 identifies common synthetic polymers employed for growth factor delivery in tissue engineering [140, 151].

8.4.2.3 Rational Design of Polymeric Delivery Systems. As mentioned, many delivery devices will incorporate multiple natural and/or synthetic polymers to achieve more desirable characteristics. Poly(ethylene glycol) (PEG) can be co-incorporated with hydrophobic polymers to create a more hydrophilic device and can be used as a surface treatment to reduce initiation of inflammation caused by protein adsorption. Natural polymers such as collagen and fibrin can be incorporated with synthetic polymers to produce a device with superior mechanical properties while retaining specific growth factor interactions. Polymers that rapidly degrade can be partnered with those that do not in order to tune overall device degradation rate. Such combinations result in a wide array of possible characteristics for growth factor delivery devices that can be tailored to the required application in attempt to mirror native growth factor delivery.

A large variety of other polymers and copolymers also exist for use in tissue engineering and growth factor delivery, with novel constructs being continuously developed. A device that is solely intended for growth factor delivery will emphasize transport and degradation properties. A device that is intended to both make growth factors accessible to cells and serve as a cell residence must in addition possess compatible biochemical and mechanical properties. Tissues with unique mechanical requirements may require scaffolds fabricated from unique polymers. Again, it is less important here to present every polymer that may be useful to growth factor delivery than to reiterate that the better a scaffold recapitulates physiological mechanical properties and growth factor presentation, the more likely the regenerated tissue will mimic the native tissue. We will next discuss different design approaches to polymeric growth factor delivery and release mechanisms associated with those designs.

8.4.3 Incorporation and Release of Growth Factors in Polymeric Delivery Systems

The method by which growth factors are incorporated into a polymeric delivery device influences the mode by which they will be released (Fig. 8.3). Growth factors can be incorporated into a construct through absorption/retention of the medium in which the

TABLE 8.3. Synthetic Polymers Commonly used for Growth Factor Delivery in Tissue Engineering

Polymer	Properties
α-Hydroxy esters	Include poly(lactic acid) (PLA), poly(glycolic acid) (PGA), copolymers of the two (PLGA), and poly(ε-caprolactone) and are the most widely used synthetic polymers in tissue engineering. They are biocompatible and can be manufactured to have a wide range of degradation rates through variation of molecular weight, copolymer ratio, and degree of crystallinity during fabrication. They degrade slowly through hydrolysis, with PLA, PLGA, and PCL exhibiting bulk erosion. PGA has been shown to degrade over 4–12 mo *in vivo* depending upon preparation, while different preparations of PLA can last 12 mo to 2 yr in the body. 50:50 PLGA copolymers degrade more rapidly than either PLA or PGA alone. PCL can have a 2 yr duration of degradation, thus is it most commonly used as a copolymer with other, more quickly degrading materials. Polyesters can also be engineered to have superior mechanical properties compared to natural materials. However, α-hydroxy ester polymers are typically hydrophobic and create acidic degradation products that can lower local pH, damaging proximal cells and accelerating their own hydrolytic degradation.
Poly(ethylene glycol) (PEG)	Highly hydrophilic polymer, forming well-swollen hydrogels when cross-linked. PEG hydrogels are very biocompatible but do not naturally degrade. Thus formulations such as PEG–fumerate have been developed which contain ester linkages for hydrolytic degradation. Furthermore, PEG resists protein adsorption and cell attachment and can be used as a copolymer with other materials to impart hydrophilicity and increase biocompatibility (PEG–PLA is a common example). Mechanical stiffness and diffusion from a PEG hydrogel can be controlled by adjusting the initial monomer MW and the cross-linking density. PEG cross-linking can be performed under mild conditions that are not damaging to cells or proteins
Polyvinyl alcohol (PVA)	A hydrophilic polymer that contains hydroxyl groups for increased protein and cell interactions. PVA hydrogels are not typically used for the delivery of proteins, but it is often incorporated as a copolymer to enhance cell and protein associations
Poly(N-isopropyl acrylamide) (PNIPAAm)	A thermoresponsive polymer that undergoes a coiling/uncoiling shift at near-physiological temperatures. Thus PNIPAAm is often used as a copolymer for the fabrication of temperature-responsive delivery constructs

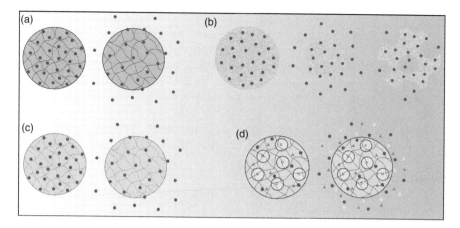

Figure 8.3. Various polymeric approaches to delivery of bioactive proteins. (a) Diffusion-based release. (b) Release by surface or bulk polymer erosion. (c) Release by cleavage of an enzymatically/chemically degradable tether molecule. (d) Cell-based delivery.

factors are dissolved, electrostatic interaction, physical entrapment, or chemical linkage of the factor either directly to the polymer itself or to a secondary molecule which interacts with the polymer. Depending upon the nature of growth factor–material interactions within the construct, release can then be diffusion controlled, erosion controlled, or exhibit mixed behavior. Additionally, a polymer that is engineered to release a factor at a specific, steady, and predetermined rate is said to exhibit controlled delivery, whereas a polymer that can initiate or halt release by stimulation from environmental cues is said to exhibit responsive delivery. Many examples of controlled and responsive release devices that deliver bioactive agents by diffusion and/or erosion currently exist in the literature and are given throughout this text. In the following sections, we will highlight several forms of growth factor incorporation into delivery matrices and discuss how they affect release of the factor.

8.4.3.1 *Constructs with Little or No Growth Factor Interaction.* For devices consisting of a nondegradable polymer with a large pore size or swelling ratio in which the incorporated growth factor does not interact with the polymer, release occurs passively in a diffusion-dominant manner. Swollen synthetic polymer hydrogels, such as those formed by cross-linked PEG, and rigid synthetic polymer scaffolds with large pores that are loaded after fabrication by immersion of the construct in a concentrated growth factor solution represent diffusion-dominant growth factor delivery devices. Reservoir-type systems are also diffusion-controlled with little association between the bioactive protein and the polymer. In these devices, the rate of delivery is governed by the initial loading concentration and the rate of diffusion of the growth factor through the polymer network, properties that are established during fabrication. In particular, diffusion rate is determined by factors that define the factor's route of diffusion, such as swelling ratio, polymer stiffness, pore/mesh size or cross-linking

density, and the interconnectivity and tortuousity of diffusional paths. As growth factors are large molecules, the mesh or pore size required for relatively unhindered diffusion is larger than for many other nonproteinous drugs. Also, it is important to consider that, depending upon the electrochemical properties of the construct material and the charge of the specific agent to be delivered, electrostatic interactions can contribute to increased agent retention and a departure from diffusion-controlled release.

Diffusion-controlled release devices that do not physically entrap an incorporated growth factor exhibit controlled release because delivery is sustained at a determined rate over time. Compared with bolus injection, this approach allows for a prolonged residence of the factor at the sight of action. However, diffusion from these devices is still fairly rapid, with an initial burst of release following implantation and full release occurring within several days or less. This time frame is shorter than the time required for the full progression of many tissue generative processes. Thus such simple diffusional delivery approaches do not readily allow delivery to be matched to the desired range of release profiles. Furthermore, they are also unable to alter delivery as cellular requirements change and have difficulty in achieving delivery of multiple growth factors at different rates.

KINETICS OF RELEASE FROM DIFFUSION-CONTROLLED DELIVERY CONSTRUCTS
Delivery is considerably easier to predict in a diffusion-controlled device than in a device that erodes or that features covalently bound growth factors. Equations that quantify diffusional mass transport of a solute from a device can be obtained from Fick's first and second laws of diffusion for constructs of various designs and geometries. For simplified modeling, these rely on geometric parameters of the device and known diffusional constants of the particular growth factor through the specific polymer material. For illustrative purposes, convenient equations for diffusion of an agent from constructs with common geometries are shown here [152].

DIFFUSION FROM A RESERVOIR CONSTRUCT For thin slab:

$$\frac{M_t}{M_\infty} = 1 - \exp\left(-\frac{ADKt}{VL}\right) \tag{8.1}$$

where M_t is the cumulative amount of agent released at time t, M_∞ is the cumulative amount released after infinite time, A is the surface area of the slab, D is the diffusion coefficient of the drug through the polymer, K is the partition coefficient of the agent between the polymer and the reservoir, V is the reservoir volume, and L is the polymer thickness.

For spheres:

$$\frac{M_t}{M_\infty} = 1 - \exp\left(-\frac{3R_o DKt}{R_i^2 R_o - R_i^3}\right) \tag{8.2}$$

where R_i is the radius of the inner surface of the polymer and R_o is the radius of the outer surface of the polymer.

DIFFUSION FROM MATRIX CONSTRUCTS For thin slab:

$$\frac{M_t}{M_\infty} = 1 - \frac{8}{\pi^2} \sum_{n=0}^{\infty} \frac{\exp\left[\frac{-D(2n+1)^2\pi^2 t}{L^2}\right]}{(2n+1)^2} \tag{8.3}$$

For spheres:

$$\frac{M_t}{M_\infty} = 1 - \frac{6}{\pi^2} \sum_{n=1}^{\infty} \frac{\exp\left[\frac{-Dn^2\pi^2 t}{R^2}\right]}{n^2} \tag{8.4}$$

where R is the total device radius.

8.4.3.2 Physical Entrapment of Growth Factors in Delivery Constructs.

Growth factors are retained longer, and thus delivery is extended, in polymers that are more highly cross-linked or exhibit a smaller pore/mesh size. If the polymer network is dense enough to physically exclude growth factor diffusion, then the factors are physically entrapped in the polymer matrix. This type of incorporation is common in solid polymers and must usually be accomplished by including dissolved growth factors during the fabrication process so that they become entrapped during polymerization/cross-linking. This illustrates the benefit of using water-soluble polymers that can be formed under mild conditions. If the growth factor is physically entrapped yet still not directly associated to the polymer, then the polymer degradation and/or polymer swelling are the methods by which the factor may be released, with the release rate dependent upon the rates of these processes. For hydrophilic polymers such as PEG, swelling occurs rapidly, and once swollen, diffusional transport will dominate (Section 8.4.3.1). For nonswelling hydrophobic polymers and polymers to which the growth factor becomes electrostatically associated, polymer erosion will be required for release. Again, devices that release growth factors by degradation commonly consist of poly(lactic acid) (PLA), poly(glycolic acid) (PGA), and poly(lactic-co-glycolic acid) (PLGA) formed through processes such as solvent casting, freeze-drying, or gas-foaming. These constructs are also controlled-release devices with the degradation rate dependent upon the susceptibility of the polymer to hydrolysis, which is determined by the polymer's chemical makeup. Degradable delivery devices are favorable because they do not require a follow up surgery to remove the depleted construct. They also exhibit growth factor release over a longer time frame than typical diffusion-dominant devices (weeks to months). However, degradable release devices still do not exhibit responsive release and also have trouble coordinating release of multiple growth factors at different rates. Nonetheless, attempts have been made to achieve multiple growth factor release by incorporating different growth factors into separate regions of the construct which have been fabricated from different polymers with various degradation rates. This can be accomplished in a layered thin film or by entrapping growth factor-laden microparticles within a larger hydrogel or scaffold.

Release kinetics for erosion controlled delivery are significantly more complex than for diffusion-controlled delivery and are similarly more difficult to model mathematically. Models for describing such behavior must take into account such factors as the rate of water infiltration, the degree of polymer chain disentanglement, surface versus bulk erosion, and geometrical parameters. The interested reader may refer to mathematical approaches put forth by Hopfenberg [153], Peppas [154], and Goepferich [155].

8.4.3.3 Direct or Indirect Binding of Growth Factors to a Delivery Scaffold.

Approaches that seek to further prolong growth factor delivery employ chemical interactions between incorporated growth factors and the polymer carrier. Specific interactions that exist between growth factors and natural polymers have already been discussed, but highlight the convenience of using natural biopolymers for growth factor delivery. Collagen and fibrin are often employed in growth factor delivery as stand-alone hydrogels and scaffolds. They have the favorable qualities of both binding growth factors for extended release/activity and being naturally degraded through enzymatic pathways that exist in the body. Collagen can be formed into a hydrogel "sponge" for growth factor delivery and scaffolds, and films can be formed from fibrin. These materials can also be used as copolymers or surface treatments of synthetic polymer constructs to enhance growth factor retention and delivery of a device. Synthetic polymers can be engineered to exhibit direct interaction with growth factors by appropriate modification of their surface charge to encourage electrostatic adsorption. In another approach, a natural secondary molecule can be employed for growth factor retention. Heparin, whose growth factor binding properties have been discussed, can be coincorporated into hydrogels and scaffolds for this purpose and is often used in fibrin scaffolds [156]. Release of the growth factor from devices constructed in this manner occurs through matrix degradation processes, such as those discussed in Section 8.3.2.3.

For synthetic polymer delivery devices, another approach includes covalently attaching growth factors by means of a chemical linker, called a tether, which can include a site for proteolytic degradation and allow for the release of a factor in response to enzymatic activity, as commonly occurs in the body. In this case, release is triggered by biochemical cues generated by the body itself, and is thus responsive. Growth factors can also be permanently bound to the polymer matrix to form an engineered microenvironment to encourage cell infiltration. This approach is most commonly employed in scaffold constructs that serve as a provisional matrix and provide structural stability as tissue formation progresses. As an example, TGF-β1 has been covalently conjugated to PEG hydrogels to achieve enhanced matrix production from vascular smooth muscle cells [157]. Such scaffolds can additionally benefit from the inclusion of integrin-binding moieties, sequences that are inherently present in many natural polymers and allow for cell attachment. For constructs engineered to contain a bound bioactive agent, it must be ensured that cells can attain access to the factor and that the factor activity is not detrimentally impacted by polymer binding.

8.4.3.4 Responsive Biopolymers. Some efforts to better control growth factor delivery have incorporated "smart" polymers that swell or degrade for release in response to variable external cues, such as local pH or temperature changes. Though it can be more difficult to control the release profile of a responsive device, it is generally accepted they have the potential to achieve growth factor release profiles that more closely match delivery as it occurs in the body, and thus could be more effective in achieving regeneration of replacement tissues. A construct that incorporates growth factors tethered to the polymer by enzymatically degradable linkers represent an example of a responsive release device because release is actively triggered by cues delivered from the local tissue microenvironment. Other responsive release construct designs include those that swell or exhibit tether degradation under specific temperature or pH conditions. Modified PEG hydrogels and PNIPAAM-containing polymers have been employed to these effects, respectively [158]. Responsive release devices have the potential to be engineered to deliver multiple bioactive agents in response to different cues by altering the identity of the tether to which each type of growth factor is bound.

8.4.4 Growth Factor Delivery Systems

The structure and geometry of a growth factor delivery device helps to tailor the system to the required therapeutic application. Delivery systems can include degradable microparticles, topical or injectable hydrogels, thin films and tubes, and solid polymer scaffolds, as well as designs that combine various features of such constructs. These designs may offer different benefits depending upon the specific intended therapy. For instance, ease of fabrication, minimalization of invasiveness during implantation, duration of factor release, mechanical strength, and provision of cell interaction can vary between different delivery designs. Additionally, most of the above systems can employ any of the different incorporation and release mechanisms that we have just discussed (Section 8.4.3). Thus, considering the number of different material polymers and (co)polymers, modes for growth factor incorporation and release, and structural and geometrical choices available, it is no wonder that polymeric systems are heavily employed in tissue engineering. In the following sections, we will provide an overview of common designs for polymeric growth factor delivery devices.

8.4.4.1 Degradable Polymeric Microparticles. Growth factor-loaded microparticles can be fabricated from natural or synthetic polymers. An aqueous solution of a natural polymer and the growth factor of interest can simply be chemically cross-linked to form microspheres. Synthetic polymer microparticles are typically fabricated by solvent extraction, whereby the dissolved growth factor is dispersed in an agitated organic solvent–aqueous solvent emulsion with subsequent evaporation of the organic solvent from the emulsion droplets yielding laden microspheres. Microparticles of various sizes can easily be formed and can be separated by sieving. Delivery of an agent from a microparticle generally occurs by particle erosion, thus polymer degradation rate is a key factor in the design of microparticle delivery systems. Coatings can also be applied to further modulate the microparticle release profile.

Degradable microparticles can be applied topically to an open wound or can be injected into the required site of action, a convenient benefit that avoids the need for an invasive implantation surgery. Microparticles remain at the site of administration providing continual release of their incorporated growth factor as they degrade. As compared to other injectable delivery matrixes, namely *in situ* forming hydrogels, microparticles maintain a defined shape/structure and are not intended to be space filling. Also, unlike delivery scaffolds, they are not intended to contribute to the mechanical stability of the regenerating tissue and typically are not engineered to promote direct cell interaction. Microspheres are most often used *in vivo* and not in tissue engineering culture.

Various microparticle systems have been described for the delivery of different bioactive factors, including IGF, nerve growth factor (NGF), TGF-β1, VEGF, BMP-2, and IL-2, and are especially useful for delivery to sensitive and hard-to-reach tissues such as brain, heart, and lung. IGF exhibited controlled release over 14–18 days from PLGA microparticles implanted in rats [159]. Hyaluronane, alginate–polylysine, and PLGA microparticles have been described for the release of NGF [160, 161], with NGF delivery from PLGA particles inducing survival of injured neurons for 6 weeks [160]. TGF-β1 could be released from blended PLGA–PEG microparticles for at least 28 days and enhanced the proliferation and osteoblastic differentiation of marrow stromal cells [162]. VEGF has been delivered from PLGA microspheres for myocardial repair [163] and from gelatin [164] and alginate [165] microparticles for the induction of tissue vascularization. BMP-2 for the enhancement of bone repair has been delivered from gelatin microparticles [166, 167]. Also, aerosolized PLGA microspheres loaded with IL-2 have been investigated for pulmonary delivery of the factor [168]. *In vivo* studies utilizing microparticles for growth factor delivery generally report enhanced growth factor effects because of prolonged delivery with an initial burst phase of release immediately following implantation followed by a sustained plateau of release for up to 30 days.

Microparticles can also be combined with polymer hydrogels and scaffolds to prepare complex delivery systems capable of more prolonged delivery or delivery of multiple growth factors. Simple incorporation of BMP-2-laden PLGA microparticles in carboxylmethylcellulose gel provided release for at least 21 days and promoted superior bone repair when implanted into a bone defect [169]. Alginate microspheres loaded with VEGF [170] and PLGA microspheres loaded with IGF-1 [171] imbedded in poly(vinyl alcohol) (PVA) hydrogels have been described for the induction of angiogenesis and cartilage repair, respectively. Dual release of BMP-2 and IGF-1 from Dex-GMA/gelatin microparticles and imbedded in a Dex-GMA/gelatin scaffold increased metabolism and proliferation of periodontal ligament fibroblasts [172]. A device incorporating the more specialized factors, brain-derived neurotrophic factor and glial cell-derived neurotrophic factor, achieved dual delivery in the brain by incorporating the factors into PLGA microspheres which were loaded into a PVA hydrogel for implantation [173].

8.4.4.2 Hydrogels. Hydrogels are cross-linked, water-soluble polymer networks notable for their hydrophilicity and ability to absorb many times their volume in water. Many natural polymers form hydrogels, including collagen, gelatin, fibrin, hyaluronic acid, alginate, and chitosan. Synthetic polymers such as PEG and PVA also form hydrogels. Despite their high water content, hydrogels maintain their shape and thus function as solids on the macroscale but act much like aqueous solutions microscopically. This facilitates the free diffusion of dissolved biochemicals within the polymer network and allows many hydrogels, particularly those formed from natural matrix polymers, to provide a framework for cell infiltration and residence. However, in general, hydrogels do not provide significant mechanical stability.

Synthetic hydrogels do not possess much capacity for innate growth factor or cellular interaction other than electrostatic association. For growth factors that are smaller than the mesh size of the polymer network, release occurs by diffusion and proceeds rapidly upon implantation. Increasing the cross-linking density of the hydrogel to decrease the mesh size can slow diffusion. Also, co-incorporation of a growth factor-binding agent, such as heparin, can increase factor retention and prolong delivery. Alternatively, covalent linkage of the factor to the polymer immobilizes it for increased retention. Release can occur by polymer erosion, or not at all, for cases in which cell invasion of the matrix is desired. On the other hand, natural polymer hydrogels often possess inherent growth factor and cellular interactions. As many natural polymers that form hydrogels are matrix components, many of the matrix–growth factor interactions that were discussed in Section 8.3.2 apply to impact delivery. Natural hydrogels are also eroded by cell-regulated processes, allowing them to be enzymatically degraded and replaced with natural matrix as tissue generation progresses.

Bioactive factors are incorporated into hydrogel constructs upon soaking the construct in an aqueous solution containing the growth factor, by physical entrapment of factors that are present in solution during cross-linking, or by covalent attachment of the factor to the precursor polymer units. Pre-formed hydrogel delivery constructs can be surgically implanted, or *in situ* cross-linking polymers can be injected for hydrogel formation within the body. The existence of relatively gentle methods for hydrogel cross-linking means that loss of growth factor activity is often minimal. Depending upon the polymer, hydrogel cross-linking can proceed in the presence of divalent cations, under mild temperature shifts or by the addition of light- or heat-activated chemical initiators.

Hydrogels have been employed for the delivery of many different growth factors in regenerative medicine and tissue engineering. Some hydrogel implants have been intended to deliver a factor into the surrounding tissue, while others are designed to encourage migration of specific cell populations into the hydrogel. In particular, natural polymer hydrogels tend to be well suited for cell invasion. Alternatively, PEG has been an extensively utilized synthetic polymer because of its biocompatibility and versatility. EGF, HGF, and bFGF have been delivered from gelatin hydrogels to promote neuronal healing of the eye [174], ear [175], and face [176]. To promote neurite ingrowth, NGF has been delivered from heparin-containing fibrin hydrogels [177]. Fibrin hydrogels containing PDGF-BB and bFGF induced increased chemotactic and mitogenic responses in smooth muscle cells that were also incorporated into the hydrogel [178]. StarPEG-heparin hydrogels have been investigated for the delivery of VEGF and bFGF to enhance endothelial cell morphogenesis and vascular formation/repair [179, 180]. BMP-2 has been incorporated into degradable PEG hydrogels for the enhancement of bone repair [181] and into hyaluronic acid and heparin–alginate hydrogels for cartilage generation [182, 183]. TGF-β3 has also been delivered via agarose hydrogels to promote cartilage growth [184]. Gradients of covalently immobilized bFGF in PEG hydrogels directed alignment and migration of smooth muscle cells within the construct [185].

An exciting class of polymers form hydrogels in physiological conditions following injection of the precursor polymer–growth factor solution. Like injectable microparticle delivery vehicles, implantation of these hydrogels does not require an invasive surgical procedure. Additionally, they can be used to fill irregularly shaped tissue voids. Some natural polymers, such as collagen, innately form hydrogels in aqueous conditions. Others, such as chitosan–polyol salt systems and specific PLGA–PEG–PLGA block polymers have been engineered to do so. Injectable collagen has been used for the delivery of EGF and bFGF for spinal cord repair [186]. Injectable PEGylated fibrin hydrogels have been shown to be useful for the delivery of TGF-β1 and PDGF-BB [187]. BMPs could be delivered from injectable chitosan–polyol salt formulations [188]. IL-2 was delivered from thermoresponsive injectable PLGA–PEG–PLGA block hydrogels [189].

8.4.4.3 Porous Polymer Scaffolds.

Scaffold delivery systems couple a means for growth factor administration with desirable mechanical properties. Even more than hydrogels, they are often specifically engineered as 3-D microenvironments designed to promote cell invasion, sustain vital cell functions, and direct cell behavior. Solid scaffolds are intended to fill lost tissue space and contribute to the mechanical properties of the regenerating tissue while providing cell signals. Though general-purpose scaffolds can be formed by many techniques, the recent need for delivery of proteins from scaffolds in tissue engineering limits feasible fabrication options to those that do not result in the loss or denaturation of growth factors. Freeze-drying, salt-leaching, gas-foaming, and electrospinning are fabrication techniques commonly applied for growth factor delivery scaffolds. In most cases, the growth factor is present in solution during scaffold fabrication for direct incorporation. As with microparticles and hydrogels, covalent binding of the factor of interest to the polymer can be employed to increase retention and prolong release/availability.

Scaffolds are intended to directly interact with host cells to promote tissue formation. The polymer(s) used to construct a scaffold may affect the way in which the device will interact with the host tissue even in the absence of growth factors. For instance, many natural polymer scaffolds can directly contribute to tissue repair; however, the addition of growth factors can greatly enhance effects on cell behavior. Synthetic scaffolds have many more tunable characteristics and a wide range of engineerable properties. Scaffold sponges represent the simplest delivery scaffolds, which are loaded by immersion in a growth factor-containing medium. Diffusional transport dominates delivery from such devices. Scaffolds can also be engineered to incorporate growth factors physically and/or chemically. In such devices, release will usually be more dependent upon scaffold degradation. Many recently developed delivery scaffolds have striven for responsive growth factor delivery, with release triggered by protease secretion from infiltrating cells. These responsive devices may be best able to mimic the natural availability of growth factors, with delivery occurring on demand in accordance with native physiological pathways.

Besides growth factor delivery, scaffolds have the intended purpose of promoting cell invasion and residence. Growth factor gradients within the scaffold can help to achieve this, but mechanical and chemical characteristics of the polymer material contribute as well. Scaffolds must be rigid enough so that cells can generate the tractional forces required for migration. Closely matching the mechanical properties of the scaffold to that of the native tissue can provide an environment that is conducive to the invasion, arrangement, and survival of appropriate tissue-specific cell types. It is also important for the scaffold to present sites for cell attachment which enable mobility and promote cell survival. For synthetic polymers, incorporation of peptide sequences, such as arginine-glycine-aspartate (RGD), can fulfill this requirement. Finally, it is important that the pore size of the scaffold matrix is large enough to allow for cell movement into and within the scaffold.

Solid polymer scaffolds can be pre-seeded with cells before implantation or can be engineered to promote invasion of specific cells from the surrounding tissue following implantation. It is generally desirable to match the rate of scaffold degradation to the rate of new matrix deposition by resident cells so that mechanical integrity is maintained while the developing tissue simultaneously integrates with the surrounding tissue. Collagen sponges have been used to deliver acidic FGF for dermal wound healing [190], and collagen–heparin scaffolds have been used to deliver FGF-2 and VEGF to promote angiogenesis [191]. Chitosan and chitosan–PLA scaffolds have been used to deliver PDGF-BB [192]. FGF-2 containing PLA scaffold disks have been used to promote angiogenesis and hepatocyte engraftment for liver regeneration [193], while gas-foamed PLA and PEG–PLA block copolymer scaffolds have been used to deliver BMP-2 for bone formation [194] and acidic FGF for spinal cord regeneration [195], respectively. PLG scaffolds have been shown to be effective in delivering BMP-2 for bone formation [196] and VEGF and PDGF for enhanced blood vessel formation and maturation [197]. Scaffolds formed by gas-foaming and particle-leaching of PLGA have been used to deliver VEGF [198, 199], EGF and HGF [199], and bFGF [200]. More specialized polymer and copolymer scaffolds can be employed for the production of specialized mechanical properties. Poly(ester urethane)urea hydrogels loaded with IGF-1 and HGF may be useful for the regeneration of various soft tissues [201], while rigid polymer and ceramic scaffolds are often utilized in bone engineering.

CHALLENGES OF INCORPORATING IMMOBILIZED GROWTH FACTOR GRADIENTS INTO SCAFFOLDS Scaffolds are intended to house cells, providing a microenvironment that exhibits the proper mechanical and biochemical properties required to regulate the cellular behaviors required for generation of a new specific tissue. In this regard, an implantable scaffold for tissue engineering represents an ECM analog. As we have discussed, natural ECM is reciprocally interactive with cells and bioactive factors

in numerous complex ways. A major way in which the ECM influences cell signaling and behavior is through association with growth factors for the formation of
3-D immobilized factor gradients. Gradients of growth factors guide many cellular
behaviors, including morphogenesis (e.g., differentiation), migration and alignment
(e.g., fibroblasts during wound healing), vessel pathfinding (e.g., capillary sprouting),
and axonal guidance (e.g., neural regeneration). In most cases, cells are guided in the
direction of increasing concentration gradient. While administration of a growth factor at a uniform concentration may elicit specific cellular responses, many processes
that require the coordinated activity of multiple cells over time cannot be satisfacto-
rily accomplished by this method. What's more, the combined signaling input from
gradients of multiple factors may be needed. Thus, it has become apparent that incorporation of spatial gradients of growth factors may be a major hurdle facing future
scaffold design approaches.

Techniques for generating immobilized growth factor gradients in 3-D degradable tissue engineering scaffolds are in their infancy [202]. Common approaches for
patterning a protein gradient onto a polymer surface are not easily adapted to 3-D
systems. On the other hand, microfluidic and microdroplet approaches can develop a
solution gradient within a hydrogel, but because of diffusion such gradients cannot
be maintained within the construct for more than a day [203]. Recent approaches for
achieving spatial control over growth factors within scaffolds involve regionalizing
the factors. For instance, microspheres loaded with different growth factors or different concentrations of the same growth factor can be embedded in a hydrogel [204,
205]. Or, a multilayered scaffold can be prepared, with each layer containing a different concentration of incorporated growth factor. However, neither approach generates
a true, continuous gradient throughout the scaffold and, additionally, the processing
involved in fabrication of multiple-component scaffolds can unintentionally alter the
intended degradation and release profiles of individual components. Moore et al. [206]
developed poly(hydroxyethyl methacrylate) scaffolds containing gradients of NGF and
neurotrophic-3 for directed neurite outgrowth using a gradient maker, and Singh et al.
[207] have described a technique for the assembly of microspheres loaded with different concentrations of dyes into a 3-D cell scaffold, though the effect of processing
on growth factor function was not evaluated . More recently, a gradient of silk microspheres loaded with IGF-1 or BMP-2 was incorporated into an alginate scaffold for
the formation of a growth factor gradient in the scaffold as the factors were released
[208]. It has been suggested that 3-D microprinting techniques that can carefully position microparticles may be beneficially applied in this approach to gradient formation
[209–211]. However, at the present, degradable bioengineered scaffolds that contain
multiple growth factors in immobilized gradients have yet to be realized, representing
a current limitation of material-based growth factor delivery systems.

8.4.4.4 Cell-Based Growth Factor Delivery as an Alternative to Material-Based Approaches.
To this point, we have discussed systems that
utilize material–growth factor interactions for the delivery of therapeutic agents
aimed at tissue regeneration and engineering. We have seen that it is desirable to
mimic the natural temporal and spatial patterns of growth factor delivery in order

to achieve the most desirable results. In light of this, we can identify two potential shortcomings of material-based growth factor delivery systems. First, material-based delivery systems are limited by their loading capacity. Although delivery rate can be adjusted so as to prolong the duration of factor release, a material-based system will inevitably become fully depleted or degraded and incapable of any further delivery. The second shortcoming is that material-based systems do not fully recapitulate the complex temporal and spatial networks of growth factors that act simultaneously in the body. Though we have discussed approaches for delivering multiple growth factors or patterning gradients within a scaffold, the fact remains that the natural processes exhibit far more complexity with some interactions that are yet to be fully understood. Even "smart" biomaterials cannot encompass the level of regulation over stability, activity, presentation (spatial and temporal), and production of the many dynamically interacting growth factors that natural cell matrix systems do.

A recent alternative approach to growth factor delivery has been to harness the natural capacity for cells to manufacture and secrete these cytokines. Such delivery approaches are termed *cell-based techniques*. The advantage of using cell-based delivery is that cells can naturally release a variety of different bioactive factors for paracrine activity, with responsive delivery of each occurring at the appropriate time and in the appropriate concentration by input from the surrounding environment. Thus natural profiles of multiple factors can be achieved without the need for complex material engineering.

While cytokine and matrix secretion from mature cells helps to maintain the identity of mature tissues, the large number of different mature phenotypes, along with their inflexibility, suggests that they may not be the ideal delivery source for tissue generation in regenerative medicine and tissue engineering. Alternatively, adult mesenchymal stem cells (MSCs) appear to be uniquely suited to the task. MSCs can be readily harvested and expanded and are capable eliciting numerous immunomodulatory and trophic effects. Most relevantly, MSCs have been shown to secrete PDGF, FGFs, TGF-βs, VEGFs, angiopoietins, NGF, HGF, IGFs, SDF-1, and IL-6, among others [212]. Furthermore, secretion profiles can be affected by local environmental factors such as dissolved biochemicals, nutrient and oxygen availability, and mechanical stimulation, as well as the stem cell source and the degree of line commitment (though differentiation is not required for secretion) [212]. This implies that various culture conditions may be used to promote different desirable secretion profiles.

MSCs and/or MSC-conditioned media have been employed in facilitation of graft acceptance, enhancement of dermal wound repair and repair of myocardial infarct, regeneration of renal tubular cells and microvasculature in kidney failure, and protection of neurons from degeneration. In these cases, they appear to exert beneficial effects by secreting cytokines that attract progenitor cells and trigger growth factor secretion by host cells [212]. MSCs can also differentiate into many mesodermal cell types, providing the potential for direct integration into the regenerating tissue and high quality tissue repair.

The primary difficulty in employing cells as a growth factor delivery system is maintaining their viability and function. To address this, encapsulation may represent an attractive method for providing a favorable cell environment while simultaneously providing cues that can influence secretion in a desirable way. For example, encapsulated pancreatic β-cells have been evaluated as means for insulin delivery for treatment of diabetes [213]. In tissue engineering, porous scaffolds may represent the most promising cell carriers. Cell-seeded scaffolds carry the same requirements as scaffolds for material-based delivery, with the added necessity that they promote the viability and function of the cells they support. Construct materials must be biocompatible, have sufficient mechanical properties, incorporate cell-binding motifs, allow for easy diffusion of dissolved factors, permit cell migration, and degrade so as to be replaced by new matrix. Natural biopolymers meet these criteria and also bind many of the growth factors that may be secreted by MSCs, allowing for the formation of immobilized gradients, unlike synthetic and material-based systems. Cell-seeded scaffolds can be implanted for tissue regeneration *in vivo* or can be maintained in culture for generation of a tissue, which is then implanted. Often times, various pretreatment culture conditions can be used to "prime" the cells to exhibit a desired functional response.

Cell-based growth factor delivery therapies represent a promising approach but are still in an early developmental stage. Nonetheless, they have attracted a growing amount of interest and attention. Careful engineering of material scaffolds, choice of appropriate cell source, and provision of appropriate microenvironmental conditions may allow cell-based delivery systems to drive high quality tissue repair and regeneration.

8.5 KEY POINTS

- Natural biological processes exist for the generation and regeneration of human tissues and are regulated by the paracrine activity of various bioactive proteins.
- Tissue engineering and regenerative medicine seek to use natural bioactive factors to modify and improve tissue healing and regeneration processes.
- The spatial and temporal presentation of growth factors, as well as cooperative action between multiple different growth factors, influences their effects on cell behavior.
- In the body, the ECM represents a material that interacts with bioactive agents to modulate their activity. Tissue engineering and regenerative medicine can apply lessons learned from these interactions to the engineering of material systems for controlled growth factor delivery.
- Polymers represent an ideal class of material for use in the delivery of bioactive proteins with natural and synthetic materials, each offering different benefits depending upon the specific application.
- Material-based systems for the delivery of bioactive proteins must incorporate the appropriate factor(s) for the application, maintain prolonged factor functionality, localize the factor to the desired target site, and provide an appropriate release profile.

- The method by which the bioactive factor is incorporated into the polymer construct affects its release. With minimal factor–material interaction, release is diffusion-controlled. Physical entrapment and direct linkage require material degradation for release.
- Delivery system designs include degradable microparticles, hydrogels, and scaffolds. As with materials, different designs offer different benefits depending on the required application.
- Immobilization of factor gradients into the material best re-creates the nature of factor presentation that occurs *in vivo* but is hard to re-create with material-based delivery systems.
- Cell-based delivery of bioactive agents represents a very recent approach in which cells are used to produce and secrete complex combinations and profiles of growth factors that cannot be achieved by material-based methods. This approach best re-creates growth factor networks as they occur in the body.

8.6 WORKED EXAMPLE

A nondegradable microsphere is fabricated from a synthetic polymer with TGF-β evenly distributed throughout. The microsphere has a diameter of 1 mm. Assuming no electrostatic interaction between TGF-β and the polymer, immediate wetting of the polymer and dissolution of TGF-β upon implantation, and negligible tissue concentration of TGF-β (release does not significantly raise tissue TGF-β levels), what percentage of the initial load of TGF-β remains in the device after 4 weeks? The diffusivity of TGF-β in the polymer is 4.0×10^{-11} cm^2 s^{-1}.

Answer:

$$\% \text{ Delivery} = 1 - \frac{6}{\pi^2} \sum_{n=1}^{\infty} \frac{\exp\left[\frac{-Dn^2\pi^2 t}{R^2}\right]}{n^2}$$

where

$D = 4.0 \times 10^{-11}$
$R = 0.05$ cm
$T = 2{,}419{,}200$ s (4 weeks)

$$\sum_{n=1}^{\infty} \frac{\exp\left[\frac{-Dn^2\pi^2 t}{R^2}\right]}{n^2} \approx 0.74$$

$$\% \text{ Delivery} = (1 - 0.45) \times 100\% = 55\%$$

$$\% \text{ Retention} = 100\% - \% \text{ Delivery} = 45\%$$

8.7 HOMEWORK PROBLEMS

1. A device consists of a 0.1 mm thick collagen membrane enclosing a reservoir containing a solution of $VEGF_{121}$ in water. The device is a 1 cm^2 sheet with a thickness of 2 mm. The diffusivity of VEGF in collagen in 5.55 × 10^{-7} cm^2 s^{-1} and the partition coefficient is 0.72. The device is implanted into a tissue containing no detectable VEGF. Calculate the percentage of VEGF that will have been delivered from the device after 5 min.

2. What are some benefits of using naturally derived polymers for the delivery of bioactive proteins? Name several growth factors whose administration might be benefitted by the use of natural polymers. What are the benefits of synthetic polymers in bioactive protein delivery? In what tissues may synthetic polymers be preferential for growth factor delivery?

3. What are important design considerations for devices that are intended to aid in the regeneration of a tissue through the delivery of bioactive proteins?

4. Compare the benefits and difficulties associated with material-based and cell-based growth factor delivery approaches.

REFERENCES

1. Lazarus GS, Cooper DM, Knighton DR, Margolis DJ, Percoraro RE, Rodeheaver G, Robson MC. Definitions and guidelines for assessment of wounds and evaluation of healing. Wound Repair Regen 1994;2:165–170.

2. Kim WLH, Gittes GK, Longaker MT. Signal transduction in wound pharmacology. Arch Pharm Res 1998;21:487–495.

3. Robson MC, Steed DL, Franz MG. Wound healing: biologic features and approaches to maximize healing trajectories. Curr Probl Surg 2001;38:71–141.

4. Monaco JL, Lawrence TL. Acute wound healing and overview. Clin Plast Surg 2003;30: 1–12.

5. Diegelmann RF, Evans MC. Wound healing: and overview of acute, fibrotic, and delayed healing. Front Biosci 2004;9:283–289.

6. Richardson M. Acute wounds: an overview of the physiological healing process. Nurs Times 2004;10:50–53.

7. Velnar T, Bailey T, Smrkolj V. The wound healing process: an overview of the cellular and molecular mechanisms. J Int Med Res 2009;37:1528–1542.

8. Bigazzi PE, Yoshida T, Ward PA, Cohen S. Production of lymphokine-like factors (cytokines) by simian virus 40-infected and simian virus 40-transformed cells. Am J Pathol 1975;80:69–78.

9. Nathan C, Sporn M. Cytokines in context. J Cell Biol 1991;113:981–986.

10. Whitaker MJ, Quirk RA, Howdle SM, Shakesheff KM. Growth factor release from tissue engineering scaffolds. J Pharm Pharmacol 2001;53:1427–1437.

11. Chen RR, Mooney DJ. Polymeric growth factor delivery strategies for tissue engineering. Pharm Res 2003;20:1103–1112.

12. Behm B, Babilas P, Landthaler M, Schreml S. Cytokines, chemokines and growth factors in wound healing. J Eur Acad of Dermatol and Venereol 2012;26:812–820.

13. Kozu A, Kato Y, Shitara Y, Hanano M, Sugiyama Y. Kinetic analysis of transcytosis of epidermal growth factor in Maden-Darby canine kidney epithelial cells. Pharm Res 1997;14:1228–1235.

14. Carpenter G, Cohen S. Epidermal growth factor. Annu Rev Biochem 1979;48:193–216.

15. Todderud G, Carpenter G. Epidermal growth factor: the receptor and its function. Biofactors 1989;2:11–15.

16. Konturek SJ, Pawlik W, Mysh W, Gustaw P, Sendur R, Mikos E, Bielański W. Comparison of organ uptake and disappearance half-time of human epidermal growth factor and insulin. Regul Pept 1990;30:137–148.

17. Jiang CK, Magnaldo T, Ohtsuki M, Freedberg IM, Bernerd F, Blumenberg M. Epidermal growth factor and transforming growth factor alpha specifically induce the activation- and hyperproliferation-associated keratins 6 and 16. Proc Natl Acad Sci U S A 1993;90: 6786–6790.

18. Mooney DJ, Kaufmann PM, Sano K, Schwendeman SP, Majahod K, Schloo B, Vacanti JP, Langer R. Localised delivery of epidermal growth factor improves the survival of transplanted hepatocytes. Biotechnol Bioeng 1996;50:422–429.

19. Chen GP, Ito Y, Imanishi Y. Photo-immobilization of epidermal growth factor enhances its mitogenic effect by artificial juxtacrine signaling. Biochim Biophys Acta 1997;1358:200–208.

20. Haller MF, Saltzman WM. Localized delivery of proteins in the brain: can transport be customized? Pharm Res 1998;15:377–385.

21. Ulubayram K, Nur Cakar A, Korkusuz P, Ertan C, Hasirci N. EGF containing gelatin-based wound dressing. Biomaterials 2001;22:1345–1356.

22. Bowen-Pope DF, Malpass TW, Foster DM, Ross R. Platelet-derived growth factor in vivo: levels, activity, and rate of clearance. Blood 1984;64:458–469.

23. Narayanan AS, Page RC. Biosynthesis and regulation of type V collagen in diploid human fibroblasts. J Biol Chem 1983;258:11694–11699.

24. Ross R, Raines EW, Bowen-Pope DF. The Biology of Platelet-Derived Growth Factor. Cell 1986;46:155–169.

25. Greenhalgh DG, Sprugel KH, Murray MJ, Ross R. PDGF and FGF stimulate wound healing in the genetically diabetic mouse. Am J Pathol 1990;136(6):1235–1246.

26. Pierce GF, Tarpley JE, Yanagihara D, Mustoe TA, Fox GM, Thomason A. Platelet-derived growth factor (BB homodimer), transforming growth factor-beta 1, and basic fibroblast growth factor in dermal wound healing. Neovessel and matrix formation and cessation of repair. Am J Pathol 1992;140:1375–1388.

27. Kim HD, Valentini RF. Human osteoblast response in vitro to platelet-derived growth factor and transforming growth factor-beta delivered from controlled-release polymer rods. Biomaterials 1997;18:1175–1184.

28. Lohmann CH, Schwartz Z, Niederauer GG, Carnes DL, Dean DD, Boyan BB. Pretreatment with platelet-derived growth factor-BB modulates the ability of costochondral resting zone chondrocytes incorporated into PLGA/PGA scaffolds to form new cartilage in vivo. Biomaterials 2000;21:49–61.

29. Deuel TF, Huang JS, Proffitt RT, Baenziger JU, Chang D, Kennedy BB. Human platelet-derived growth factor. Purification and resolution into two active protein fractions. J Biol Chem 1981;256:8896–8899.

30. Bauer EA, Cooper TW, Huang JS, Altman J, Deuel TF. Stimulation of in vitro human skin collagenase expression by platelet-derived growth factor. Proc Natl Acad Sci U S A 1985;82:4132–4136.

31. Edelman ER, Nugent MA, Karnovsky MJ. Perivascular and intravenous administration of basic fibroblast growth factor: vascular and solid organ deposition. Proc Natl Acad Sci U S A 1993;90:1513–1517.

32. Bikfalvi A, Klein S, Pintucci G, Rifkin DB. Biological roles of fibroblast growth factor-2. Endocr Rev 1997;18:26–45.

33. Shireman PK, Hampton B, Burgess WH, Greisler HP. Modulation of vascular cell growth kinetics by local cytokine delivery from fibrin glue suspensions. J Vasc Surg 1999;29:852–861.

34. Tabata Y, Miyao M, Inamoto T, Ishii T, Hirano Y, Yamaoki Y, Ikada Y. De novo formation of adipose tissue by controlled release of basic fibroblast growth factor. Tissue Eng 2000;250:97–103.

35. Sogabe Y, Abe M, Yokoyama Y, Ishikawa O. Basic fibroblast growth factor stimulates human keratinocyte motility by Rac activation. Wound Repair Regen 2006;14:457–462.

36. Yu PJ, Ferrari G, Galloway AC, Mignatti P, Pintucci G. Basic fibroblast growth factor (FGF-2): the high molecular weight forms come of age. J Cell Biochem 2007;100:1100–1108.

37. Schreiber AB, Winkler ME, Derynck R. Transforming growth factor-α: a more potent angiogenic mediator than epidermal growth factor. Science 1986;232:1250–1253.

38. Derynck R. Transforming growth factor α. Cell 1988;54:593–595.

39. Ebner R, Derynck R. Epidermal growth factor and transforming growth factor-α: differential intracellular routing and processing of ligand-receptor complexes. Cell Reg 1991;2:599–612.

40. Philip A, O'Connor-McCourt MD. Interaction of transforming growth factor-beta 1 with alpha 2-macroglobulin. Role in transforming growth factor-beta 1 clearance. J Biol Chem 1991;266:22290–22296.

41. McCartney-Francis NL, Wahl SM. Transforming growth factor β: a matter of life and death. J Leukoc Biol 1994;55:401–409.

42. Roberts AB, Sporn MB, Assoian RK, Smith JM, Roche NS, Wakefield LM, Heine UI, Liotta LA, Falanga V, Kehrl JH, Fauci AS. Transforming growth factor type beta: rapid induction of fibrosis and angiogenesis in vivo and stimulation of collagen formation in vitro. Proc Natl Acad Sci U S A 1986;83:4167–4171.

43. Postlethwaite AE, Keski-Oja J, Moses HL, Kang AH. Stimulation of the chemotactic migration of human fibroblasts by transforming growth factor beta. J Exp Med 1987;165:251–256.

44. Massagué J. The transforming growth factor-β family. Annu Rev Cell Biol 1990;6:597–641.

45. Desmouliere A, Geinoz A, Gabbiani F, Gabbiani G. Transforming growth factor-beta 1 induces alpha-smooth muscle actin expression in granulation tissue myofibroblasts and in quiescent and growing cultured fibroblasts. J Cell Biol 1993;122:103–111.

46. Gailit J, Welch MP, Clark RA. TGF-beta 1 stimulates expression of keratinocyte integrins during re-epithelialization of cutaneous wounds. J Invest Dermatol 1994;103:221–227.

47. Lin M, Overgaard S, Glerup H, Søballe K, Bünger C. Transforming growth factor-beta1 adsorbed to tricalciumphosphate coated implants increases peri-implant bone remodeling. Biomaterials 2001;22:189–193.

48. Mann BK, Schmedlen RH, West JL. Tethered-TGF-beta increases extracellular matrix production of vascular smooth muscle cells. Biomaterials 2001;22:439–444.

49. Barrientos S, Stojadinovic O, Golinko MS, Brem H, Tomic-Canic M. Growth factors and cytokines in wound healing. Wound Repair Regen 2008;16:585–601.

50. Munger JS, Sheppard D. Cross talk among TGF-β signaling pathways, integrins, and the extracellular matrix. Cold Spring Harb Perspect Biol 2011;3.

51. Lazarous DF, Shou M, Scheinowitz M, Hodge E, Thirumurti V, Kitsiou AN, Stiber JA, Lobo AD, Hunsberger S, Guetta E, Epstein SE, Unger EF. Comparative effects of basic fibroblast growth factor and vascular endothelial growth factor on coronary collateral development and the arterial response to injury. Circulation 1996;94:1074–1082.

52. Senger DR, Perruzzi CA, Feder J, Dvorak HF. A highly conserved vascular permeability factor secreted by a variety of human and rodent tumor cell lines. Cancer Res 1986;46:5629–5632.

53. Klagsbrun M, D'Amore PA. Vascular endothelial growth factor and its receptors. Cytokine Growth Factor Rev 1996;7:259–270.

54. Weatherford DA, Sackman JE, Reddick TT, Freeman MB, Stevens SL, Goldman MH. Vascular endothelial growth factor and heparin in a biologic glue promotes human aortic endothelial cell proliferation with aortic smooth muscle cell inhibition. Surgery 1996;120:433–439.

55. Zachary I. Vascular endothelial growth factor. Int J Biochem Cell Biol 1998;30:1169–1174.

56. Ferrera N. Role of vascular endothelial growth factor in the regulation of angiogenesis. Kidney Int 1999;56:794–814.

57. Ferrara N, Gerber HP, LeCouter J. The biology of VEGF and its receptors. Nat Med 2003;9:669–676.

58. Woolard J, Bevan HS, Harper SJ, Bates DO. Molecular diversity of VEGF-A as a regulator of its biological activity. Microcirculation 2009;16:572–592.

59. Whang K, Tsai DC, Nam EK, Aitken M, Sprague SM, Patel PK, Healy KE. Ectopic bone formation via rhBMP-2 delivery from porous bioabsorbable polymer scaffolds. J Biomed Mater Res 1998;42:491–499.

60. Boden SD. Bioactive factors for bone tissue engineering. Clin Orthop Relat Res 1999;367(Suppl):S84–S94.

61. Valentin-Opran A, Wozney J, Csimma C, Lilly L, Riedel GE. Clinical evaluation of recombinant human bone morphogenetic protein-2. Clin Orthop Relat Res 2002;395:110–120.

62. Sekiya I, Larson BL, Vuoristo JT, Reger RL, Prockop DJ. Comparison of effect of BMP-2, -4, and −6 on in vitro cartilage formation of human adult stem cells from bone marrow stroma. Cell Tissue Res 2005;320:269–276.

63. Knippenberg M, Helder MN, Zandieh Doulabi B, Wuisman PI, Klein-Nulend J. Osteogenesis versus chondrogenesis by BMP-2 and BMP-7 in adipose stem cells. Biochem Biophys Res Commun 2006;342:902–908.

64. Xiao YT, Xiang LX, Shao JZ. Bone morphogenetic protein. Biochem Biophys Res Commun 2007;362:550–553.

65. Burks MV, Nair L. Long-term effects of bone morphogenic protein-based treatments in humans. J Long Term Eff Med Implants 2010;20:277–293.

66. Rider CC, Mulloy B. Bone morphogenetic protein and growth differentiation factor cytokine families and their protein antagonists. Biochem J 2010;429:1–12.

67. Boon MR, van der Horst G, van der Pluijm G, Tamsma JT, Smit JW, Rensen PC. Bone morphogenetic protein 7: a broad-spectrum growth factor with multiple target therapeutic potency. Cytokine Growth Factor Rev 2011;22:221–229.

68. Davis S, Aldrich TH, Jones PF, Acheson A, Compton DL, Jain V, Ryan TE, Bruno J, Radziejewski C, Maisonpierre PC, Yancopoulos GD. Isolation of angiopoietin-1, a ligand for the TIE2 receptor, by secretion-trap expression cloning. Cell 1996;87:1161–1169.

69. Xu Y, Yu Q. Angiopoietin-1, unlike angiopoietin-2, is incorporated into the extracellular matrix via its linker peptide region. J Biol Chem 2001;276:34990–34998.

70. Kim I, Kim HG, Moon SO, Chae SW, So JN, Koh KN, Ahn BC, Koh GY. Angiopoietin-1 induces endothelial cell sprouting through the activation of focal adhesion kinase and plasmin secretion. Circ Res 2000;86:952–959.

71. Kim I, Kim HG, So JN, Kim JH, Kwak HJ, Koh GY. Angiopoietin-1 regulates endothelial cell survival through the phosphatidylinositol 3'-Kinase/Akt signal transduction pathway. Circ Res 2000;86:24–29.

72. Chae JK, Kim I, Lim ST, Chung MJ, Kim WH, Kim HG, Ko JK, Koh GY. Coadministration of angiopoietin-1 and vascular endothelial growth factor enhances collateral vascularization. Arterioscler Thromb Vasc Biol 2000;20:2573–2578.

73. Dallabrida SM, Zurakowski D, Shih SC, Smith LE, Folkman J, Moulton KS, Rupnick MA. Adipose tissue growth and regression are regulated by angiopoietin-1. Biochem Biophys Res Commun 2003;311:563–571.

74. Pizurki L, Zhou Z, Glynos K, Roussos C, Papapetropoulos A. Angiopoietin-1 inhibits endothelial permeability, neutrophil adherence and IL-8 production. Br J Pharmacol 2003;139:329–336.

75. Fiedler U, Augustin HG. Angiopoietins: a link between angiogenesis and inflammation. Trends Immunol 2006;27:552–558.

76. Thomas M, Augustin HG. The role of angiopoietins in vascular morphogenesis. Angiogenesis 2009;12:125–137.

77. Tria MA, Fusco M, Vantini G, Mariot R. Pharmacokinetics of nerve growth factor (NGF) following different routes of administration to adult rats. Exp Neurol 1994;127:178–183.

78. Cattaneo E, McKay R. Proliferation and differentiation of neural stem cells regulated by neural growth factor. Nature 1990;347:762–765.

79. Haller MF, Saltzman WM. Nerve growth factor delivery systems. J Control Release 1998;53:1–6.

80. Sakiyama-Elbert SE, Hubbell JA. Controlled release of nerve growth factor from a heparin-containing fibrin-based cell ingrowth matrix. J Control Release 2000;69:149–158.

81. Skaper SD. Nerve growth factor. Mol Neurobiol 2001;24:183–199.

82. Kingham PJ, Terenghi G. Bioengineered nerve regeneration and muscle reinnervation. J Anat 2006;209:511–526.

83. Appasamy R, Tanabe M, Murase N, Zarnegar R, Venkataramanan R, Van Thiel DH, Michalopoulos GK. Hepatocyte growth factor, blood clearance, organ uptake, and biliary excretion in normal and partially hepatectomized rats. Lab Invest 1993;68:270–276.

84. Nakamura T. Structure and function of hepatocyte growth factor. Prog Growth Factor Res 1991;3:67–85.

85. Mizuno K, Nakamura T. Molecular characteristics of HGF and the gene, and its biochemical aspects. EXS 1993;65:1–29.

86. Zioncheck TF, Richardson L, DeGuzman GG, Modi NB, Hansen SE, Godowski PJ. The pharmacokinetics, tissue localization, and metabolic processing of recombinant human hepatocyte growth factor after intravenous administration in rats. Endocrinology 1994;134:1879–1887.

87. Matsumoto K, Nakamura T. Emerging multipotent aspects of hepatocyte growth factor. J Biochem 1996;119:591–600.

88. Miller KJ, Thaloor D, Matteson S, Pavlath GK. Hepatocyte growth factor affects satellite cell activation and differentiation in regenerating skeletal muscle. Am J Physiol Cell Physiol 2000;278:C174–C181.

89. Toyoda M, Takayama H, Horiguchi N, Otsuka T, Fukusato T, Merlino G, Takagi H, Mori M. Overexpression of hepatocyte growth factor/scatter factor promotes vascularization and granulation tissue formation in vivo. FEBS Lett 2001;509:95–100.

90. Yoshida S, Yamaguchi Y, Itami S, Yoshikawa K, Tabata Y, Matsumoto K, Nakamura T. Neutralization of hepatocyte growth factor leads to retarded cutaneous wound healing associated with decreased neovascularization and granulation tissue formation. J Invest Dermatol 2003;120:335–343.

91. Rahman S, Patel Y, Murray J, Patel KV, Sumathipala R, Sobel M, Wijelath ES. Novel hepatocyte growth factor (HGF) binding domains on fibronectin coordinate a distinct and amplified Met-integrin induced signaling pathway in endothelial cells. BMC Cell Biol 2005;6:8.

92. Grahnén A, Kastrup K, Heinrich U, Gourmelen M, Preece MA, Vaccarello MA, Guevara-Aguirre J, Rosenfeld RG, Sietnieks A. Pharmacokinetics of recombinant human insulin-like growth factor I given subcutaneously to healthy volunteers and to patients with growth hormone receptor deficiency. Acta Paediatr 1993;82(391 Suppl):9–13.

93. Jones JI, Gockerman A, Busby WH Jr, Camacho-Hubner C, Clemmons DR. Extracellular matrix contains insulin-like growth factor binding protein-5: potentiation of the effects of IGF-I. J Cell Biol 1993;121:679–687.

94. Jones JI, Clemmons DR. Insulin-like growth factors and their binding proteins: biological actions. Endocr Rev 1995;16:3–34.

95. Aria T, Busby W Jr, Clemmons DR. Binding of insulin-like growth factor (IGF) I or II to IGF-binding protein-2 enables it to bind to heparin and extracellular matrix. Endocrinology 1996;137:4571–4575.

96. Florini JR, Ewton DZ, Coolican SA. Growth hormone and the insulin-like growth factor system in myogenesis. Endocr Rev 1996;17:481–517.

97. Kim H, Barton E, Muja N, Yakar S, Pennisi P, Leroith D. Intact insulin and insulin-like growth factor-I receptor signaling is required for growth hormone effects on skeletal muscle growth and function in vivo. Endocrinology 2005;146:1772–1779.

98. Fourtier LA, Barker JU, Strauss EJ, McCarrel TM, Cole BJ. The role of growth factors in cartilage repair. Clin Orthop Relat Res 2011;469:2706–2715.

99. Bleul CC, Fuhlbrigge RC, Casasnovas JM, Aiuti A, Sprigner TA. A highly efficacious lymphocyte chemoattractant, stromal cell-derived factor 1 (SDF-1). J Exp Med 1996;184: 1101–1109.

100. Netelenbos T, Zuijderduijn S, van den Born J, Kessler FL, Zweegman S, Huijgens PC, Dräger AM. Proteoglycans guide SDF-1-induced migration of hematopoietic progenitor cells. J Leukoc Biol 2002;72:353–362.

101. Jaszczyñska-Nowinka K, Markowska A. New cytokine: stromal derived factor-1. Eur J Gynaecol Oncol 2009;30:124–127.

102. Kimura Y, Tabata Y. Controlled release of stromal-cell-derived factor-1 from gelatin hydrogels enhances angiogenesis. J Biomater Sci Polym Ed 2010;21:37–51.

103. Henderson PW, Singh SP, Krijgh DD, Yamamoto M, Rafii DC, Sung JJ, Rafii S, Rabbany SY, Spector JA. Stromal-derived factor-1 delivery via hydrogel drug-delivery vehicle accelerates wound healing in vivo. Wound Repair Regen 2011;19:420–425.

104. Lau TT, Wang DA. Stromal cell-derived factor-1 (SDF-1): homing factor for engineered regenerative medicine. Expert Opin Biol Ther 2011;11:189–197.

105. Ratanavaraporn J, Furuya H, Kohara H, Tabata Y. Synergistic effects of the dual release of stromal cell-derived factor-1 and bone morphogenetic protein-2 from hydrogels on bone regeneration. Biomaterials 2011;32:2797–2811.

106. De Falco S, Gigante B, Persico MG. Structure and function of placental growth factor. Trends Cardiovasc Med 2002;12:241–246.

107. Gabhann FM, Popel AS. Model of competitive binding of vascular endothelial growth factor and placental growth factor to VEGF receptors on endothelial cells. Am J Physiol Heart Circ Physiol 2004;286:H153–H164.

108. Ribatti D. The discovery of the placental growth factor and its role in angiogenesis: a historical review. Angiogenesis 2008;11:215–221.

109. Mizel SB, Dukovich M, Rothstein J. Preparation of goat antibodies against interleukin 1: use of an immunoadsorbent to purify interleukin 1. J Immunol 1983;131:1834–1837.

110. Auron PE, Warner SJ, Webb AC, Cannon JG, Bernheim HA, McAdam KJ, Rosenwasser LJ, LoPreste G, Mucci SF, Dinarello CA. Studies on the molecular nature of human interleukin 1. J Immunol 1987;138:1447–1456.

111. Mizel SB. The interleukins. FASEB J 1989;3:2379–2388.

112. Liles WC, Van Voorhis WC. Review: nomenclature and biological significance of cytokines involved in inflammation and host immune response. J Infect Dis 1995;172: 1573–1580.

113. Barrientos S, Stojadinovic O, Golinko MS, Brem H, Tomic-Canic M. Growth factors and cytokines in wound healing. Wound Repair Regen 2003;16:585–601.

114. Lin ZQ, Kondo T, Ishida Y, Takayasu T, Mukaida N. Essential involvement of IL-6 in the skin wound-healing process as evidenced by delayed wound healing in IL-6-deficient mice. J Leukoc Biol 2003;73:713–721.

115. Ishida Y, Kondo T, Kimura A, Matsushima K, Mukaida N. Absence of IL-1 receptor antagonist impaired wound healing along with aberrant NF-kappaB activation and a reciprocal suppression of TGF-beta signal pathway. J Immunol 2006;176:5598–5606.

116. Hu Y, Liang D, Li X, Liu HH, Zhang X, Zheng M, Dill D, Shi X, Qiao Y, Yeomans D, Carvalho B, Angst MS, Clark JD, Peltz G. The role of interleukin-1 in wound biology. Part II: in vivo and human translational studies. Anesth Analg 2010;111:1534–1542.

117. Flaumenhaft R, Rifkin DB. The extracellular regulation of growth factor action. Mol Biol Cell 1992;3:1057–1065.

118. Cao L, Mooney DJ. Spatiotemporal control over growth factor signaling for therapeutic neovascularization. Adv Drug Deliv Rev 2007;59:1340–1350.

119. Schönherr E, Hausser HJ. Extracellular matrix and cytokines: a functional unit. Dev Immunol 2000;7:89–101.

120. Taipale J, Keski-Oja J. Growth factors in the extracellular matrix. FASEB J 1997;11:51–59.

121. Schultz GS, Wysocki A. Interaction between extracellular matrix and growth factors in wound healing. Wound Repair Regen 2009;17:153–162.

122. Gospodarowicz D, Cheng J. Heparin protects basic and acidic FGF from inactivation. J Cell Physiol 1986;128:475–484.

123. Flaumenhaft R, Moscatelli D, Saksela O, Rifkin DB. Role of extracellular matrix in the action of basic fibroblast growth factor: matrix as a source of growth factor for long-term stimulation of plasminogen activator production and DNA synthesis. J Cell Physiol 1989;140:75–81.

124. Rapraeger AC, Krufka A, Olwin BB. Requirement of heparin sulfate for bFGF-mediated fibroblast growth and myoblast differentiation. Science 1991;252:1705–1708.

125. Yayon A, Klagsbrun M, Esko JD, Leder P, Ornitz DM. Cell surface, heparin-like molecules are required for binding of basic fibroblast growth factor to its high affinity receptor. Cell 1991;64:841–848.

126. Lyon M, Deakin JA, Mizuno K, Nakamura T, Gallagher JT. Interaction of hepatocyte growth factor with heparan sulfate. Elucidation of the major heparan sulfate structural determinants. J Biol Chem 1994;269:11216–11223.

127. Zioncheck TF, Richardson L, Liu J, Chang L, King KL, Bennett GL, Fugedi P, Chamow SM, Schwall RH, Stack RJ. Sulfated oligosaccharides promotes hepatocyte growth factor association and govern its mitogenic activity. J Biol Chem 1995;270:16871–16878.

128. Murphy-Ullrich JE, Poczatek M. Activation of latent TGF-beta by thrombospondin-1: mechanisms and physiology. Cytokine Growth Factor Rev 2000;11:59–69.

129. Roberts R, Gallagher J, Spooncer E, Allen TD, Bloomfield F, Dexter TM. Heparin sulfate bound growth factors: a mechanism for stromal cell mediated haemopoiesis. Nature 1988;332:376–378.

130. Houck KA, Leung DW, Rowland AM, Winer J, Ferrera N. Dual regulation of vascular endothelial growth factor bioavaiability by genetic and proteolytic mechanisms. J Biol Chem 1992;267:26031–26037.

131. Soyombo AA, DiCorleto PE. Stable expression of human platelet-derived growth factor B chain by bovine aortic endothelial cells. Matrix association and selective proteolytic cleavage by thrombin. J Biol Chem 1994;269:17734–17740.

132. Park JE, Keller GA, Ferrara N. The vascular endothelial growth factor (VEGF) isoforms: differential deposition into the subepithelial extracellular matrix and bioactivity of extracellular matrix-bound VEGF. Mol Biol Cell 1993;4:1317–1326.

133. Taipale J, Keski-Oja J. Hepatocyte growth factor releases epithelial and endothelial cells from growth arrest induced by transforming growth factor-beta1. J Biol Chem 1996;271:4342–4348.

134. Benezra M, Vlodavsky I, Ishai-Michaeli R, Neufeld G, Bar-Shavit R. Thrombin-induced release of active basic fibroblast growth factor-heparan sulfate complexes from subendothelial extracellular matrix. Blood 1993;81:3324–3331.

135. Werb Z. ECM and cell surface proteolysis: regulating cellular ecology. Cell 1997;91:439–442.

136. Mott JD, Werb Z. Regulation of matrix biology by matrix metalloproteinases. Curr Opin Cell Biol 2004;16:558–564.

137. Eppler SM, Combs DL, Henry TD, Lopez JJ, Ellis SG, Annex BH, McCluskey ER, Zioncheck TF. A target-mediated model to describe the pharmacokinetics and hemodynamic effects of recombinant human vascular endothelial growth factor in humans. Clin Pharmacol Ther 2002;72:20–32.

138. Silva EA, Mooney DJ. Spatiotemporal control of vascular endothelial growth factor delivery from injectable hydrogels enhances angiogenesis. J Thromb Haemost 2007;5:590–598.

139. Fu Y, Kao WJ. Drug release kinetics and transport mechanisms of non-degradable and degradable polymeric delivery systems. Expert Opin Drug Deliv 2010;7:429–444.

140. Langer R. New methods of drug delivery. Science 1990;249:1527–1533.

141. Manning MC, Patel K, Borchardt RT. Stability of protein pharmaceuticals. Pharm Res 1989;6:903–918.

142. Krishnamurthy R, Manning MC. The stability factor: importance in formulation development. Curr Pharm Biotechnol 2002;3:361–371.

143. Maquet V, Jerome R. Design of macroporous biodegradable polymer scaffolds for cell transplantation. Mater Sci Forum 1997;250:15–42.

144. Übersax L, Merkle HP, Meinel L. Biopolymer-based growth factor delivery for tissue repair: from natural concepts to engineered systems. Tissue Eng-B 2009;15:263–289.

145. Saari H, Konttinen YT, Friman C, Sorsa T. Differential effects of reactive oxygen species on native synovial fluid and purified human umbilical cord hyaluronate. Inflammation 2000;17:403–415.

146. Paulsson M, Mörgelin M, Wiedemann H, Beardmore-Gray M, Dunham D, Hardingham T, Heinegård D, Timpl R, Engel J. Extended and globular protein domains in cartilage proteoglycans. Biochem J 1987;245(3):763–772.

147. Suh KY, Yang JM, Khademhosseini A, Berry D, Tran TN, Park H, Langer R. Characterization of chemisorbed hyaluronic acid directly immobilized on solid substrates. J Biomed Mater Res-B 2005;72(2):292–298.

148. Drury JL, Dennis RG, Mooney DJ. The tensile properties of alginate hydrogels. Biomaterials 2004;25:3187–3199.

149. Aggarwal D, Matthew HW. Branched chitosans: effects of branching parameters on rheological and mechanical properties. J Biomed Mater Res-A 2007;82:201–212.

150. Radu FA, Bause M, Knabner P, Lee GW, Friess WC. Modeling of drug release from collagen matrices. J Pharm Sci 2002;91:94–972.

151. Sokolsky-Papkov M, Agashi K, Olaye A, Shakesheff K, Domb AJ. Polymer carriers for drug delivery in tissue engineering. Adv Drug Deliv Rev 2007;59:187–206.

152. Siepmann J, Siepmann F. Modeling of diffusion controlled drug delivery. J Control Release 2012;161:351–362.

153. Hopfenberg HB. Controlled release from erodible slabs, cylinders, and spheres. In: Paul DR, Harris FW, editors. Controlled Release Polymeric Formulations. ACS Symposium Series. Vol. 22. Washington: American Chemical Society; 1976. p 26–32.

154. Ritger PL, Peppas NA. A simple equation for description of solute release. I. Fickian and non-Fickian release from non-swellable devices in the form of slabs, spheres, and cylinders or discs. J Control Release 1987;5:23–36.

155. Goepferich A, Langer R. Modeling of polymer erosion in three dimensions—rotationally symmetric devices. AIChE J 1995;41:2292–2299.

156. Sakiyama-Elbert SE, Hubbell JA. Development of fibrin derivatives for controlled release of heparin-binding growth factors. J Control Release 2000;65:389–402.

157. Mann BK, Schmedlen RH, West JL. Tethered-TGF-beta increases extracellular matrix production of vascular smooth muscle cells. Biomaterials 2001;22:439–444.

158. Kim S, Kim JH, Jeon O, Kwon IC, Park K. Engineered polymers for advanced drug delivery. Eur J Pharm Biopharm 2009;71:420–430.

159. Singh M, Shirley B, Bajwa K, Samara E, Hora M, O'Hagan D. Controlled release of recombinant insulin-like growth factor from a novel formulation of polylactide-co-glycolide microparticles. J Control Release 2001;70:21–28.

160. Benoit JP, Faisant N, Venier-Julienne MC, Menei P. Development of microspheres for neurological disorders: from basics to clinical applications. J Control Release 2000;65:285–296.

161. Péan JM, Menei P, Morel O, Montero-Menei CN, Benoit JP. Intraseptal implantation of NGF-releasing microspheres promote the survival of axotomized cholinergic neurons. Biomaterials 2000;21:2097–2101.

162. Lu L, Yaszemski MJ, Mikos AG. TGF-beta1 release from biodegradable polymer microparticles: its effect on marrow stromal osteoblast function. J Bone Joint Surg Am 2001;83-A(1 Suppl):S82–S91.

163. Formiga FR, Pelacho B, Garbavo E, Abizanda G, Gavira JJ, Simon-Yarza T, Mazo M, Tamayo E, Jauquicoa C, Ortiz-de-Solorzano C, Prósper F, Blanco-Prieto MJ. Sustained release of VEGF through PLGA microparticles improves vasculogenesis and tissue remodeling in an acute myocardial ischemia-reperfusion model. J Control Release 2010;147:30–37.

164. Patel ZS, Ueda H, Yamamoto M, Tabata Y, Mikos AG. In vitro and in vivo release of vascular endothelial growth factor from gelatin microparticles and biodegradable composite scaffolds. Pharm Res 2008;25:2370–2378.

165. Jay SM, Saltzman WM. Controlled delivery of VEGF via modulation of alginate microparticle ionic crosslinking. J Control Release 2009;134:26–34.

166. Patel ZS, Yamamoto M, Ueda H, Tabata Y, Mikos AG. Biodegradable gelatin microparticles as delivery systems for the controlled release of bone morphogenetic protein-2. Acta Biomater 2008;4:1126–1138.

167. Solorio L, Zwolinski C, Lund AW, Farrell MJ, Stegemann JP. Gelatin microspheres crosslinked with genipin for local delivery of growth factors. J Tissue Eng Regen Med 2010;4:514–523.

168. Devrim B, Bozkir A, Canefe K. Preparation and evaluation of poly(lactic-co-glycolic acid) microparticles as a carrier for pulmonary delivery of recombinant human interleukin-2: I. Effects of some formulation parameters on microparticle characteristics. J Microencapsul 2011;28:582–594.

169. Woo BH, Fink BF, Page R, Schrier JA, Jo YW, Jiang G, DeLuca M, Vasconez HC, DeLuca PP. Enhancement of bone growth by sustained delivery of recombinant human bone morphogenetic protein-2 in a polymeric matrix. Pharm Res 2001;18:1747–1753.

170. Wie L, Lin J, Cai C, Fang Z, Fu W. Drug-carrier/hydrogel scaffold for controlled growth of cells. Eur J Pharm Biopharm 2011;78:346–354.

171. Spiller KL, Liu Y, Holloway JL, Maher SA, Cao Y, Liu W, Zhou G, Lowman AM. A novel method for the direct fabrication of growth factor-loaded microspheres within porous nondegradable hydrogels: controlled release for cartilage tissue engineering. J Control Release 2012;157:39–45.

172. Chen FM, Chen R, Wang XJ, Sun HH, Wu ZF. In vitro cellular responses to scaffolds containing two microencapsulated growth factors. Biomaterials 2009;30:5215–5224.

173. Lampe KJ, Kern DS, Mahoney MJ, Bjugstad KB. The administration of BDNF and GDNF to the brain via PLGA microparticles patterned within a degradable PEG-based hydrogel: protein distribution and the glial response. J Biomed Mater Res-A 2011;96:595–607.

174. Hori K, Sotozono C, Hamuro J, Yamasaki K, Kimura Y, Ozeki M, Tabata Y, Kinoshita S. Controlled-release of epidermal growth factor from cationized gelatin hydrogel enhances corneal wound healing. J Control Release 2007;118:169–176.

175. Inaoka T, Nakagawa T, Kikkawa YS, Tabata Y, Ono K, Yoshida M, Tsubouchi H, Ido A, Ito J. Local application of hepatocyte growth factor using gelatin hydrogels attenuates noise-induced hearing loss in guinea pigs. Acta Otolaryngol 2009;129:453–457.

176. Komobuchi H, Hato N, Teraoka M, Wakisaka H, Takahashi H, Gyo K, Tabata Y, Yamamoto M. Basic fibroblast growth factor combined with biodegradable hydrogel promotes healing of facial nerve after compression injury: an experimental study. Acta Otolaryngol 2010;130:173–178.

177. Sakiyama-Elbert SE, Hubbell JA. Controlled release of nerve growth factor from a heparin-containing fibrin-based cell ingrowth matrix. J Control Release 2000;69:149–158.

178. Ucuzian AA, Brewster LP, East AT, Pang Y, Gassman AA, Greisler HP. Characterization of the chemotactic and mitogenic response of SMCs to PDGF-BB and FGF-2 in fibrin hydrogels. J Biomed Mater Res-A 2010;94:988–996.

179. Chwalek K, Levental KR, Tsurkan MV, Zieris A, Freudenberg U, Werner C. Two-tier hydrogel degradation to boost endothelial cell morphogenesis. Biomaterials 2001;32:9649–9657.

180. Zieris A, Chwalek K, Prokoph S, Levental KR, Welzel PB, Freudenberg U, Werner C. Dual independent delivery of pro-angiogenic growth factors from starPEG-heparin hydrogels. J Control Release 2011;156:28–36.

181. Hänsler P, Jung UW, Jung RE, Choi KH, Cho KS, Hämmerle CH, Weber FE. Analysis of hydrolysable polyethylene glycol hydrogels and deproteinized bone mineral as delivery systems for glycosylated and non-glycosylated bone morphogenetic protein-2. Acta Biomater 2012;8:116–123.

182. Patterson J, Siew R, Herring SW, Lin AS, Guldberg R, Stayton PS. Hyaluronic acid hydrogels with controlled degradation properties for oriented bone regeneration. Biomaterials 2010;31:6772–6781.

183. Jeon O, Powell C, Solorio LD, Krebs MD, Alsberg E. Affinity-based growth factor delivery using biodegradable, photocrosslinked heparin-alginate hydrogels. J Control Release 2011;145:258–266.

184. Huang AH, Stein A, Tuan RS, Mauck RL. Transient exposure to transforming growth factor beta 3 improves the mechanical properties of mesenchymal stem cell-laden cartilage constructs in a density-dependent manner. Tissue Eng-A 2009;15:3461–3472.

185. Delong SA, Moon JJ, West JL. Covalently immobilized gradients of bFGF on hydrogel scaffolds for directed cell migration. Biomaterials 2005;26:3227–3234.

186. Jimenez Hamann MC, Tator CH, Shoichet MS. Injectable intrathecal delivery system for localized administration of EGF and FGF-2 to the injured rat spinal cord. Exp Neurol 2005;194:106–119.

187. Drinnan CT, Zhang G, Alexander MA, Pulido AS, Suggs LJ. Multimodal release of transforming growth factor-β1 and the BB isoform of platelet derived growth factor from PEGylated fibrin gels. J Control Release 2010;147:180–186.

188. Chenite A, Chaput C, Wang D, Combes C, Buschmann MD, Hoemann CD, Leroux JC, Atkinson BL, Binette F, Selmani A. Novel injectable neutral solutions of chitosan form biodegradable gels in situ. Biomaterials 2000;21:2155–2161.

189. Qiao M, Chen D, Hao T, Zhao X, Hu H, Ma X. Injectable thermosensitive PLGA-PEG-PLGA triblock copolymers-based hydrogels as carriers for interleukin-2. Pharmazie 2008;63:27–30.

190. Pandit A, Ashar R, Feldman D, Thompson A. Investigation of acidic fibroblast growth factor delivered through a collagen scaffold for the treatment of full-thickness skin defects in a rabbit model. Plast Reconstr Surg 1998;101:766–775.

191. Nilleson ST, Geutjes PJ, Wismans R, Schalkwijk J, Daamen WF, van Kuppevelt TH. Increased angiogenesis and blood vessel maturation in acellular collgen-heparin scaffolds containing both FGF2 and VEGF. Biomaterials 2007;28:1123–1131.

192. Lee JY, Nam SH, Im SY, Park YJ, Lee YM, Seol YJ, Chung CP, Lee SJ. Enhanced bone formation by controlled growth factor delivery from chitosan-based biomaterials. J Control Release 2002;78:187–197.

193. Lee H, Cusick RA, Browne F, Kim TH, Ma PX, Utsunomiya H, Langer R, Vacanti JP. Local delivery of basic fibroblast growth factor increases both angiogenesis and engraftment of hepatocytes in tissue-engineered polymer devices. Transplantation 2002;73:1589–1593.

194. Yang XB, Whitaker MJ, Sebald W, Clarke N, Howdle SM, Shakesheff KM, Oreffo RO. Human osteoprogenitor bone formation using encapsulated bone morphogenetic protein 2 in porous polymer scaffolds. Tissue Eng 2004;10:1037–1045.

195. Maquet V, Martin D, Scholtes F, Frazen R, Schoenen J, Moonen G, Jérôme R. Poly(D,L-lactide) foams modified by poly(ethylene oxide)-block-poly(D,L-lactide) copolymers and a-FGF: in vitro and in vivo evaluation for spinal cord regeneration. Biomaterials 2001;22:1137–1146.

196. Whang K, Tsai DC, Aitken M, Sprague SM, Patel PK, Healy KE. Ectopic bone formation via rhBMP-2 delivery from porous bioabsorbable polymer scaffolds. J Biomed Mater Res 1998;42:491–499.

197. Chen RR, Silva EA, Yuen WW, Mooney DJ. Spatio-temporal VEGF and PDGF delivery patterns blood vessel formation and maturation. Pharm Res 2007;24:258–264.

198. Murphy WL, Peters MC, Kohn DH, Mooney DJ. Sustained release of vascular endothelial growth factor from mineralized poly(lactide-co-glycolide) scaffolds. Biomaterials 2000;21:2521–2527.

199. Smith MK, Riddle KW, Mooney DJ. Delivery of hepatotrophic factors fails to enhance long-term survival of subcutaneously transplanted hepatocytes. Tissue Eng 2006;12:235–244.

200. Yoon JJ, Chung HJ, Lee HJ, Park TG. Heparin-immobilized biodegradable scaffolds for local and sustained release of angiogenic growth factor. J Biomed Mater Res-A 2006;79: 934–942.

201. Nelson DM, Baraniak PR, Ma Z, Guan J, Mason NS, Wagner WR. Controlled release of IGF-1 and HGF from a biodegradable polyurethane scaffold. Pharm Res 2011;28:1282–1293.

202. Singh M, Tech B, Berkland C, Detamore MS. Strategies and applications for incorporating physical and chemical signal gradients in tissue engineering. Tissue Eng-B 2008;14:341–366.

203. Rosoff WJ, McAllister R, Esrick MA, Goodhill GJ, Urbach JS. Generating controlled molecular gradients in 3D gels. Biotechnol Bioeng 2005;91:754–759.

204. Richardson TP, Peters MC, Ennett AB, Mooney DJ. Polymeric system for dual growth factor delivery. Nat Biotechnol 2001;19:1029–1034.

205. Suciati T, Howard D, Barry J, Everitt NM, Shakesheff KM, Rose FR. Zonal release of proteins within tissue engineering scaffolds. J Mater Sci Mater Med 2006;17:1049–1056.

206. Moore K, MacSween M, Shoichet M. Immobilized concentration gradients of neurotrophic factors to guide neurite outgrowth of primary neurons in macroporous scaffolds. Tissue Eng 2006;12:267–278.

207. Singh M, Morris CP, Ellis RJ, Detamore MS, Berkland C. Microsphere-based seamless scaffolds containing macroscopic gradients of encapsulated factors for tissue engineering. Tissue Eng-C Methods 2008;14:299–309.

208. Wang X, Wenk E, Zhang X, Meinel L, Vunjak-Novakovic G, Kaplan DL. Growth factor gradients via microsphere delivery in biopolymer scaffolds for osteochondral tissue engineering. J Control Release 2009;134:81–90.

209. Quaglia F. Bioinspired tissue engineering: the great promise of protein delivery technologies. Int J Pharm 2008;364:281–297.

210. Biondi M, Ungaro F, Quaglia F, Netti PA. Controlled drug delivery in tissue engineering. Adv Drug Deliv Rev 2008;60:229–242.

211. Chen FM, Zhang M, Wu ZF. Toward delivery of multiple growth factors in tissue engineering. Biomaterials 2010;31:6279–6308.

212. Doorn J, Moll G, Le Blanc K, van Blitterswijk C, de Boer J. Therapeutic applications of mesenchymal stromal cells: paracrine effects and potential improvements. Tissue Eng-B Rev 2012;18:101–115.

213. Shapiro AM, Lakey JR, Ryan EA, Korbutt GS, Toth E, Warnock GL, Kneteman NM, Rajotte RV. Islet transplantation in seven patients with type 1 diabetes mellitus using a glucocorticoid-free immunosuppressive regimen. N Engl J Med 2000;343:230–238.

PART IV

ORAL POLYMERIC DRUG DELIVERY SYSTEMS

9

ORAL CONTROLLED-RELEASE POLYMERIC DRUG DELIVERY SYSTEMS

James W. McGinity

Pharmaceutics Division, College of Pharmacy, The University of Texas at Austin, Austin, TX, USA

James C. DiNunzio

Pharmaceutics Division, College of Pharmacy, The University of Texas at Austin, Austin, TX, USA; Hoffmann-La Roche, Inc., Nutley, NJ, USA

Justin M. Keen

Pharmaceutics Division, College of Pharmacy, The University of Texas at Austin, Austin, TX, USA

9.1 INTRODUCTION

During the past two decades, there has been a prolific increase in the number of new polymeric controlled-release products entering the marketplace [1]. Scientists have employed new polymers and combinations of polymers to optimize drug absorption, modify drug release, and target drug delivery to specific sites in the gastrointestinal (GI) tract. Significant advances in materials science and processing technologies have led to the development of unique compositions to solve challenging solubility

Engineering Polymer Systems for Improved Drug Delivery, First Edition.
Edited by Rebecca A. Bader and David A. Putnam.
© 2014 John Wiley & Sons, Inc. Published 2014 by John Wiley & Sons, Inc.

and absorption problems presented by very potent BCS II and BCS IV (biopharmaceutics classification system II and IV) compounds. Many drugs present problems in absorption and chemical stability in the GI tract when administered in an oral controlled-release dosage form. For drugs that have a narrow absorption window, the design of the controlled drug delivery system for that particular active pharmaceutical ingredient (API) must be developed with both bioavailability and efficacy in mind.

The drug release rate from a polymeric drug delivery system can be influenced by many factors, including the particle size of the drug substance, the hydrophilic and hydrophobic properties of the retardant polymer, other functional excipients in the oral dosage form, and the processing method to manufacture the final dosage form. In addition to this text, a number of reviews have recently been published detailing the fundamentals of oral controlled release [2–4]. Direct compression, wet granulation, and thermal processes such as hot-melt extrusion and melt granulation have all been used to prepare controlled-release polymeric dosage forms. In addition to their use as matrix retardants in tablets and pellets, pharmaceutical polymers have been effectively used by scientists to regulate the release of drug from the oral dosage form by dissolving at a particular pH in the GI tract, by diffusion, or by other erosion-based mechanisms.

For a drug to be absorbed from an oral dosage form, the active substance must first pass into solution. The rate at which the dosage form transits down the GI tract and the absorption rate for that particular API. For some drugs, the presence of enzymes and the hostile acidic environment in the stomach will influence both drug stability and bioavailability. As a result, the design of a successful controlled-release polymeric drug delivery system requires detailed understanding of both the drug absorption process and the factors influencing the transit of the delivery system in the different regions of the GI tract.

Oral controlled-release dosage forms have been shown to have numerous advantages over conventional tablet and capsule formulations. Both hydrophilic and hydrophobic polymers have been widely used in controlled-release oral dosage forms when the blood level of the drug substance must be maintained in a desired and stable therapeutic range over an extended period. Such dosage forms can then be administered to the patient either once or twice a day, depending upon the particular absorption behavior and pharmacokinetic properties of the active ingredient. By maintaining drug levels within a particular therapeutic range, controlled-release preparations eliminate time periods where drug levels in the bloodstream are either subtherapeutic or have exceeded the minimum toxic concentration. Studies have also shown decreased side effects and increased patient compliance with these dosage forms since the patient need take only one or two units per day versus three or four tablets or capsules. Intra- and intersubject variability in blood levels may still be seen in particular patient populations as a result of physiological factors including GI pH variations, changes in metabolic rates, and different transit times seen within specific subpopulations [5].

In addition to the chemical stability of the drug substance in the GI tract, formulation scientists must design a chemically stable system that will meet specifications throughout the shelf life of the product. Besides chemical stability, dissolution storage stability must also be maintained. Dissolution stability has been defined as the retention of the dissolution characteristics of a solid oral dosage form from the time of manufacture up to the expiration date [6]. Significant changes in the *in vitro* release profiles of a drug product during storage may alter its bioavailability. The physical stability of a product can also be influenced by processing variables including coating conditions, drying, and curing of polymeric film coats applied to tablets and pellets. Murthy and Ghebre-Sellassie reported that the excipients in the composition can also interact with drug substances and that residual moisture in the excipients can affect the release rate of drug from the product during storage [6]. Acid-labile compounds such as the proton pump inhibitors, for example, omeprazole and lanoprazole, rapidly degrade when in contact with enteric polymers. The factors that impact the chemical stability of drugs and the dissolution storage stability of controlled-release oral dosage forms can also be influenced by environmental factors including light, oxygen, temperature, and humidity.

For drugs that undergo first-pass metabolism when given by the oral route, slowly eroding lozenges in the buccal cavity and bioadhesive buccal tablets for drugs such as testosterone have been successfully utilized to deliver the drug substance over an extended period. Matrix pellets and coated pellets have been formulated into capsule delivery systems and have also been compressed into tablets. For drugs having different pharmacokinetic and absorption properties, bilayered tablets with different drugs in each layer have been utilized to release each API at different rates in the GI tract. Osmotic-based formulations have been successfully used for a wide variety of medicines, and ion-exchange resins have been employed in oral controlled-release suspension formulations to treat symptoms of the common cold. Since most of the absorption of the API from a controlled-release dosage form takes place in the small intestine, numerous attempts to extend the residence time in the small intestine have been reported in the literature. These approaches include: utilizing floating pellets, floating tablets and the inclusion of bioadhesive polymers in pellets and tablet formulations. The objective with such formulations is to maintain the dosage form in the small intestine to increase systemic absorption of the active moiety from the dosage form. A multiparticulate floating-pulsatile drug delivery system was developed using porous calcium silicate and sodium alginate for the time- and site-specific release of the drug meloxicam [7]. Davis and coworkers had previously reported that attempts to modify GI transit by pharmaceutical means using bioadhesives and adjusting the density of the product were less than successful in humans despite promising results in animal models [8, 9]. These findings were similar to those reported by Sangekar et al. [10].

Extensive studies have been reported in the literature regarding the influence of ingested food on GI transit times for the dosage form and of food on oral bioavailability. The presence of food will influence the gastric emptying time of the drug from the stomach into the small intestine, as well as the pH of the stomach, which could influence the performance of enteric polymers that are designed to be insoluble in the acidic environment of the stomach. For poorly water-soluble drugs, prolonged gastric residence may promote drug dissolution, which would account for higher blood levels of poorly soluble compounds when administered with certain foods.

Gamma scintigraphy has been used extensively to follow the transit of a pharmaceutical dosage form through the GI tract. Transit time in the small intestine has been reported in the literature to be in the 3–5 h range. This may vary depending upon the age of the patient and disease state, which could influence normal GI motility. The residence time for multiparticulate drug delivery systems has been shown to be less than that of matrix tablets, and there is a reduced risk of dose dumping with multiparticulates. For certain drugs that are not well absorbed in the colon, the rapid transit of the dosage form through the small intestine may lead to poor absorption or variable bioavailability of the API from the dosage form. Controlled drug delivery systems for colonic delivery are generally delayed-release dosage forms utilizing enteric polymers that are designed to release the drug at close to the neutral pH of the colon to provide a sustained prolonged release in the colon. Alternatively, products are designed such that a burst-release of the API occurs once the dosage form reaches the colon. The drugs in these colonic formulations are utilized to treat several diseases, including colon cancer, Crohn's disease, ulcerative colitis, and irritable bowel syndrome. Gastric retention of a controlled-release product intended for colonic drug delivery may result in the bulk of the drug being released in the stomach and in the small intestine before its arrival in the large intestine. Davis and coworkers reported that the propulsion of preparations through the colon is highly variable and that the transit of large units through the proximal colon tends to be faster than that of the released contents [11, 12].

The following sections focus on the drug release mechanisms of oral dosage forms, polymers for controlled-release formulation, manufacturing technologies, and industrial applications of controlled release.

9.2   RELEASE MECHANISMS OF ORAL POLYMERIC DOSAGE FORMS

An understanding of the physicochemical properties of the polymer and the dosage form structure are of critical importance in investigating the mechanism of drug release from a polymeric dosage form. Polymers may be selected on the basis of many properties including the propensity to hydrate or degrade [13, 14], water permeability [15], or their ability to solubilize the drug [16]. When polymers are used for oral controlled release, commonly employed dosage forms may be broadly classified as (i.) matrix or monolithic systems, (ii.) membrane-controlled reservoir systems, or (iii.) osmotic pumps [17]. Membrane systems have the advantage of time-independent release rates but may suffer from dose dumping if the membrane fails. Matrix systems are less prone to dose dumping but release rates typically vary with time [17]. However, when polymer swelling and hydration dominates release, matrix systems will have near-time-independent release rates. It should be noted that combination matrix/membrane systems, drug-containing film coatings, and other variations are also well known in the field.

A matrix system is formed by dispersing or dissolving the drug homogeneously in the polymer carrier. Drug release may occur by diffusion of the drug through the matrix or by erosion of the polymer matrix surface. Eroding systems may proceed by dissolution of the outer polymer layer or by degradation of the polymer chains.

While degrading systems have been demonstrated for oral use, the timescale for degradation is usually too long for the oral route. In the case of diffusion, the drug release rate may be affected by the formation of pores, swelling of the polymer, or by molecular interactions between the drug and polymer. The release kinetics will be determined by the physical form of the drug in the matrix. Dissolved drug matrices proceed by diffusion, whereas dispersed drug matrices, containing drug loadings exceeding the saturation solubility in the matrix, involve a dissolution step before diffusion, which alters the time dependence of release.

A reservoir system consists of a drug core encapsulated by a polymer film which acts as a rate-controlling membrane. Reservoir systems release the drug either by diffusion through the macromolecular network or through cracks or pores in the film. Mechanistically, water penetration through the film occurs, allowing crystalline drug to dissolve. A concentration gradient results and diffusion occurs through the rate-controlling film, the overall diffusion rate a function of solute size, polymer molecular weight, viscosity, intermolecular interactions, and layer integrity. For an ideal film, this process is controlled purely by diffusion, allowing the control of release rates through manipulation of material properties which impact mass transport through the layer. For real systems, layer integrity is also a critical aspect, which can be controlled through proper formulation. If needed, materials may actually be incorporated into the drug product to disrupt mechanical integrity of the layer, resulting in pore formation or complete rupture. By the creation of pores or cracks in the system, release rates can be increased. Through careful design, unique release behaviors can be achieved, including pulsatile release and nonlinear release. In general, however, these controlled-release system will be engineered to achieve zero-order drug release, at least during the initial phase of release before substantial drug depletion within the reservoir.

Osmotic pumps utilize a semipermeable membrane and an osmotic agent to absorb water and generate hydrostatic pressure, which pumps a drug solution through a small orifice in the membrane. The semipermeable membrane allows the dosage form to imbibe water. Salts and other osmotic agents present in the core dissolve and generate osmotic pressure. A laser-drilled or other similarly formed orifice releases a drug solution at a constant rate.

9.2.1 Modeling Drug Release

Modeling drug release from controlled-release dosage forms is complicated because of the many geometric and environmental factors that likely vary with time and influence drug dissolution and diffusion. For example, to model the drug release from a simple reservoir system, one must understand the rate at which water penetrates the reservoir, the osmotic pressure generated in the core, the degree and rate of swelling of the reservoir skin, the permeability of the drug in the swollen skin, and if and when the skin forms cracks or pores.

Nevertheless, many researchers have extensively characterized various release modalities developing systems of partial differential equations to explain their behavior and solving them by analytical or numerical methods [14, 18–22]. In general, drug release occurs in three phases.

The initial phase is the burst or lag; a reservoir system will lag initially as drug saturates the membrane. Matrix systems may burst-release initially as the surface drug easily accessible to the release medium is dissolved [23]. Following the initial phase, the polymer becomes a barrier and controls the drug release. Finally, the drug release rate will tail off as drug is depleted from the dosage form.

In the case of oral controlled-release formulations, drug release occurs in a matter of hours, and pseudo-steady-state mechanistic models as well as empirical and semiempirical models are useful for this timescale to understand the underlying release mechanism. Determination of the release mechanism is a prerequisite for tailoring a release profile to target *in vivo* blood levels or for troubleshooting release rate variations from batch to batch. In this section, the basic models are described. The interested reader is encouraged to consult the many reviews available in the literature for more detail [14, 19–21, 23–33].

9.2.2 Fickian Release

The simple case of drug release from a nonswelling, noneroding matrix containing dispersed drug was first studied by Higuchi, who created a drug release equation to quantify the release of drug from a slab of ointment containing the dispersed drug at an initial concentration, Cini [27]. Higuchi recognized that the release would occur as a moving front, in which the drug would dissolve up to the saturation concentration C_s and diffuse out of the slab. As the drug diffuses from the slab, additional drug would dissolve at the moving front and maintain saturation (Fig. 9.1). Using Fig. 9.1, it is possible to define a pseudo-steady-state mathematical model of the amount of drug released at time t per unit area A on the basis of the geometry and a mass balance.

From the geometry shown in Fig. 9.1, the amount of drug released at any given time, M_t, is

$$\frac{M_t}{A} = h\left(c_{ini} - \frac{c_s}{2}\right) \tag{9.1}$$

A mass balance on the moving boundary, having moved an incremental amount dh, yields the following equation:

$$\frac{dM}{A} = c_{ini}dh - \frac{c_s}{2}dh \tag{9.2}$$

Furthermore, assuming that the skin in contact with the ointment is a perfect sink, the driving force for drug release will be the magnitude of the saturation concentration, and the release rate will be dependent on the diffusivity D of the drug in the matrix. Fick's first law is defined for this system as

$$\frac{dM}{dt} = AD\frac{c_s}{h} \tag{9.3}$$

Substitution and integration of Eqs. 9.2 and 9.3, combined with the assumption that $c_{ini} \gg c_s$ results in the well-known Higuchi equation defining the cumulative

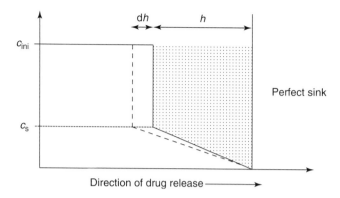

Figure 9.1. Schematic presentation of the drug concentration versus distance profile within the ointment base after exposure to perfect sink conditions at time t (solid line) and at time $t + dt$ (dashed line). The variables have the following meanings: c_{ini} and c_s denote the initial drug concentration and drug solubility, respectively; h represents the distance of the front, which separates ointment free of nondissolved drug excess from ointment still containing nondissolved drug excess, from the "ointment–skin" interface at time t; dh is the distance this front moves inwards during the time interval dt. Reprinted from the International Journal of Pharmaceutics, [26], Copyright (2008), with permission from Elsevier.

amount of drug release as a function of the square root of time:

$$\frac{M_t}{A} = \sqrt{2c_{ini}Dc_s t} \tag{9.4}$$

A first-pass approximation for diffusivity may be calculated from the Stokes–Einstein relation. This is an idealized relation for spherical particles and assumes no interactions between the particles and the medium. This relation may be useful in determination of experimental starting points, such as polymer molecular weights or dosage-form dimensions. The diffusivity varies with temperature T, medium viscosity η, and drug radius r, and can be calculated using π and the Boltzmann constant k:

$$D = \frac{kT}{6\pi r\eta} \tag{9.5}$$

The presence of hydrophilic excipients may result in a porous matrix, in which case the diffusivity of the drug must be considered for that of the solution filling the pores. A porous network may also be formed upon dissolution of the drug when the drug loading is high. In such cases, the diffusivity is no longer unidirectional and an adjustment must be made for the tortuosity τ and porosity ε of the network [31]. The tortuosity and porosity may be analytically determined and used to determine an effective diffusion term for substitution into Eq. 9.5:

$$D_{eff} = \frac{\varepsilon D}{\tau} \tag{9.6}$$

From a practical perspective, the saturation solubility and/or the diffusivity of the drug in the matrix may not be known. A more general form of the equation may be used for fitting experimental intrinsic dissolution data to evaluate whether a diffusion mechanism is responsible for drug release:

$$M_t = kt^{1/2} \tag{9.7}$$

While this solution is widely applied in the pharmaceutical literature because of its simplicity, many assumptions were applied to derive this result. Violation of these assumptions may incorrectly imply a diffusion mechanism [28]. An exact solution to this system was derived by Paul and McSpadden in 1976 [34].

The Higuchi equation, Eq. 9.4 or 9.7, is not valid once 60% of the drug has been released from the matrix [17] or once the dispersed drug has all dissolved. Diffusion from dissolved matrices is modeled by first-order release kinetics. In this case, the modeling equation will take the following form and relates to the initial drug loading M_0, with k varying with geometry:

$$M_t = M_0(1 - e^{-kD_t}) \tag{9.8}$$

For reservoir systems, the drug release will also be first order and take the form of Eq. 9.8 when drug loading within the core is below the saturation solubility of the core. However, a highly desirable zero-order release profile will result when the core consists of a dispersed drug matrix. Such systems are termed *constant activity reservoirs* because the concentration gradient across the membrane is constant. As drug partitions into the membrane, more drug is dissolved, maintaining a saturated concentration, assuming that the dissolution rate exceeds the rate of diffusion through the membrane. The solution is easily derived for different geometries, with k being dependent on the actual geometry:

$$M_t = kDc_st \tag{9.9}$$

Similar to the case of porous matrix systems, the diffusion coefficients may be adjusted to account for porosity or cracking and may require adding the contributions of diffusion through the macromolecular network and the pores. Additional modifications must be made if internal hydrostatic pressure is generated by osmosis [35]. Furthermore, statistical treatments may be required for modeling multiunit dosage forms, such as a capsule containing coated pellets, that likely vary in coating thicknesses and core diameters from pellet to pellet [29].

9.2.3 Swelling Controlled Release

Polymeric dosage forms for oral delivery must have some capacity to absorb water in order to release drug. The previous equations model systems in which the rate-controlling polymer does not swell in the presence of water; instead, water displaces the dissolved drug or other excipients or fills the existing free volume between the

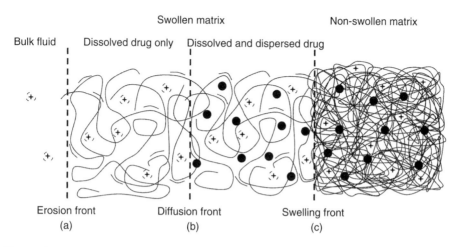

Figure 9.2. Schematic presentation of a swelling-controlled drug delivery system containing dissolved and dispersed drug (stars and black circles, respectively), exhibiting the following moving boundaries: (a) an "erosion front", separating the bulk fluid from the delivery system; (b) a "diffusion front", separating the swollen matrix containing dissolved drug only and the swollen matrix containing dissolved and dispersed drug; and (c) a "swelling front", separating the swollen and nonswollen matrix. Reprinted from the International Journal of Pharmaceutics, [26], Copyright (2008), with permission from Elsevier.

polymer backbones. Matrix systems based on hydrophilic polymers will swell and erode (Fig. 9.2). The rate at which water can penetrate the matrix will affect the time dependence of release because of a change in release mechanism that can be characterized into three regimes, Fickian, Case II, and anomalous.

The simplest case occurs when the rate of water penetration into the matrix is rapid compared to polymer erosion. An increased degree of swelling will increase the rate of drug diffusion. If the hydration dependence of the drug diffusivity can be determined and the dosage form water concentration measured, the previously defined equations may still be applied. An effective diffusion coefficient D_{eff} may be calculated from the degree of swelling v [36]:

$$D_{eff} = D\left(\frac{1-v}{1+v}\right)^2 \qquad (9.10)$$

The second scenario is commonly referred to as *Case II* transport [17], first studied in the field of drug delivery by Ritger and Peppas [37, 38], which occurs when the rate of water penetration into the polymer matrix is controlled by the time required for relaxation of the polymer network and is characterized by having a diffusion coefficient dependent on both time and water concentration. In Case II transport, the drug release rate is controlled by the hydration rate of the polymer, which for glassy polymers may be limited by the rate of transition to the rubbery state. Ritger and Peppas proposed a

TABLE 9.1. Drug Release Mechanism as Defined by the Peppas Power law[a]

	n		Mechanism
Slab	Cylinder	Sphere	
0.5	0.45	0.43	Fickian
0.5 < n < 1.0	0.45 < n < 0.89	0.43 < n < 0.85	Anomalous
1.0	0.89	0.85	Case II

[a]Equation reprinted from the International Journal of Pharmaceutics, [26] Copyright (2008), with permission from Elsevier.

semiempirical model, commonly referred to as the *Peppas Equation*, that is routinely used in the literature to determine whether Case II transport or Fickian diffusion dominates the drug release:

$$\frac{M_t}{M_0} = kt^n \qquad (9.11)$$

Dissolution data may be fitted to Eq. 9.11 to determine the power n, and together with the dosage geometry the release mechanism can be determined, Table 9.1 [26]. It is notable that in the case of slab geometry, first studied by Higuchi, a pure Fickian release has a value of 0.5 and Eq. 9.11 collapses to Eq. 9.7. When Case II transport dominates, drug release is zero-order for a slab geometry and near-zero-order for cylindrical and spherical geometries.

The third scenario for transport of drug from a swelling polymer matrix is referred to as *anomalous transport*, signifying that a combination of Fickian diffusion and Case II transport is occurring.

9.2.4 Osmotic Release

Osmotic systems for oral use represent a special subset of reservoir-controlled systems. The reservoir membrane is selected such that it is rigid and semipermeable; water may be transported into the dosage form but the drug and osmotic agents will not transport out of the dosage form through the macromolecular network [39]. The result is an internal osmotic pressure π in the presence of water, which may be estimated by the van't Hoff relation using the molarity n of the osmotic agent, the ideal gas constant R, and the temperature T:

$$\pi = nRT \qquad (9.12)$$

A mechanical or laser-drilled hole in the membrane will release a drug solution at a rate proportional to the osmotic pressure gradient across the membrane. A zero-order release rate will be maintained as long as a solid osmotic agent, such as salt or sugar, and drug are available to maintain the internal osmotic pressure and constant drug concentration in the expelled fluid [17].

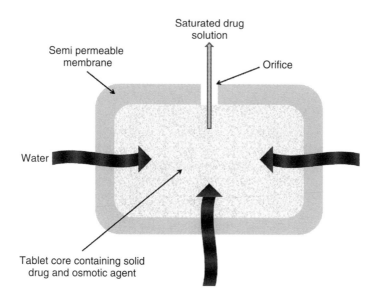

Figure 9.3. An elementary osmotic tablet. Reprinted from the Journal of Controlled Release, [39], Copyright (1995), with permission from Elsevier.

Osmotic pumps were originally developed such that the osmotic agent and drug were maintained in different compartments, separated by flexible membranes or pistons. Theeuwes and Higuchi, on behalf of the Alza Corporation, developed an elegant, simplified osmotic tablet (Fig. 9.3). Subsequently, Bend Research and Pfizer collaborated to develop asymmetric membranes with increased water permeability, making them suitable for poorly soluble compounds. The asymmetric membranes are prepared by a phase-inversion process and include pore formers, obviating the need for a mechanical or laser-drilled hole.

The release rate from a simple osmotic tablet is dependent on the water permeability P of the membrane, the membrane thickness l, the membrane area A, the osmotic gradient, and the drug concentration in the expelled fluid.

$$\frac{\mathrm{d}M_t}{\mathrm{d}t} = \frac{AP(\pi_{int} - \pi_{\text{ext}})C_s}{l} \tag{9.13}$$

9.3   ORAL POLYMERIC RELEASE MODIFIERS

During the development of an oral controlled-release formulation, polymer selection may be driven by the need to target a specific area of the GI tract, chemical compatibility with the drug, drug dose, failure mode, or ability to solubilize the drug. For example, for drug substances with a narrow therapeutic window, the dosage form should have a zero-order release rate, little or no initial burst, and a small failure rate. In this case, a reservoir system could be problematic if the membrane fails, so a matrix tablet that rapidly surface-hydrates would be desirable. Knowledge of the polymer chemistry effects on solubility, drug diffusion, and hydration rate is essential in development of a safe and efficacious dosage form.

9.3.1 Hydrophobic Polymers

Insoluble polymers are desirable for diffusion-based systems such as nonerodible matrix tablets and reservoir systems. Ethylcellulose is a directly compressible cellulose derivative that releases drug by diffusion. At low drug loadings, interstitial drug diffusion and polymer relaxation control release, whereas at high drug loadings a porous diffusion mechanism dominates [40]. Alternatively, ethylcellulose or other hydrophobic polymers such as the neutral poly(methyl methacrylate) copolymers (Eudragit RL/RS, Eudragit N) are diffusion barriers when used as reservoir membranes. In order to achieve permeation rates suitable for oral release, hydrophilic material may be incorporated to create pores for diffusion [41]. Eudragit N will impart flexibility and elasticity to a membrane, while Eudragit RL and RS may be varied to increase or decrease the permeability, respectively. Cellulose acetate and cellulose acetate butyrate form rigid semipermeable films that permeate water at rates suitable for use in elementary oral osmotic pumps [42].

9.3.2 Water-Soluble Polymers

As previously noted, water-soluble polymers may be used in conjunction with insoluble polymers to create porous networks for diffusion. Hydrophilic polymers such as poly(vinyl alcohol), pluronics, or soluble cellulose ethers have surface-active properties that may alter the solubility or dissolution rate of poorly soluble drugs within the porous channels of a matrix. Other hydrophilic polymers may be of interest for their mucoadhesive properties, which may be useful for controlled release in the oral cavity or for reducing gastric transit time. Polymers with hydroxyl, carboxyl, or amine groups, such as chitosan, sodium alginate, carboxymethyl cellulose, and polycarbophil, are capable of hydrogen bonding and have been used historically for this purpose; however, biopolymers such as glycoproteins and lectins may be more effective because of additional secondary binding interactions [43].

Hydrophilic polymers such as polyethylene oxide, xanthan gum, and the cellulose ethers form eroding matrices upon direct compression, allowing inexpensive and reproducible production of matrix tablets. When used as rate-controlling matrix formers, hydrophilic polymers should be selected on the basis of their rate of hydration, gel strength, ionic strength sensitivity, and drug solubility. For example, slowly hydrating polymers may be prone to burst-release, and strong gelling polymers may erode slowly resulting in square-root-of-time kinetics. Polymer mixtures may offer synergies in achieving zero-order drug release with minimal lag or burst effect, as was observed for release of diltiazam hydrochloride from matrices prepared from a combination of sodium carboxymethylcellulose, which forms a strong gel, and hydroxypropylmethylcellulose, which hydrates rapidly [44].

9.3.3 pH-Dependent Polymers

pH-dependent polymers relevant to the GI tract, such as acidic polymethylmethacrylates (Eudragits®), polymethacrylic acid cross-linked hydrogels (carbomers), cellulose acetate phthalate, hydroxypropylmethylcellulose acetate succinate, and hydroxypropylmethylcellulose phthalate, have solubilities or swelling potentials that vary between the stomach (pH 1) and that of the intestines (pH 5–7). Eudragits and modified cellulose ethers are suitable for enteric coating for modified drug release. These coatings are not soluble at the pH of the stomach and are effective for preventing gastric irritation or protection of acid-labile drugs [45].

pH-dependent polymers swell when ionized above their pK_a and may ionically interact with cationic drugs. The interaction of cationic diphenhydramine and the anionic carboxylic acids of Eudragit L was observed to produce zero-order release of diphenhydramine from a combination acrylic/wax matrix tablet [46].

9.4 MANUFACTURING TECHNOLOGIES AND INDUSTRIAL APPLICATIONS OF CONTROLLED RELEASE

Oral drug delivery is one of the simplest modes of administration and preferred by patients when compared to other more complicated and invasive approaches. Table and capsule-based dosage forms tend to be the most common systems and have been routinely manufactured by the pharmaceutical industry for more than a century. In modern commercial manufacturing, production of oral delivery systems is achieved through the combination of multiple, well-characterized unit operations as part of a validated process, typically run as discrete batches based on global regulatory requirements for quality control and traceability. Manufacturing techniques for oral controlled-release products rely on unit operations similar to those used in conventional immediate-release products, along with several advanced technologies to achieve the desired delivery profile. This section highlights the formulation, manufacturing, and characterization of controlled-release drug products, focusing on monolithic matrices, coated reservoir systems, and osmotic delivery products. Detailed discussion of delivery mechanism, manufacturing technology, and formulation design is provided, along with key aspects related to the *in vitro* characterization of such systems.

9.4.1 Drug Substance Properties and Selection of Delivery System

Formulation scientists are presented with a range of technologies for oral delivery, and these platforms can provide an array of release profiles. Selection of the appropriate dosage form is driven by the molecular properties of the moiety being developed, in conjunction with considerations of the disease state, desired biopharmaceutical performance, and manufacturing efficiency [47]. Selection of the appropriate dosage form will result in the optimum performance of all major functional attributes.

Driven by the chemical structure of the compound, properties such as solubility and stability will play a major role in the ability to formulate a controlled-release system. Many pharmaceutical actives are ionizable, resulting in pH-dependent solubility and oral bioavailability. Similarly, long-term chemical stability and solution stability are also a direct result of the molecular structure. These are intrinsic properties of the system and cannot be modified without changing the nature of the compound. While strategies such as salt form selection, prodrug development, or amorphous formulation may improve performance, these strategies represent monumental tasks that cannot be quickly incorporated in the later stages of development for controlled-release products. Therefore, early assessment of controlled-release viability based on physicochemical properties is essential to address any major structural limitations of the compound.

In general, compounds requiring low to moderate doses of less than about 300 mg can be formulated effectively. Larger doses may not be able to be accommodated along with controlled-release excipients in a dosage form of suitable size, although some newer technologies are helping to raise this limit. In many cases, dosage size restriction may become a further function of disease state either due to progression or population. This becomes particularly critical when looking at products intended for pediatric, disabled, or elderly groups, where swallowing may be difficult. Solubility of the compound is also an important factor in developing a controlled-release product. Many pharmaceutical compounds exhibit low solubility, which is defined as any compound where the dose cannot be dissolved in 250 ml of water. In reality, controlled-release systems can be developed for compounds containing much lower solubilities; however, the challenge becomes ever greater as the volume required to dissolve the dose exceeds 1000 ml. Consideration must also be given to the pH dependence of compound solubility, especially where products would be expected to exhibit significant increases or decreases in solubility due to environmental changes that occur during the GI transit. Some level of compensation for this behavior can be achieved through the incorporation of microenvironmental pH modifiers or the use of pH-sensitive release agents; however, such approaches do not always ensure success. Similarly, compounds intended for oral controlled release should exhibit acceptable solid-state and solution stability.

Biopharmaceutical properties also factor into the viability of a controlled-release approach as a result of the molecule's biological activity. To effectively elicit the activity of the compound, it is necessary to achieve and maintain therapeutic concentrations by balancing the absorption, distribution, and elimination behavior *in vivo*. Absorption of active compounds is critical to achieving the needed oral bioavailability, and is a function of regional biological factors, absorption mechanism, metabolism, and efflux. It is well known that surface area, liquid content, pH and distribution of biological transporters and enzymes change throughout the length of the GI tract. Compounds having low permeability may exhibit low oral bioavailability and, in certain cases, site-specific absorption, which limit the effectiveness of a controlled-release system. This behavior may become even more exaggerated if the molecule exhibits strong pH-dependent solubility or is an active transport substrate. Substrate affinity for efflux and metabolic mechanisms may also have a negative impact on absorption and, therefore, the ability to produce a suitable dosage form. Rapid elimination of the compound can further limit the ability to develop a controlled-release product, particularly for compounds that exhibit a half-life ($t_{1/2}$) less than 3 h.

Given the extensive number of properties that impact the ability to produce a controlled-release system, it is possible to define the properties of a suitable compound. Such a molecule would have a dose less than 300 mg, solubility of 100 μg ml^{-1}, no major substrate behavior ($t_{1/2} > 3$ h), high permeability via passive diffusion with no regional limitations, and good stability. For cases in which compounds exhibit deficiencies, it is critical to assess these limitations as early as possible in development so that a derisking strategy may be developed and molecular intervention initiated.

Manufacturing efficiency will also factor into the decision of final product dosage form. The production process will need to be as simple and cost effective as possible, yielding an efficient and highly robust manufacturing train. Considerations for each of the major types of controlled-release products are discussed below.

9.4.2 Design Considerations for Monolithic Matrix Systems

Monolithic controlled-release drug delivery systems are products consisting of a homogeneous drug containing a release-controlling phase [48]. With two unique types based on the nature of the polymers, these systems are classified as hydrophilic matrices or insoluble matrices. These systems provide unique opportunities for formulation development and different mechanisms of release, which can be exploited to develop novel controlled-release systems.

For hydrophilic systems, drug particles are uniformly dispersed within a hydratable polymer, such as hydroxypropyl methylcellulose (hypromellose), which results in the formation of a gel layer at the interface with the aqueous environment [48]. Chemical composition and molecular weight of the material impact the hydration rates and gel viscosities, contributing to the release rate from the system. Mechanistically, as the dosage form is exposed to the aqueous environment, the polymer hydrates, transitioning from a glassy state to a higher mobility state. Drug release begins as the active material on the outer periphery of the tablet dissolves and diffuses through the thin gel layer. This behavior contributes to the burst behavior frequently seen in these systems. As the gel layer increases and the characteristic diffusion lengths grow, the release rate slows. Over extended periods, the polymer chains swell and disentangle, leading to erosion and reducing the integrity of the system. This behavior contributes to changes in the release mechanism over time as erosion plays a more dominant factor in the later stages. Solubility of the drug substance also influences the release mechanism of the product. Soluble drugs are released as a result of diffusion or anomalous transport due to the higher diffusive driving force. Compounds exhibiting low solubility may be prepared as controlled-release products in hydrophilic matrices; however, the mechanism of release becomes predominately erosion-based.

For manufacturing these systems, conventional technologies, including granulation, blending, compression, and coating, can be employed, providing a robust platform for production. In addition to the drug and the controlled-release polymer, formulations will consist of diluents, binders, glidants, and lubricants to support manufacturing of the drug product. Selection and sequence of the unit operations will depend largely on the properties of the drug substance and the desired release profile. Identification of the controlled-release polymer type and grade will depend on the properties of the drug substance and the desired release profile. In general, as slower release rates are desired, higher molecular weight grades of polymer are used. Conversely, for systems exhibiting low solubility, it will be necessary to use lower molecular weight grades to increase the rate of erosion. Chemistry of the polymer also plays a role, influencing hydration and gel formation of the material [48]. For example, with hypromellose, the grade of the material is described by the level of methoxyl and hydroxypropyl substitutions. For improved hydration and wetting characteristics, grades with higher hydroxypropyl content and lower methoxyl substitutions will be used.

Exploiting the benefits of conventional processing, these dosage forms can be produced using basic equipment available in most commercial manufacturing sites. Common manufacturing trains will consist of granulation, milling, blending, compression, and coating. Advanced technologies, such as hot-melt extrusion, may also be applied to the manufacture of hydrophilic controlled-release products; however, the use is limited by the nonthermoplastic nature of the most commonly used excipient, hypromellose. It should also be noted that other cellulosics, such as hydroxypropyl cellulose, are thermoplastic and can be processed by extrusion. In addition to achieving the desired release characteristics, primary challenges in developing these products relate to uniformity of the blending process, powder flowability, drug product compressibility, and stability of the dosage form. As a detailed discussion of basic pharmaceutical unit operations is outside the scope of this chapter, the reader is referred to the *Encyclopedia of Pharmaceutical Technology* [49] for more information on routine production technologies.

Selection of formulation additives is based not only on the need to achieve the target release profile but also to support dosage form production. A list of commonly used pharmaceutical excipients for controlled-release products is provided in Table 9.2.

Insoluble monolithic matrices are produced using inert materials that lack solubility in GI fluids, allowing the drug to dissolve and slowly diffuse from the system via

TABLE 9.2. Commonly Used Excipients for Water-Soluble/Swellable Controlled-Release Matrices

Function and common levels	Materials
Controlled-release matrix 10–80%	Hypromellose, hydroxypropylcellulose, hydroxyethylcellulose, methylcellulose, xanthan gum, polyethylene oxide, acrylic acid polymers, sodium alginate, xanthan gum, guar gum
Diluent as needed	Microcrystalline cellulose, starch, dicalcium phosphate, lactose, mannitol
Disintegrant 0–10%	Croscarmellose sodium, crospovidone, sodium carboxymethylcellulose, sodium starch glycolate
Binder 0–5%	Poly(vinyl pyrrolidone), vinylacetate:vinylpyrrolidone copolymer, hydroxypropyl cellulose
Wetting agent 0–2%	Poloxamer, polysorbate 80, sodium lauryl sulfate
Glidant/lubricant 0.25–1.0%	Magnesium stearate, sodium stearyl fumarate, colloidal silicon dioxide, stearic acid

TABLE 9.3. Commonly Used Excipients for Insoluble Controlled-Release Matrices

Function and common levels	Materials
Controlled-release matrix 10–80%	Ethylcellulose, cellulose acetate, poly(vinyl acetate), shellac, carnuba wax, glyceryl behenate, glyceryl monostearate, stearyl alcohol, paraffin wax
Pore former as needed	Lactose, mannitol, polyvinylpyrrolidone
Diluent as needed	Microcrystalline cellulose, starch, dicalcium phosphate, lactose, mannitol
Binder 0–5%	Poly(vinyl pyrrolidone), vinylacetate:vinylpyrrolidone copolymer, hydroxypropyl cellulose
Wetting agent 0–2%	Poloxamer, polysorbate 80, sodium lauryl sulfate
Glidant/lubricant 0.25–1.0%	Magnesium stearate, sodium stearyl fumarate, colloidal silicon dioxide, stearic acid

water penetration and pore formation [48]. These systems are limited by drug loading and solubility requirements of the active moiety, which impact matrix integrity and driving force; however, they can provide greater robustness against hydrodynamic influences than the hydrophilic systems because of the integrity of the composition. In certain cases, this can lead to the presence of "ghosts", materials that transit through the GI tract and are excreted intact even though they have delivered their payload. These types of systems also rely on different excipients, which inherently lack solubility in aqueous media. Such materials include ethylcellulose, cellulose acetate, poly(vinyl acetate), methycrylic acid copolymer, stearyl alcohol, and glycerol monostearate. Formulation design of an insoluble matrix, summarized in Table 9.3, will consist of the drug substance, an insoluble matrix former, pore-forming additive, and additional functional excipients to support the manufacturing technology. Based on the nature of the formulation, which relies on tortuosity and pore dimensions to regulate release, conventional manufacturing techniques may not provide the best mode for production. Technologies such as melt extrusion, injection molding, and calendaring may be used to prepare insoluble matrix systems. By providing a more uniform matrix with smaller domain sizes, it is possible to provide enhanced controlled-release properties. Crowley et al. [50] compared the difference between directly compressed ethylcellulose tablets and melt-extruded tablets, showing lower porosity of the crystalline solid dispersion product.

9.4.3 Coated Reservoir Systems

Coated reservoir systems are designed to provide controlled drug delivery through the use of diffusion from a reservoir of drug through a permeable membrane layer and into the bulk media, where the drug is able to be absorbed by the body. Drug products of this type are also prepared as both tablets and multiparticulates; however, the higher risk for individual dose failure has driven most of these systems to be prepared as multiparticulates. Dating back to the 1950s with the launch of Spansules, a number of inert coating materials have been used, including waxes, fatty acids, cellulosic polymers, and methacrylic polymers. Also falling under this umbrella is the enteric coated product, where the dosage form is intended to protect the payload from the acidic environment of the stomach. Using pH-sensitive polymers, acidic functionalities unionized in gastric conditions create an insoluble coating which is then dissolved as the environmental pH of the system is elevated and the acidic functionalities of the polymer become ionized. Several extensively used materials include methacrylic acid copolymer, hypromellose acetate succinate, cellulose acetate phthalate, and poly(vinyl acetate) phthalate. Another application is for continuous diffusive release from the reservoir. In these cases, systems are designed with a coating layer of insoluble material having a defined structure that regulates drug release. Modulation of release rates is achieved by tuning the diffusivity via addition of soluble or insoluble additives, as dictated by the needs of the product. Final product design is also strongly governed by the properties of the drug substance. Solubility of the compound establishes the diffusive driving force. For high solubility compounds, lower diffusivity and greater diffusion lengths will be needed to extend the release rates. For low solubility compounds, it may be necessary to include solubilizing excipients into the core of the system to provide sufficient driving force. An example of this strategy is the incorporation of weak acids to lower the microenvironmental pH and maintain a constant solubility and diffusive driving force throughout the GI tract [51]. Multiparticulates also present unique opportunities for contouring the release profiles by easily combining different types of pellets of unique compositions to achieve the target composite dissolution behavior. For example, the degree of burst can be tuned by combining immediate-release pellets with controlled-release pellets, increasing dissolution during the early stage of profile.

Commercial drug products are produced as reservoir systems using tablet and multiparticulate dosage forms. Tablets provide a simple and well-accepted delivery route that is also most cost effective to manufacture on a commercial scale; however, the application of tablet reservoir systems is not common for products having a narrow therapeutic index because of the risks associated with dose dumping. Enteric systems, intended only to provide protection from the stomach, are still an excellent option for tablets. Often, the enteric coating is more important for protection of the drug substance from the external environment, where exposure would be reduced by the degradation process of the drug substance. Since this would not result in potentially fatal dose dumping, enteric tablets are a viable and preferred method for delivery. Variable retention and transit can also limit the use of individual dosage forms, particularly for compounds that are not well absorbed throughout the GI tract [52, 12]. Specific surface area limitations of tablets compared to multiparticulate products can also be a factor when considering the type of reservoir dosage form to develop.

The more common delivery system of reservoir-type controlled-release products is the multiparticulate. These products can be made by drug layering onto nonpareils or via extrusion and spheronization. As a detailed description of these unit operations is outside the scope of this chapter, the reader is referred to the *Encyclopedia of Pharmaceutical Technology* [49] for additional information. In general, selection of the manufacturing method will be determined by the drug loading, where core drug loadings of less than 40% w/w can be obtained using drug layering and greater than 60% w/w can be produced through wet mass extrusion. Although both methods can be applied to all drug loadings, at levels greater than 40% the binder in the drug layer may need to be reduced, which can impact coating efficiency, as well as the simple time requirement needed to prepare the multiparticulates. Similarly, wet mass extrusion can be applied almost independently of drug loading, noting a strong dependence on drug substance properties. Owing to the greater time and cost associated with the process, as well as the lower yields, it is not economically feasible at the commercial scale for developing products with low drug loadings when compared to drug layering. At higher drug loadings where the time required for drug layering becomes exorbitant, the lower yields and costs for specialized equipment that characterize wet mass extrusion can be justified. It is important to note that the process of extrusion and spheronization is strongly dependent on the drug properties, where the process may become limited at extremely high drug loadings.

Following production of the reservoir, the functional coatings may be applied. When designing these systems, boundary-layer interactions between the drug and functional coating polymer can occur. This is particularly important in the case of acid-sensitive drug substances and enteric polymers, where the acidic functionalities of the polymer can interact to degrade the drug substance. For multiparticulate coating, fluid-bed layering of the functional coating as either a solution or suspension in aqueous or organic media will be conducted. Using a Wurster column insert inside the fluid bed, as shown in Fig. 9.4, up-bed and down-bed regions can be established based on material flow within the chamber [53–56]. In the up-bed region, the high velocity air propels the individual particles through a coating zone where a fine mist of coating materials is sprayed onto the particles and subsequently dried by the hot air stream, propelling the material through the coating zone. As the particles move through the coating zone, they enter the expansion chamber where the diameter of the fluid bed increases and the linear air velocity decreases. At a critical point, the particles can no

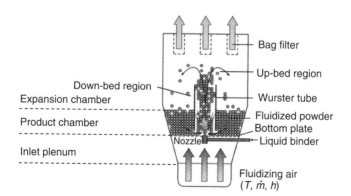

Figure 9.4. Schematic diagram of a fluid bed containing a Wurster insert. Reprinted from Chemical Engineering Science [56] with permission from Elsevier.

longer be entrained in the air stream and return to the product bed via the down-bed region which also has a lower air velocity due to the diffuser (bottom) plate geometry below the product bed. During the transit, newly coated material dries and the process is repeated continuously until the final coating thickness has been achieved. Ideally, coatings will also be able to coalesce during the process, yielding uniform films across the particles. The level of coalescence is a strong function of the formulation and the type of solvent used. For solvent-based coatings, uniform films may be directly attained during the process because of the dissolved nature of the polymer. In the case of aqueous dispersions, coalescence is required for the dispersed particles to fuse together and create a uniform film. This often does not occur during the coating process, but can be achieved through the continued heat treatment of the pellets after spraying. This process, referred to as *curing*, allows for complete coalescence of the film, which would otherwise occur during storage and alter the dissolution profile during stability.

Formulation design for controlled-release reservoir systems focuses on the design of the coating system. Coating systems consist typically of the polymer, plasticizer, pore former, opacifier, antisticking agent, and colorant, with the key ingredient types summarized in Table 9.4. Polymers are the key ingredient in the composition, representing the major component and also determining the rate of release. As a result of the polymer production process, residual components may also be incorporated into the system. Such is the case for materials produced using emulsion polymerization, where the residual surfactant from the production process is present at low levels. Combinations of polymers may also be developed to provide optimum release characteristics. Release characteristics are further modified through the incorporation of pore-forming agents and secondary polymer additives. These help to increase the porosity of the coated membrane, enhancing mass flux through the layer. The type

TABLE 9.4. Summary of Key Excipients Used for Controlled-Release Coatings

Function and common levels	Materials
Controlled-release polymers 10–40%	Ethylcellulose, cellulose acetate, poly(vinyl acetate), poly(vinyl acetate phthalate), cellulose acetate phthalate, hypromellose acetate succinate, hypromellose phthalate, methacrylic acid copolymer
Pore former as needed	Lactose, mannitol, poly(vinyl pyrrolidone), pectin
Stabilizer as needed	Colloidal silicon dioxide, albumin
Plasticizer 0–5%	Poly(ethlene glycol), dibutyl sebecate, diethyl phthalate, dibutyl phthalate, triethyl citrate, tributyl citrate
Wetting agent 0–5%	Poloxamer, polysorbate 80, sodium lauryl sulfate
Antisticking agent 0.25–5%	Magnesium stearate, sodium stearyl fumarate, colloidal silicon dioxide, stearic acid
Solvent, remainder of formulation	Water, methanol, ethanol, acetone, isopropanol

of material selected will depend on the chemical stability and mechanical integrity of the film. The level to which additives are dispersed within the film can also provide unique attributes for drug release. Continuous and uniform distribution within the film can impact the glass transition temperature, enhancing molecular mobility and diffusion. As a result, permeability through the layer increases, which impacts drug release and moisture uptake by the system, a key aspect for pharmaceutical stability. Macroscopic, heterogeneous distribution allows for the formation of pores and voids within the layer. The presence of discrete domains within the system may lower the mechanical integrity of the film, potentially causing issues for storage stability. Plasticizers are incorporated into film formulations to reduce the glass transition temperature of the polymer and enhance film-forming efficiency during manufacture. Their incorporation is of particular importance for aqueous coating dispersions, where micronized solid polymer particles are layered onto the substrate during the process. By lowering the glass transition temperature, more complete coalescence is achieved, which can reduce release rates from the drug product. In extreme cases, high levels of plasticizer can provide faster dissolution rates because of the dissolution of the plasticizer, which leaves voids in the film layer. Antisticking agents are included into the coating to enhance processability of the formulation. Low-mass particles, which have a high surface area to volume ratio, are more influenced by surface phenomena. As the surface is in a wet state during coating, capillary forces can cause particles to adhere during the process. The nature of fluid-bed processing helps to minimize the duration during which the particles are wet; however, some direct contact will result from the random collisions that occur because of high velocities and large populations in the coating region. Antisticking agents help to reduce the level of particle bonding that occurs, allowing each spheroid to remain individual throughout the process. Mechanical agitation of the product bed during the process and maintainenance of a high drying capacity also help to reduce sticking. Opacifiers and colors are included into the formulation to provide cosmetic functions. Opacifiers work to block the color of the substrate from showing through the coating, providing a neutral color pallet for further differentiation through the addition of pigments. Although multiparticulate products are incorporated into larger dosage forms (i.e., tablets or capsules), the pellets may be colored to facilitate brand identification and support manufacturing. Multiparticulate products may actually be a combination of several types of pellets that are filled into the same unit dose. To distinguish pellets during production, unique colors may be incorporated into the systems to identify formulations. In select cases, the capsule body may be transparent, requiring color addition for branding purposes. A similar need for color may also be recommended if capsules could be opened to facilitate dosing by combining with food.

Formulation design of these types of systems is also infinite. In theory, there is no limit to the number of layers that can be produced on the product or restrictions on the sequence of the layers, as is illustrated in Fig. 9.5. This allows for multiple release properties to be achieved from the same pellet. It also allows for the separation of different layers. For example, it is possible to separate the functional coating layer from the core layer when interactions are present by adding a separating layer of soluble excipient. This approach was used in Prilosec®, where omeprazole would degrade as

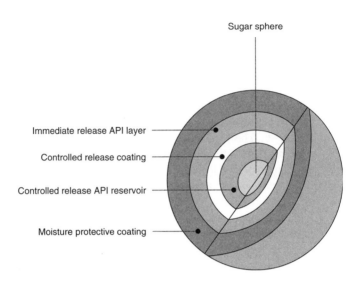

Figure 9.5. Multifunctional controlled-release pellet cross section.

a result of direct contact with the enteric polymer [57]. Multiple layering can also be designed to achieve an immediate release burst of the active ingredient before reaching the controlled-release layer, which then delivers the drug to sustain plasma levels *in vivo*. Combinations of different pellets having unique release characteristics can also be combined within the same dosage form to achieve the desired release characteristics. Assuming that sink conditions are maintained in the bulk, these profiles will be additive.

9.4.4 Osmotic Systems

Osmotic dosage forms are some of the most complex oral formulations currently manufactured commercially. These systems rely on the coating of a semipermeable membrane around a core containing an osmotic agent designed to "pull" water into the device and expel the formulation through an orifice in the device. An image of an osmotic system in action is shown in Fig. 9.6, illustrating the discharge of material from the orifice. Capable of being manufactured at different degrees of complexity, these systems can contain different layers of varying functionals and compositions as well as multiple openings to achieve unique release profiles. Production of these systems, as well as formulation, presents unique challenges and opportunities, relying on a combination of novel and traditional strategies to achieve the desired target profile. The key advantages for osmotic products are that they release at a constant rate over an extended duration independent of environmental factors such as patient physiology and food effect. Using a multilayer strategy, it is possible contour the release profile while also meeting the requirements of poorly soluble compounds.

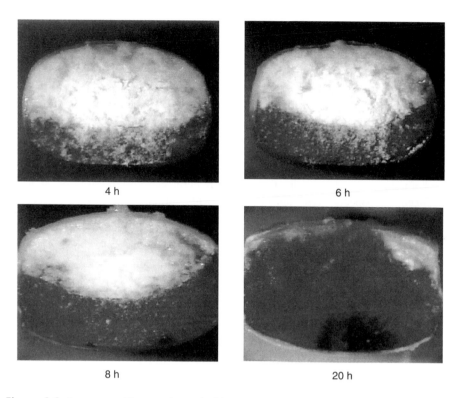

Figure 9.6. Sequence of images for a dual-layer osmotic tablet courtesy of Bend Research. White: drug-containing layer; Dark: osmotic push layer. Reprinted from Journal of Controlled Release [58] with permission from Elsevier.

Mechanistically, release of the drug from the device is controlled by the osmotic pressure. As the osmotic agent, commonly termed *osmagen* [58], is dissolved within the limited internal volume of the tablet, the osmotic pressure builds. The predrilled orifice within the device allows for equilibration of the pressure through the expulsion of the formulation through the channel. By carefully defining the formulation, it becomes possible to provide the desired release characteristics.

The production of osmotic tablets relies on a combination of traditional and nonconventional manufacturing technologies [59]. The core strategy will determine the number of layers. For simple, homogeneous osmotic systems, the osmotic agent and formulation are combined in a single matrix. These systems can easily be produced using conventional rotary tablet presses. More advanced systems define unique layers to the core tablet. These consist of an osmotic push layer and a drug-loaded formulation layer, requiring the use of a bilayer press. Systems can also be produced using three layers on a tri-layer press; however, the degree of complexity for core production increases significantly. Coating of the semipermeable membrane is also a critical step in the process. For single-layer systems, conventional coating processes may be used, but process parameters must be optimized to ensure a uniform coating layer.

More complex coating procedures are required for multilayer formulations. Since it is necessary to identify the formulation layer for laser-drilling in multilayer systems, dip-coating processes using color are applied or clear coatings are produced onto colored core tablets. This allows for the identification of the appropriate layer using a vision system. Drilling of the orifice is conducted by a series of focused lasers which produce diameters of 600–1000 μm at rates of up to 100,000 tablets per hour [60]. Extensive use of vision and detection systems ensures an appropriate degree of quality control during production. Owing to the complicated nature of the drilling process, illustrated in Fig. 9.7, production costs for osmotic products are higher than those of conventional dosage forms.

Formulation design of osmotic systems requires careful consideration of multiple functional aspects. Core tablets must provide sufficient mechanical integrity to survive the coating and handling process while also providing the required release characteristics. For multilayer products, bonding between layers is a key attribute of the formulation and must be taken into account during development. Push layers will generally consist of soluble materials, such as sodium chloride, which generate the required osmotic driving force. Osmotic pressure within the device will be a function of solute concentration. Higher osmotic pressure contributes to a greater influx of water, leading to larger hydrostatic pressure within the system and faster drug release [61].

Other soluble excipients, such as hypromellose and poly(ethylene glycol) are frequently used in the formulation of the core layers. Coating materials are insoluble and semipermeable, allowing for a consistent rate of water penetration throughout the administration period. The most common material used for preparation of the semipermeable membrane is cellulose acetate, although the use of ethylcellulose-based systems have also been reported. A list of common formulation components for use in osmotic systems is provided in Table 9.5.

A number of coating strategies have been developed to improve water uptake and drug release characteristics of osmotic systems. In the simplest form, a coating may be directly applied to the substrate by use of spray coating. This typically results in a dense membrane with low water permeability. While effective for high solubility compounds, limitations exist for low solubility drugs because of the water flux rates. Coating systems including water-leachable materials have also been developed. This allows for the formation drug delivery ports *in situ*. Again, these systems are applicable to high solubility molecules, but may be limited for low solubility compounds. Asymmetric membrane coatings, similar to those used in reverse osmosis, have also been developed [61]. Using phase inversion, it is possible to prepare low density membranes with a continuous external skin, which allows for greater permeability. For addressing systems with solubility limitations, multilayer systems, referred to as *swellable core osmotic tablets*, are utilized.

Using osmotic technology, over 30 commercial products have been developed [58]. These systems include Concerta™, Invega™, Fortamet ER™, and Altocor™. In all cases, these products use cellulose acetate as the semipermeable membrane, facilitating water absorption and subsequent drug release.

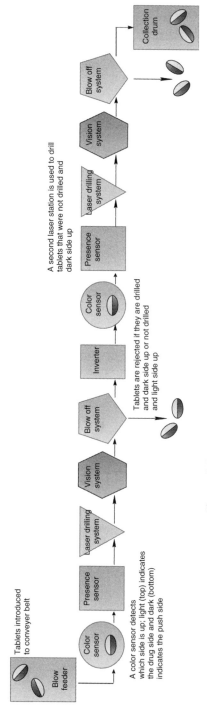

Figure 9.7. Flowchart showing the laser-drilling production line.

Tablets introduced to conveyer belt

A color sensor detects which side is up; light (top) indicates the drug side and dark (bottom) indicates the push side

Tablets are rejected if they are drilled and dark side up or not drilled and light side up

A second laser station is used to drill tablets that were not drilled and dark side up

Blow feeder

Color sensor

Presence sensor

Laser drilling system

Vision system

Blow off system

Inverter

Color sensor

Presence sensor

Laser drilling system

Vision system

Blow off system

Collection drum

TABLE 9.5. Key Commonly Used Excipients for Osmotic Controlled-Release Systems

Function	Materials
Osmotic coating	Cellulose acetate, cellulose acetate butyrate ethylcellulose,
Osmagen	Sodium chloride, cyclodextrin, dextrose, mannitol

9.4.5 Testing of Controlled-Release Formulations

Controlled-release formulations are designed to provide a desired drug release profile to yield the target *in vivo* behavior. Characterization of this behavior is necessary in development and also in routine manufacturing. Dissolution testing is the primary means of characterizing this behavior, ideally having established an *in vitro in vivo* correlation (IVIVC) to evaluate the impact of formulation and process changes to drug product performance. For characterization purposes, most such methods are too complicated and costly for routine testing. As such, methods are classified into two types: biorelevant tests and quality control tests. Biorelevant methods are used to assess formulation performance and set the basis for IVIVC determination. Data evaluation requires the implementation of comparative tests to assess similarity of dissolution profiles. This is performed using the f_2-test. This section will discuss some of the general considerations for *in vitro* evaluation of controlled-release products.

Compendial methodologies for dissolution testing identify four apparatuses for analysis. These are the basket method (apparatus I), the paddle method (apparatus II), the reciprocating cylinder method (apparatus III), and the flow-through cell method (apparatus IV). For quality control testing, apparatus I and II are routinely used. They provide a platform for simple testing capable of evaluating durations up to and exceeding 12 h. The downside to these types of methods is a limited ability to alter environmental conditions in a method analogous to the environmental changes observed *in vivo*. Using apparatus III, it is possible to simulate a number of environmental changes as a function of time. This allows for more accurate simulation of the *in vivo* situation; however, the method is generally considered too complex and time consuming for routine use. Utilization of this methodology is also supplemented with the use of biorelevant media [62]. More complex and higher cost than traditional buffers used for quality control methods, biorelevant media simulate intestinal media with the presence of phospholipids that mimic those found in the fed and fasted states. By using more detailed testing methods supported with biosimilar media, it is possible to model the *in vivo* condition. Data from these methods may be used to optimize formulations and also establish an IVIVC.

According to regulatory guidelines, there are four levels to IVIVC [63]. Level A correlation is a point-to-point relationship between *in vitro* dissolution and *in vivo* exposure. These correlations can be used to directly assess the impact of formulation changes on oral bioavailability. Level B correlation is a comparison of mean *in vitro* dissolution time to *in vivo* residence time. Level C correlation refers to a single-point relationship between *in vitro* dissolution and exposure, while a multiple level C correlation refers to a relationship between one or more pharmacokinetic parameters and several dissolution time points. For comparative purposes, the Level A correlation is the most desired relationship, as it provides a direct correlation between *in vitro* dissolution and *in vivo* exposure. Level B and C correlations provide insight into the formulation but are less preferred from a regulatory perspective.

Comparison of dissolution profile similarity is achieved using the f_2-test [64, 65]. Presented in Eq. 9.14, where n represents the number of time points used in the evaluation, T_t indicates the test value at time t, and R_t indicates the reference value at time t, similarity is assigned to systems having values from 50 to 100. For proper implementation, it is necessary that both the test and reference formulations are evaluated under the same conditions, with the same time points sampled. Furthermore, low variation (coefficient of variation (CV) < 20% at each time point) should be observed for all time points used, and only one time point greater than 85% dissolution should be included in the evaluation. Preferably, testing should also be conducted on large sample populations, where the number of tested samples is greater than or equal to 12. By applying this strategy, either using a stringent quality control method or appropriately correlated biorelevant method, it becomes possible to assess the impact of formulation and process changes that occur during development or are necessitated in the post-approval stage.

$$f_2 = 50 \cdot \log \left(100 \cdot \left(1 + n^{-1} \sum_{t=1}^{n} \left(R_t - T_t \right)^2 \right)^{-1/2} \right) \tag{9.14}$$

9.5 WORKED EXAMPLE

Example Problem 1

A series of immediate-release and controlled-release pellets have been developed, and the dissolution data for 100 mg doses are shown below. For a 1:1 blend of immediate-release and controlled-release pellets at a total dose of 100 mg, estimate the resulting release profile. Assume the API is freely soluble in the dissolution media.

Time (min)	Immediate-release (IR) formulation 100 mg Dose in 900 ml		Controlled-release (CR) formulation 100 mg Dose in 900 ml	
	%	mg	%	mg
15	35	35	10	10
30	65	65	15	15
45	90	90	20	20
60	100	100	25	25
120	100	100	50	50
180	100	100	75	75
240	100	100	100	100

Solution

Noting that the dissolution profiles for the combination will be additive and that the ratio of each formulation is 1:1 at the same dose, the amount released at each time point can be calculated as follows:

$$AMT_{t=15} = f_{IR} \cdot AMT_{IR} + f_{CR} \cdot AMT_{CR}$$

$$AMT_{t=15} = 0.5 \cdot 35 \ \text{mg} + 0.5 \cdot 10 \ \text{mg}$$

$$AMT_{t=15} = 22.5 \ \text{mg}$$

Noting that the total dose is 100 mg, the percentage released is 22.5%. The values for the remaining time points can be calculated in a similar manner. The resulting release profile is given in Fig. 9.8.

Time (min)	Combination 100 mg dose in 900 ml	
	%	mg
15	22.5	22.5
30	40.0	40.0
45	55.0	55.0
60	62.5	62.5
120	75.0	75.0
180	87.5	87.5
240	100.0	100.0

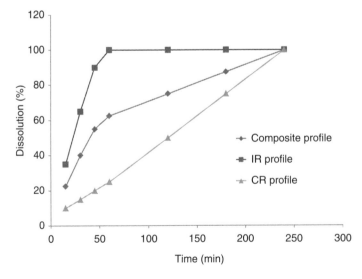

Figure 9.8. Release profile for a 1:1 blend of immediate-release and controlled-release pellets.

Example Problem 2

During clinical development, Good Manufacturing Practices (GMP) batches of a formulation were manufactured at two locations and evaluated for dissolution using the same biorelevant test. Batch 1 was manufactured at the same site and was superimposable to historical batches. Batch 2 was manufactured at a new location. Dissolution data for each formulation is provided in the table below. What is the f_2 value for the formulation?

Time (min)	Reference	Test
15	2.5	5.1825
30	5	10.23
45	7.5	15.1425
60	10	19.92
90	15	29.07
120	20	37.68
150	25	45.75
180	30	53.28
240	40	66.72
300	50	78
360	60	87.12
480	80	98.88
600	100	100

Solution

Noting that the calculation can only use one point where the value is greater than 85, all points after 360 min will not be used for the calculation. The first step is determining $\sum_{t=1}^{n} (R_t - T_t)^2$. The resulting value is calculated as 3907.884. Based on the 11 time points used in the calculation, the value for n can be defined as $n = 11$. Substituting the values for n and $\sum_{t=1}^{n} (R_t - T_t)^2$, it is possible to calculate the f_2 value.

$$f_2 = 50 \cdot \log \left(100 \cdot \left(1 + n^{-1} \sum_{t=1}^{n} (R_t - T_t)^2 \right)^{-1/2} \right)$$

$$f_2 = 50 \cdot \log \left(100 \cdot \left(1 + 11^{-1} (3907.884) \right)^{-1/2} \right)$$

$$f_2 = 36.2$$

The f_2 value is found to be 36.2, and the two batches are not similar ($f_2 < 50$).

9.6 KEY POINTS

- Oral dosage forms must be chemically and physically stable within the GI tract.
- Depending upon the desired release profile, a matrix or reservoir system can be used for oral controlled release.
- Before *in vivo* testing, oral controlled-release dosage forms must be evaluated by a dissolution test.

9.7 HOMEWORK PROBLEMS

1. Estimate the diffusivity of a drug substance having a molecular radius of 0.35 nm through a gel with a viscosity of 10^4 cps at 25 and 37 °C.

2. Compound A is a un-ionizable drug with a solubility of 10 mg ml^{-1} and molecular radius of 0.2 nm. Compound B has a molecular radius of 0.10 nm. If the compounds have the same flux from the device, what is the solubility of compound B assuming the release mechanism is pure diffusion.

3. Compounds C and D need to be manufactured as a combination product having identical release rates. The solubility of Compound C is 13 mg ml^{-1} and the molecular radius is 0.28 nm. Compound D has a solubility of 150 mg ml^{-1} and molecular radius of 0.11 nm. Will a diffusion-controlled monolithic matrix system be acceptable?

4. Calculate the f_2 value for the test formulation.

Time (min)	Reference	Test
15	5.9	5.1
30	11.6	10.2
45	17.2	15.1
60	22.7	19.8
90	33.0	28.9
120	42.8	37.3
150	51.9	45.3
180	60.3	52.6
240	75.2	65.5
300	87.6	76.2
360	97.3	84.5
480	100.0	94.2
600	100.0	100.0

5. Three cylindrical tablet formulations were prepared for drug E. Plot the percent released for each formulation. Using the Peppas equation, determine the

mechanism of drug transport. For each formulation, what polymer would give this result? Assume the drug to be soluble.

Time (min)	Formulation 1	Formulation 2	Formulation 3
0	0.0	0.0	0.0
15	6.7	17.2	33.0
30	12.4	25.7	50.7
45	17.8	32.4	57.0
60	22.9	38.3	61.9
120	42.5	57.2	75.6
240	78.8	85.5	92.4
480	100.0	99.8	99.9

REFERENCES

1. Florence AT. A short History of controlled drug release and an introduction. In: Wilson CG, Crowley PJ, editors. Controlled Release in Oral Drug Delivery. New York: Springer; 2011. p 1–26.

2. Omidian H, Fesharaki S, Park K. Oral controlled delivery mechanisms and technologies in controlled release in oral drug delivery. In: Wilson CG, Crowley PJ, editors. Controlled Release in Oral Drug Delivery. New York: Springer; 2011. p 109–130.

3. Colombo P, Colombo G, Cahyadi C. Geometric release systems: principles, release mechanisms, kinetics, polymer science, and release-modifying material in controlled release in oral drug delivery. In: Wilson CG, Crowley PJ, editors. Controlled Release in Oral Drug Delivery. New York: Springer; 2011. p 221–238.

4. Martini LG, Crowley PJ. Controlling drug release in oral product development programs: an industrial perspective in controlled release in oral drug delivery. In: Wilson CG, Crowley PJ, editors. Controlled Release in Oral Drug Delivery. New York: Springer; 2011. p 49–70.

5. Wilson CG. The Organization of the gut and the oral absorption of drugs: anatomical, biological and physiological considerations in oral formulation development in oral drug delivery. In: Wilson CG, Crowley PJ, editors. Controlled Release in Oral Drug Delivery. New York: Springer; 2011. p 27–48.

6. Murthy KS, Ghebre-Sellassie I. Current perspectives on the dissolution stability of solid oral dosage forms. J Pharm Sci 1993;82(2):113–126.

7. Sharma S, Pawar A. Low density multiparticulate system for pulsatile release of meloxicam. Int J Pharm 2006;313(1–2):150–158.

8. Davis SS, Stockwell AF, Taylor MJ, Hardy JG, Whalley DR, Wilson CG, Bechgaard H, Christensen FN. The effect of density on the gastric emptying of single- and multiple-unit dosage forms. Pharm Res 1986;3(4):208–213.

9. Khosla R, Davis SS. The effect of polycarbophil on the gastric emptying of pellets. J Pharm Pharmacol 1987;39:47–49.

10. Sangekar S, Vadino WA, Chaudry I, Parr A, Beihn R, Digenis G. Evaluation of the effect of food and specific gravity of tablets on gastric retention time. Int J Pharm 1987;35:187–191.

11. Davis SS, Hardy JG, Taylor MJ, Stockwell A, Whalley DR, Wilson CG. The in-vitro evaluation of an osmotic deliver (osmet) using gamma scintigraphy. J Pharm Pharmacol 1984;36:740–742.

12. Davis SS, Hardy JG, Fara JW. Transit of pharmaceutical dosage forms through the small intestine. Gut 1986;27:886–892.

13. Miller-Chou BA, Koenig JL. A review of polymer dissolution. Prog Polym Sci 2003; 28(8):1223–1270.

14. Siepmann J, Göpferich A. Mathematical modeling of bioerodible, polymeric drug delivery systems. Adv Drug Deliv Rev 2001;48(2–3):229–247.

15. Siepmann F et al. Polymer blends for controlled release coatings. J Control Release 2008;125(1):1–15.

16. Craig DQM. The mechanisms of drug release from solid dispersions in water-soluble polymers. Int J Pharm 2002;231(2):131–144.

17. Baker R. Controlled Release of Biologically Active Agents. New York: John Wiley & Sons, Inc; 1987.

18. Siepmann J, Siepmann F. Modeling of diffusion controlled drug delivery. J Control Release 2012;161(2):351–62.

19. Arifin DY, Lee LY, Wang C-H. Mathematical modeling and simulation of drug release from microspheres: Implications to drug delivery systems. Adv Drug Deliv Rev 2006;58(12–13): 1274–1325.

20. Lao LL et al. Modeling of drug release from bulk-degrading polymers. Int J Pharm 2011;418(1):28–41.

21. Lee PI. Modeling of drug release from matrix systems involving moving boundaries: approximate analytical solutions. Int J Pharm 2011;418(1):18–27.

22. Mitragotri S et al. Mathematical models of skin permeability: an overview. Int J Pharm 2011;418(1):115–129.

23. Sackett CK, Narasimhan B. Mathematical modeling of polymer erosion: consequences for drug delivery. Int J Pharm 2011;418(1):104–114.

24. Huang X, Brazel CS. On the importance and mechanisms of burst release in matrix-controlled drug delivery systems. J Control Release 2001;73(2–3):121–136.

25. Colombo P et al. Swellable matrices for controlled drug delivery: gel-layer behaviour, mechanisms and optimal performance. Pharm Sci Technol Today 2000;3(6):198–204.

26. Siepmann J, Siepmann F. Mathematical modeling of drug delivery. Int J Pharm 2008;364(2):328–343.

27. Siepmann J, Peppas NA. Higuchi equation: derivation, applications, use and misuse. Int J Pharm 2011;418(1):6–12.

28. Paul DR. Elaborations on the Higuchi model for drug delivery. Int J Pharm 2011;418(1):13–17.

29. Kaunisto E et al. Mechanistic modelling of drug release from polymer-coated and swelling and dissolving polymer matrix systems. Int J Pharm 2011;418(1):54–77.

30. Yin C, Li X. Anomalous diffusion of drug release from a slab matrix: fractional diffusion models. Int J Pharm 2011;418(1):78–87.

31. Frenning G. Modelling drug release from inert matrix systems: from moving-boundary to continuous-field descriptions. Int J Pharm 2011;418(1):88–99.

32. Dokoumetzidis A, Kosmidis K, Macheras P. Monte Carlo simulations and fractional kinetics considerations for the Higuchi equation. Int J Pharm 2011;418(1):100–103.

33. Maderuelo C, Zarzuelo A, Lanao JM. Critical factors in the release of drugs from sustained release hydrophilic matrices. J Control Release 2011;154(1):2–19.

34. Paul DR, McSpadden SK. Diffusional release of a solute from a polymer matrix. J Membr Sci 1976;1(0):33–48.

35. Amsden BG, Cheng Y-L. Enhanced fraction releasable above percolation threshold from monoliths containing osmotic excipients. J Control Release 1994;31(1):21–32.

36. Paul DR. Diffusive transport in swollen polymer membranes. In: Hopfenberg HB, Editor. Permeability of plastic films and coatings to gases, vapors, and liquids. New York: Plenum Pub; 1974. p 481 pp.

37. Ritger PL, Peppas NA. A simple equation for description of solute release I. Fickian and non-fickian release from non-swellable devices in the form of slabs, spheres, cylinders or discs. J Control Release 1987;5(1):23–36.

38. Ritger PL, Peppas NA. A simple equation for description of solute release II. Fickian and anomalous release from swellable devices. J Control Release 1987;5(1):37–42.

39. Santus G, Baker RW. Osmotic drug delivery: a review of the patent literature. J Control Release 1995;35(1):1–21.

40. Neau SH et al. The effect of the aqueous solubility of xanthine derivatives on the release mechanism from ethylcellulose matrix tablets. Int J Pharm 1999;179(1):97–105.

41. Lin AY et al. A study of the effects of curing and storage conditions on controlled release diphenhydramine HCl pellets coated with eudragitw NE30D. Pharm Dev Technol 2003;8(3):277–287.

42. Verma RK, Krishna DM, Garg S. Formulation aspects in the development of osmotically controlled oral drug delivery systems. J Control Release 2002;79(1–3):7–27.

43. Smart JD. The basics and underlying mechanisms of mucoadhesion. Adv Drug Deliv Rev 2005;57(11):1556–1568.

44. Conti S et al. Matrices containing NaCMC and HPMC: 2. 2007;333(1–2):143–151.

45. McGinity JW, Felton LA. Aqueous Polymeric Coatings for Pharmaceutical Dosage Forms. New York: Informa healthcare; 2008.

46. Huang H-P et al. Mechanism of drug release from an acrylic polymer-wax matrix tablet. J Pharm Sci 1994;83(6):795–797.

47. Thombre AG. Assessment of the feasibility of oral controlled release in an exploratory development setting. Drug Discov Today 2005;10:1159–1166.

48. Tiwari SB, DiNunzio J, Rajabji-Siahboomi A. Drug-polymer matrices for extended release. In: Wilsonand CG, Crowley PJ, editors. Controlled Release in Oral Drug Delivery. New York, NY: Springer; 2011. p 131–159.

49. Encyclopedia of Pharmaceutical Technology. 3rd edn. New York: Informa Healthcare; 2007. http://informahealthcare.com/doi/abs/10.3109/9780849393983.

50. Crowley MM, Schroeder B, Fredersdorf A, Obara S, Talarico M, Kucera S, McGinity JW. Physicochemical properties and mechanism of drug release from ethyl cellulose matrix tablets prepared by direct compression and hot-melt extrusion. Int J Pharm 2004;269: 509–522.

51. Farag Badaway SI, Hussain MA. Microenvironmental pH modulation in solid dosage Forms. J Pharm Sci 2007;96:948–959.

52. Coupe AJ, Davis SS, Wilding IR. Variation in gastrointestinal transit of pharmaceutical dosage forms in healthy subjects. Pharm Res 1991;8:360–364.

53. Jones D. Air suspension coating for multiparticulates. Drug Dev Ind Pharm 1994;20:3175–3206.

54. Teunou E, Poncelet D. Batch and continuous fluid bed coating - review and state of the art. J Food Eng 2002;53:325–340.

55. Norring Christensen F, Bertelsen P. Qualitative description of the Wurster-based fluid-bed coating process. Drug Dev Ind Pharm 1997;23:451–463.

56. Fries L, Antonyuk S, Heinrich S, Dopfer D, Palzer S. Collision dynamics in fluidized bed granulators: A DEM-CFD study. Chem Eng Sci 2013;86(108–123).

57. Stroyer A, McGinity JW, Leopold CS. Solid state interactions between the proton pump inhibitor omeprazole and various enteric coating polymers. J Pharm Sci 1995;95:1342–1353.

58. Thombre AG et al. Osmotic drug delivery using swellable-core technology. J Control Release 2004;94(75–89).

59. Verma RK, Arora S, Garg S. Osmotic pumps in drug delivery. Crit Rev Ther Drug Carrier Syst 2004;21:477–520.

60. Gaebler F, Coffee G. . Laser Drilling Enables Advanced Drug Delivery Systems. White Paper, 2007.

61. Herbig SM, Cardinal JR, Korsmeyer RW, Smith KL. Asymmetric-membrane tablet coatings for osmotic drug delivery. J Control Release 1995;35:127–136.

62. Dressmanand JB, Krämer J. Pharmaceutical Dissolution Testing. New York: Taylor & Francis; 2005.

63. FDA. Guidance for Industry: Extended Release Oral Dosage Forms: Development, Evaluation and Application of In Vitro / In Vivo Correlations, 1997.

64. Shah VP, Tsong Y, Sathe P, Liu J-P. In vitro dissolution profile comparison - statistics and analysis of the similarity factor, f2. Pharm Res 1998;15:889–896.

65. Polli JE, Rekhi GS, Augsburger LL, Shah VP. Methods to compare dissolution profiles. Drug Inf J 1996;30:1113–1120.

10

MUCOADHESIVE DRUG DELIVERY SYSTEMS

Srinath Muppalaneni, David Mastropietro, and Hossein Omidian

Department of Pharmaceutical Sciences, College of Pharmacy, Nova Southeastern University, Fort Lauderdale, FL, USA

10.1 INTRODUCTION

In drug delivery, bioadhesion or mucoadhesion refers to the attachment of a delivery system to a biological lining. As described in Chapter 2, these linings are the surfaces of epithelial tissues or mucous membranes found covering areas such as the buccal, sublingual, vaginal, rectal, nasal, ocular, and gastrointestinal (GI) tract. The application of mucoadhesion for drug delivery purposes was first introduced in 1947 when Scrivener and Schantz used tragacanth to administer penicillin to the oral mucosa [1]. However, it was not until the early 1980s that potential applications of mucoadhesion were fully recognized [2]. Enhancements to drug delivery using the concept of mucoadhesion have been developed to increase the dosage form residence time [3–5], modify tissue permeability, improve drug bioavailability, reduce the frequency of administration, and promote intimate contact of the drug to targeted biological absorptive membranes. To achieve these benefits, the drug is often dispersed into a polymeric material, which when in contact with mucosal medium acts as an adhesive drug-carrying system. From a structural standpoint, polymers which are hydrophilic in

Engineering Polymer Systems for Improved Drug Delivery, First Edition.
Edited by Rebecca A. Bader and David A. Putnam.
© 2014 John Wiley & Sons, Inc. Published 2014 by John Wiley & Sons, Inc.

nature and capable of interacting with mucin through its carboxyl, amine, or hydroxyl groups and of certain molecular weight and topology would serve as ideal bioadhesive materials in the carrier systems.

10.2 FACTORS AFFECTING MUCOADHESION

The mucoadhesive properties of a polymer are largely based on how it interacts with a particular mucus membrane. The mucosa (another term for mucus membrane) secretes mucus and lines body passages open to the outside environment, such as the nose, mouth, lungs, and digestive and urinary tracts. Mucus is viscous and translucent, and forms a thin gel structure (50–450 μm) attached to the mucosal epithelial surface [6]. Mucus is generally composed of water, glycoproteins, lipids, and inorganic salts [3, 7, 8]. The glycoproteins are responsible for the mucus's gelatinous structure, cohesion, and anti-adhesive properties [9]. The mucus layer has several functional roles, which include a protective function, a barrier role, an adhesive function, and a lubricant function [10]. For example, mucus in the GI tract facilitates movement of food by allowing it to pass smoothly throughout the digestive canal [11].

Because of its dynamic, nonstagnant environment, mucin turnover remains as the most challenging biological factor that formulation scientists face in achieving prolonged mucoadhesion. The rate and extent of mucin turnover controls the retention of the drug delivery system on the mucus layer, which in turn determines the pharmacokinetic feature of the drug (its release and absorption). Mucin turnover also releases soluble mucin molecules, which can interact with the adhesive system before it makes contact with the mucus layer [3]. Moreover, the mucus layer also acts as a potential barrier for drug absorption by causing a decrease in the diffusion rate of a drug or possibly binding to the drug itself limiting absorption, and varies in thickness depending on fed or fasted state conditions [12, 13].

In addition, diseases such as peptic ulcer disease, ulcerative colitis, and the presence of bacterial or fungal infections may affect mucin behavior by changing its physiological properties. If the mucoadhesive dosage form is intended for therapy under such conditions and disease states, the efficacy of the dosage form should be studied under similar conditions.

10.3 POLYMER–MUCUS INTERACTIONS

To be successful and effective as a mucoadhesive formulation, the polymer of the drug formulation and the mucin of the biological medium should provide adequate interaction, which can vary by factors such as polymer type, nature of the surrounding system, and physiological variables [14].

10.3.1 Polymer Molecular Weight

Several studies indicate that maximum bioadhesion occurs at certain polymer molecular weights, which are dependent on the polymer type, degree of swelling, size, and configuration. Low and high molecular weight polymers favor interpenetration or entanglement of the polymer chains, respectively [3, 15]. In general, bioadhesion strength increases with an increase in molecular weight up to 100,000 Da with no sensible effect beyond this point. However, polymers such as poly(ethylene oxide) have shown enhanced bioadhesiveness with molecular weights up to 4,000,000 Da.

10.3.2 Concentration of Active Polymer

Apart from optimum molecular weight, an optimum concentration of the polymer is also required to achieve maximum mucoadhesion. At high concentrations, the coiled polymer chains become less soluble and have less interpenetrating ability, resulting in weaker mucoadhesion [16].

10.3.3 Flexibility of Polymer Chains

Rigid polymers are characterized by limited mobility of their chains, and hence reduced interpenetration length into the mucus layer, which results in lower mucoadhesive strength [10].

10.3.4 Spatial Conformation

Polymer chains with linear conformations have higher adhesive strength than chains with helical conformations. For example, dextran at 19,500,000 Da molecular weight may display the same strength as that of poly(ethylene glycol) at 200,000 Da molecular weight. The helical conformation of dextran blocks the active adhesive groups responsible for promoting adhesion [10].

10.3.5 pH Value

The net charge on the mucus surface and polymer varies with the pH of the surrounding medium. The environmental pH affects the dissociation of carbohydrate and amino acid functional groups on the mucus polypeptides [17]. With cross-linked poly(acrylic acid) polymers, the degree of hydration is critically dependent on the pH of the hydrating medium: in general, increasing up to pH 7 and then decreasing at higher pH values. Similarly, the maximum adhesive strength of Polycarbophil can be observed at pH 3, with no bioadhesion beyond pH 5. A general effect of the degree of polymer chain hydration on the mucoadhesion strength can be seen in Fig. 10.1.

10.3.6 Applied Pressure

For solid mucoadhesive systems, it is important to apply pressure in order to achieve a desirable level of mucoadhesion. Bioadhesive strength increases at higher pressure and longer loading [1], as the depth of the mucosal interpenetration depends on the applied pressure.

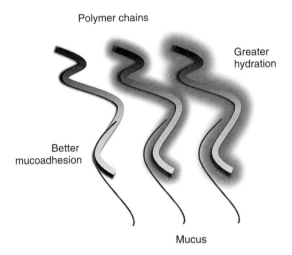

Figure 10.1. Degree of polymer hydration and mucoadhesion strength.

10.3.7   Initial Contact Time

The extent of swelling and polymer interpenetration into mucosal layer is time dependent; therefore, longer initial contact time along with the applied pressure can promote polymer–mucus adhesion [18].

10.3.8   Swelling

Swelling of mucoadhesive polymers depends on the polymer structure, pH, and temperature of the gastric medium. Apparently, environmental conditions favoring higher swelling of the mucoadhesive polymer result in lower bioadhesive strength.

10.4   MUCOADHESION MECHANISMS

Mucoadhesion is a complex phenomenon, for which several general theories based on electrical charge, wetting, adsorption, diffusion, mechanical, and fracture have been proposed.

10.4.1   Electronic Theory

Mucus membrane and adhesive material both possess electrical charge on their surface, and transfer of electrons at the site of contact leads to formation of an electrical double layer at their interface [3].

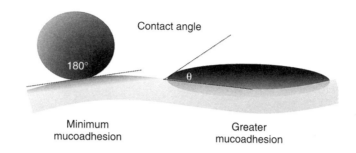

Figure 10.2. Correlation between contact angle and mucoadhesion force.

10.4.2 Wetting Theory

This is applicable only to liquid systems and occurs when a liquid spreads instantaneously on a mucus surface. The mucoadhesion strength is measured by the contact angle, spreadability coefficient, and the work of adhesion. For instance, at smaller contact angles, the adhesion strength is improved as a result of increased contact area, as shown in Fig. 10.2. Spreadability coefficient (the difference in the surface energies of the solid and the liquid) and the work of adhesion (the energy required to separate the two phases) are dependent on the surface energies of the liquid and the solid as well as their interfacial energy. The higher the individual surface energies, the greater the adhesive strength of the interface [19].

10.4.3 Adsorption Theory

Adhesive materials adhere to mucus membranes via hydrogen-bonding, van der Waals, or hydrophobic interactions. Even though the individual interactions are weak, the combined effect can be strong [2].

10.4.4 Diffusion Theory

It assumes that the polymer chains penetrate across the adhesive interface. The depth of penetration depends mainly on the polymer diffusion coefficient, mucin chain flexibility and mobility, and the polymer–mucus contact time [20, 21]. Other factors, such as mutual solubility and similar chemical structure, can facilitate the diffusion of the adhesive polymer into the mucus layer.

10.4.5 Mechanical Theory

It assumes that the adhesive material fills irregularities on a rough surface. Surface roughness increases the surface area available for interaction and favors the adhesion process along with viscoelastic and plastic dissipation of energies [9, 18, 19, 22].

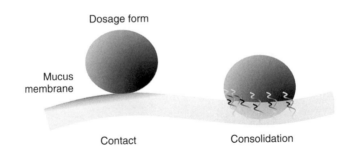

Figure 10.3. Contact and consolidations steps in mucoadhesion process.

10.4.6 Fracture Theory

It relates the adhesive strength to the force required to detach two attached surfaces. This theory does not take interpenetration of polymer chains into account and is only applicable to rigid or semirigid bioadhesive materials.

Although the process of mucoadhesion is too complex to be explained by any of these theories, there are two steps involved in the process, namely contact and then consolidation, as shown in Fig. 10.3. The adhesive polymer and the mucus come freely into contact with each other, sometimes under an external force such as the peristaltic motions of the GI tract, motions of organic fluids, or Brownian motion. As a result, both repulsive and attractive electrostatic forces would act, and adhesion initiates only when the repulsive forces are overcome. During consolidation, moisture activates and plasticizes the adhesive material, and facilitates the formation of van der Waals and hydrogen bonds. Diffusion and dehydration theories can explain the consolidation step. With the former, the adhesive material and glycoprotein of the mucus interact by interdiffusion of their chains and form secondary bonds. With the latter, the adhesive material forms an instantaneous gel once placed in an aqueous environment as a result of dehydration. As expected, the mucoadhesion mechanism in solid and hydrated dosage forms should be explained by other theories than dehydration.

10.5 MUCOADHESIVE POLYMERS

Ideally, a mucoadhesive polymer should be nontoxic and incapable of being absorbed from the GI tract. It should also possess adequate spreadability, wetting, swellability, solubility, and biodegradability. Moreover, it should quickly adhere to mucosa, and provide adequate stability and cumulative mechanical strength with adequate peeling, tensile, and shear strengths at a bioadhesive range. Availability, cost, bioadhesive properties especially in the wet state, local enzyme inhibition, and penetrability are also factors worth considering [18, 23].

Generally speaking, an adhesive polymer in contact with mucosa should be safe and nonirritating to the cells and lining. Once contacted, the polymer should be able to make a sustainable but temporary bond with the mucus as quickly as possible in order to provide a stationary platform for the dispersed drug to be released. From a polymer–drug standpoint, the polymer should be compatible with the drug, and the whole composition should remain stable in the service environment for an intended period. This requires a mucoadhesive formulation to be thermodynamically and kinetically optimized to fulfill the requirements.

Mucoadhesive polymers are typically anionic and hydrophilic, and have numerous sites available for forming hydrogen bonds. They are also flexible and have surface wetting properties, so they can penetrate into mucus tissue crevices. The first generations of mucoadhesive polymers are generally anionic, cationic, or nonionic in structure, and have been studied with many drugs, as shown in Table 10.1. The most common first-generation mucoadhesive polymers include natural-based cellulosics (carboxymethyl cellulose, hydroxyethyl cellulose, hydroxypropyl methylcellulose), natural-based hydrocolloids (sodium alginate, guar gum, pectin, gum Arabic, hyaluronic acid, gelatin, chitosan, psyllium), synthetic-based acrylic derivatives (Carbopol, Polycarbophil, hydroxyethyl methacrylate), and other synthetic such as polyvinylpyrrolidone and poly(ethylene glycol). Mucoadhesive materials can be categorized on the basis of various properties, for instance, molecular charge, solubility, source, etc. (Table 10.1) [8, 24].

10.5.1 Anionic Polymers

The interactions seen between anionic polymers and the mucus layer are hydrophilic, hydrogen-bonding, and van der Waals in nature [22, 25]. Because of their carboxyl content and its potential to interact with oligosaccharide chains of mucin, poly(acrylic

TABLE 10.1. First-Generation Mucoadhesive Systems

Property	Category	Examples
Molecular charge	Cationic	Chitosan, aminodextran, quaternized chitosan
	Anionic	Polycarbophil, Carbopol, pectin, sodium alginate
	Nonionic	Hydroxypropyl cellulose, hydroxyethylated starch, polyvinylpyrrolidone, poly(vinyl alcohol)
	Amphoteric	Gelatin, N-carboxymethyl chitosan
Solubility	Water-soluble	CMC, thiolated CMC, hydroxypropyl methylcellulose, hydroxypropyl cellulose
	Water-insoluble	Ethyl cellulose, polycarbophil
Specificity	Site-specific	Lectins, bacterial invasins, B12
	Nonspecific	Polyacrylates, CMC
Source	Natural and semisynthetic	Agarose, chitosan, carrageenan, pectin
	Synthetic	Carbopol, polyacrylates, methyl cellulose, cellulose derivatives

CMC, carboxymethyl cellulose.

acid), carboxymethyl cellulose, and alginates have been studied for their mucoadhesive properties [14]. Anionic polymers have better mucoadhesive properties at lower pH, as the carboxyl groups form hydrogen bonds. Polymers such as Carbopol form a gel upon changes in pH, this is useful in the designing of *in situ* gelling dosage forms with mucoadhesive properties [26]. Using allyl sucrose or allyl pentaerythritol, acrylic acid is copolymerized and cross-linked into a high molecular weight, lightly cross-linked product (Carbopol) with good mucoadhesive properties [18, 27]. The product is also used as a thickener, emulsifier, gelling agent, and suspending agent in pharmaceutical dosage forms. Park and Robinson [28] examined the effect of pH on Carbopol's mucoadhesive property, and found that maximum mucoadhesiveness appears under acidic conditions. Most commonly used Carbopol are CP934 and CP934P. Polycarbophil is a synthetic polymer based on lightly cross-linked poly(acrylic acid) with divinyl glycol (0.5–1% w/w). Polycarbophil's mucoadhesion is mainly due to entanglement of the polymer chains with surface mucus and from hydrogen bonds between nonionized carboxylic acid groups and mucin molecules [17].

Sodium carboxymethylcellulose is soluble in water and insoluble in most organic solvents [29]. It has commonly been used as emulsifying, gelling, and binding agents. It has good mucoadhesive properties and several studies were conducted in preparing mucoadhesive dosage forms based on this cellulosic polymer [30]. The interaction of sodium carboxymethyl cellulose is due to formation of hydrogen bonds with oligosaccharides of mucin via carboxyl groups.

Sodium alginate is a natural hydrocolloid obtained by purifying the alkaline extract of carbohydrate product of brown seaweed. It is slightly soluble in water and insoluble in organic solvents. It has several applications in the pharmaceutical field and is typically used as an emulsion stabilizer, suspending agent, disintegrating agent, and hemostatic agent. It is anionic in nature and its interaction with mucus is mainly electrostatic, and hence depends on the ionic strength of the medium.

10.5.2 Cationic Polymers

Cationic polymers can offer mucoadhesion by generating electrostatic forces with negatively charged amino groups in the mucin molecules [8]. Most commonly used cationic polymers are chitosan, poly(amino methacrylate)s, glycol chitosan, and chitosan derivatives. Chitosan, a nontoxic, biodegradable, biocompatible cationic hydrocolloid is obtained by alkaline deacetylation of chitin [31]. Chitosan possesses good mucoadhesive properties [25] and unique physicochemical and biological characteristics, such as being polyatomic in nature, is capable of forming films, has antimicrobial and wound-healing properties, binds to lipids and fatty acids, and can enhance penetration through mucosal membranes [2]. The mucoadhesive nature of chitosan is mainly due to the electrostatic interactions between chitosan and the negatively charged mucin [2]. Chitosan derivatives such as trimethyl chitosan, glycol chitosan, thiolated chitosan, carboxymethyl chitosan are commonly used as mucoadhesive polymers [32]. Studies by Bogataj et al. [33] showed that chitosan has better mucoadhesive properties than carboxymethyl cellulose and Polycarbophil.

10.5.3 Nonionic and Amphoteric Polymers

Compared to ionic polymers, nonionic polymers have poor mucoadhesive properties because of the lack of very hydrophilic functional groups in their structure [34]. Hydroxypropyl cellulose, hydroxypropyl methylcellulose, hydroxyethyl cellulose, and ethyl cellulose are commonly used cellulose derivatives for such applications. Interactions of nonionic polymers with mucin are mainly through diffusion and interpenetration into the mucus layer. On the other hand, very few studies have been carried out on the mucoadhesive properties of amphoteric polymers such as gelatin and N-carboxymethyl chitosan. Polyampholytes can be positively charged, noncharged, or negatively charged depending on their isoelectric point and the solution pH (Table 10.2).

10.6 NOVEL MUCOADHESIVE MATERIALS

Rapid mucin turnover, nonspecific site adhesion, and adhesion to soluble mucin are major drawbacks of the first-generation or conventional mucoadhesive materials. To overcome these drawbacks, novel materials such as lectins, invasins, thiomers, synthetic glycopolymers, dendrimers, and different derivatives of poly(acrylic acid) have been investigated for their mucoadhesive properties.

10.6.1 Thiomers

Thiomer polymers are prepared by cross-linking a thiol-bearing functional group to a conventional polymer to increase its mucoadhesive property [48]. Some thiomers are conjugates of poly(acrylic acid)/cysteine, chitosan/N-acetyl cysteine, alginate/cysteine, or chitosan/thioglycolic acid. As explained by Bernkop-Schurch et al., the interaction between thiomers and the mucus layer results in disulfide covalent bonds with glycoprotein of mucin molecules [48, 49], which results in their improved mucoadhesive properties over conventional polymers.

10.6.2 Lectins

Lectins are proteins or glycoproteins from plants, bacteria, or invertebrates having special affinity to carbohydrates [50]. Based on their molecular structure, lectins are classified into three groups: (i) merolectins (lectins with only one carbohydrate recognizing domain), (iii) hololectins (lectins with two or more carbohydrate recognizing domains), and (iii) chimolectins (lectins with additional nonrelated domains) [51]. Lectins that are noncovalently bound to glycosilated components of the cellular membrane attach to the cell and may stay on the surface or be taken into the cell by endocytosis. Lectins are used to target specific sites in the gut via a bioinvasive mechanism [51]. Commonly used lectins are *Abrus precatroius*, *Agaricus bisporus*, *Anguilla anguilla*, *Arachis hypogaea*, *Pandeiraea simplicifolia*, and *Bauhinia purpurea* [52].

TABLE 10.2. Polymers Used in Mucoadhesive Drug Delivery Studies

Polymer	Drug incorporated	Features	References
Anionic			
Carbopol 974P with poly(ethylene oxide)	Acyclovir or acyclovir derivatives	Tablet swelled rapidly without disintegration; retained in gastric tract and released the drug in a controlled manner	35
Poly(acrylic acid) with PEG	Botulinum toxin	Botulinum toxin for oral administration; prolonged gastric retention of toxin due to mucoadhesion	36
Sodium alginate	Captopril	Captopril microcapsules coated with alginate and other mucoadhesive polymers; alginate–Carbopol 934P microparticles displayed better mucoadhesive properties than other polymers	37
Carbopol 934P and Polycarbophil	Clarithromycin	Clarithromycin microspheres for better eradication of *Helicobacter pylori*; microspheres showed better mucoadhesive properties and improved drug entrapment properties	38
Polycarbophil	Chlorthiazide	Polycarbophil–albumin beads remained in stomach, whereas ordinary albumin beads moved away from the small intestine	39
CMCNa	Famotidine	Improved mucoadhesive properties of famotidine microspheres with an increase in CMCNa concentration	40
Carbopol 974P	Lamotrigine	Bilayer lamotrigine tablets formulated with a controlled release polymer in the upper layer and mucoadhesive Carbopol 974P in the lower layer	41
Cationic			
Chitosan	Amoxicillin or antibiotic to treat *H. pylori*	Chitosan encapsulated in a surface-modified network of nanoparticles of colloidal silica; drug bound to chitosan nanoparticles when added during *in situ* gelation of colloidal silica	42
Chitosan and guar gum	Itraconazole	Combined chitosan and guar gum to provide mucoadhesion and controlled release of Itraconazole	43

TABLE 10.2. (*Continued*)

Polymer	Drug incorporated	Features	References
Chitosan or chitosan derivatives	Acyclovir or its derivatives	Microspheres adhered to gastric mucosa and released the drug in a controlled manner	35
Positively charged gelatin	Amoxicillin	Biodegradable microspheres prepared using aminated gelatin via surfactant-free emulsification in olive oil and cross-linking with glutaraldehyde; improved mucoadhesive properties of modified gelatin microspheres over gelatin spheres	44
Nonionics			
PGEFs	Furosemide	Mucoadhesive microspheres to increase bioavailability	45
PGEFs coated with Eudragit S 100	Vancomycin	Increase in vancomycin absorption without using absorption enhancers	46
Poly(ethylene oxide)	Famotidine	Mucoadhesive effect of poly(ethylene oxide) on famotidine nanosuspension	47

CMCNa, sodium carboxymethyl cellulose; PGEFs, polyglycerol esters of fatty acids.

10.6.3 Fimbrial Proteins/Bacterial Adhesions

Fimbriae are long proteins similar to lectins located on the surfaces of many bacterial strains. Fimbriae help bacteria to adhere to epithelial surfaces of the enterocytes [53]. Fimbrial presence is correlated to pathogenicity; for example, in production and uptake of *Escherichia coli* enterotoxin K99, fimbriae aided in adherence of *E. coli* to the brush border of the epithelial cells [18]. Haltner et al. used Invasin, a membrane protein from *Yersinia pseudotuberculosis*, in studying cellular uptake of polymeric nanospheres [54]. Drug delivery systems with bacterial invasion factors help in improving adhesion.

10.6.4 Polymers with Acrylate End Groups

Davidovich-Pinhas and Bianco-Peled [55] introduced a new class of mucoadhesive polymers capable of forming covalent bonds with mucin molecules. Studies showed that poly(ethylene glycol) diacrylate reacts with thiol groups of mucin, and follows the same mechanism carried by thiolated polymers. Mucoadhesion of poly(ethylene glycol) diacrylate has been measured under tension, and was found comparable to that of thiolated alginate. More studies are required to assess the mucoadhesive properties of polymers with numerous acrylate and methacrylate end groups [2].

10.6.5   Synthetic Glycopolymers

Glycopolymers are polymers having sugar moieties as pendant groups [56]. Because of their behavior as both polysaccharides and synthetic polymers, they have several advantages over conventional water-soluble polysaccharides. Their applications as mucoadhesives have been studied by Rathi et al. [57]. Glycopolymers have been synthesized by free-radical copolymerization of N-(2-hyroxypropyl)methyl acrylamide with various sugar-containing monomers such as fucosylamine, glucosamine, and mannosamine bearing the methacryloyl functionality. The mucoadhesive properties of these polymers were studied *in vitro* using guinea pigs' small intestinal and colonic tissues. Polymers with larger sugar moieties displayed better mucoadhesive properties compared to others. Fucosylamine copolymers showed specific adhesion to colon.

Dendrimers and boronic acid copolymers have also been investigated for their mucoadhesive properties. Vandamme et al. [58] studied the mucoadhesive properties of polyamidoamine dendrimers of different functional groups such as carboxyl, hydroxyl, and amino surface groups. A rheometer was used to measure the interactions of dendrimers with mucin, which found that amino dendrimers offered stronger mucoadhesive properties at neutral pH. Ivanov and his group [59] worked on preparing a new group of mucoadhesives, boronic acid copolymers. N-acryloyl-m-aminophenylboronic acid with N,N-dimethyl acrylamide copolymers formed insoluble complexes with porcine stomach mucin at pH 9.

10.7   MUCOADHESION TESTING

In vitro and *in vivo* testing are both utilized to characterize the strength and the mechanism of adhesion in polymers. *In vitro* tests are primarily conducted to screen potential bioadhesives and generally performed using mechanical and rheological testers [18].

10.7.1   Tensile Strength

In this method, the force required to break the adhesive bond between the mucoadhesive and the mucus membrane is measured by tensile testers and balances [9]. Robinson and his group [17] used the same principle to measure the force required to separate a bioadhesive sample from fresh rabbit tissue.

10.7.2   Shear Strength

In this method, the force required for the mucoadhesive to slide with respect to the mucus layer is measured in the direction parallel to the plane of the contact area. In a modified Wilhelmy plate method, as reported by Smart et al., a glass plate suspended from a microbalance is dipped into mucus solution, and the force needed to pull the plate out of the solution is determined [23, 60].

10.7.3 Falling Liquid Film Method

In this method, proposed by Teng and Buri [61], small intestine segments from rats are placed on a tygon tube flute with an inclination. The particle suspensions are passed over the mucous surface, and the adhesion strength is determined by the fraction of particles adhering to the mucus surface. In the modified method by Nielson, Schubert, and Hansen [62], a 37 °C isotonic solution was first pumped over the mucus surface and then followed by particulate systems. The amount remaining on the mucus surface could generally be quantified using a Coulter counter [52]. For semisolid systems, liquid chromatography is utilized to quantify the portion unattached to the mucus surface.

10.7.4 Rheological Methods

A simple viscometric method has been used by Hassan and Gallo to measure the mucin–bioadhesive bond strength. The force of mucoadhesion is measured on the basis of rheological changes of the polymer/mucin mixtures [63]. Mucoadhesive polymers/mucin mixtures will display a higher viscosity than the sum of viscosities of the individual components of the mixture. The interaction between the mucin and the mucoadhesive polymer generally results in enhanced viscosity depending on the polymer used in developing mucoadhesion.

10.7.5 Colloidal Gold Staining Method

In this technique, proposed by Park et al. [64], red colloidal gold particles are stabilized onto mucin molecules, and the interaction between a bioadhesive and the mucin gold conjugates will develop a red color on the mucoadhesive surface. The strength of the mucoadhesive interaction can then be measured by the change in color intensity on the mucin molecules.

10.7.6 Mechanical Spectroscopic Method

This method was first used by Kerr et al. [65] to study the interaction between glycoprotein gels and poly(acrylic acid). Rheological properties of the mixture were studied utilizing mechanical spectroscopy. With this technique, they studied the effect of pH and polymer chain length on mucoadhesion. A similar method was used by Mortazavi et al. [66] to investigate the effect of carbopol 934P on rheological properties of mucus gel. The difference between the storage modulus of the mixture and of the individual components at same concentration is an indication of the extent of interaction between the polymer and mucin. The greater this difference, the stronger is the presumed interaction.

Several other methods, including the fluorescent probe method [67], the flow channel method [68], the adhesion weight test [69], electrical conductance [70], and the adhesion number test, have also been used for *in vitro* mucoadhesive studies.

Compared to *in vitro* tests, very few *in vivo* methods are available for testing mucoadhesion. Radioisotopes [71], gamma scintigraphy [52], pharmacoscintigraphy

[72], X-ray studies [73], and electron paramagnetic resonance oximetry [74] have been used to measure the residence time of the bioadhesive at the mucus membrane. The GI transit time of many bioadhesives can be measured by radioisotopes and scintigraphy methods.

10.8   DRUG RELEASE STUDIES

Since no standard method is available to study drug release from mucoadhesive systems, other official United States Pharmacopeia (USP) methods have been reported in the literature. The USP apparatus I, II, and III are respectively used for capsules, tablets, and bead-type formulations. Ahmed et al. studied the *in vitro* release of Captopril-entrapped mucoadhesive beads by using USP 23 TDT-06T dissolution testing (Electrolab-paddle method) at 50 rpm [75]. Krishna et al. [76] used the USP II dissolution apparatus at 50 rpm to study the release of rosiglitazone maleate from a mucoadhesive tablet.

10.9   MUCOADHESIVE DOSAGE FORMS

Most commonly studied mucoadhesive drug delivery systems are tablets, multilayered tablets, semisolid forms, powders, microparticles, microspheres, nanoparticles, microcapsules, and capsules. Mucoadhesive tablets are primarily used to extend the release of the drug, to reduce frequency of drug administration, to improve patient compliance, and to facilitate localized action of the drug in the GI tract [77]. Decrosta et al. formulated Captopril sustained release tablets using carbopol 934P as mucoadhesive polymer [78]. In another study, multilayered tablets with acrylic acid polymers and cellulose derivatives provided immediate and sustained drug release as well as greater mucoadhesion [79]. Mucoadhesive microparticles, in the form of pellets, beads, microspheres, microcapsules, and lipospheres, offer efficient drug absorption and enhanced bioavailability, greater interpenetrated contact with the mucus layer, and specific targeting of drugs to the absorption site [80]. Table 10.3 shows the advantage of using mucoadhesive dosage forms compared to their regular non-mucoadhesive counterparts.

There as several methods of achieving mucoadhesion and formulating mucoadhesive drug delivery systems. Some of these technologies include the use of multilayered drug delivery devices, erodible drug delivery devices, microparticles, and liquid systems.

10.9.1   Multilayer Mucoadhesive Drug Delivery Systems

One of the patented technologies used in preparing mucoadhesive drug delivery systems is the multilayer system. The system consists of a mucoadhesive layer and a non-mucoadhesive layer. The former is water-soluble, which releases the drug in a controlled manner, whereas the latter is primarily used for immediate release purposes. The residence time of the whole system can be modified by the non-mucoadhesive layer [90, 91].

TABLE 10.3. Bioavailability Studies of Mucoadhesive Systems

Drug/Mucoadhesive system	Polymer	Site of action	Features	References
Amoxicillin/microspheres	Carboxyvinyl polymer	GIT	Increased bioavailability compared to oral suspension and improved drug absorption helping to reduce dose	81
Alendronate/liposomal delivery system	Chitosan	GIT	Improvement of stability, mucoadhesiveness, and oral drug absorption in rats	82
Acetaminophen/suppository	Polycarbophil	Rectal	Sustained release and prolonged plasma levels of acetaminophen compared to conventional formulation	83
Valsartan/pellets	Hydroxypropyl methylcellulose and carbomer	GIT	Compared to non-mucoadhesive pellets and suspension, it has fast drug release, delayed GI transit, and improved bioavailability	84
Pilocarpine nitrate/liposomes	Carbopol 1342	Ophthalmic	Longer duration of action and larger AUC compared to a non-mucoadhesive system and drug suspension	85
Gentamycin/microparticulate system	Chitosan/hyaluronan	Nasal	Prolonged drug release and improved drug absorption	86
Bupravaquone/ nano suspension	Carbopol/chitosan	GIT	Prolonged retention time and increased absorption	87
Buserelin/suspension	Carbomer/Chitosan	GIT	Improved intestinal absorption of peptide drug	88
Acyclovir/microspheres	Carbopol 974 P	GIT	Enhanced bioavailability and increased residence time compared to drug suspension	89

10.9.2 Liquid Mucoadhesive Systems

The most commonly used liquid mucoadhesive systems are emulsions and suspensions used for oral, peroral, and intranasal routes of administration. These systems utilize gums and hydrocolloids to improve mucoadhesion of the drug. Liquid mucoadhesive systems not only offer longer periods of action but also allow localized drug delivery, especially in the GI tract [92, 93].

10.9.3 Mucoadhesive Microparticulate Systems

Microparticulate systems such as granules and microgranules can be used to achieve mucoadhesion. Drug release is controlled by spraying a mucoadhesive coat onto a lipophilic material [94]. For example, targeted delivery to the gastric mucosa was described using mucoadhesive granules composed of carbomer and drug [95].

Despite the fact that mucoadhesive dosage forms of different nature are now being studied, such formulations for oral and buccal delivery can primarily be found in the market in the form of tablets, lozenges, films, and powders, as summarized in Table 10.4.

10.10 CONCLUSION

In this chapter, we have tried to provide an overview of mucoadhesion, mucoadhesive polymers, mucoadhesive drug products, and tests used to measure mucoadhesion. Even though several mucoadhesive dosage forms are available on the market, this area of research is still new. Future efforts are most likely to be focused on mucoadhesive drug delivery systems that are designed using novel mucoadhesive materials with enhanced adhesion and specificity. Additionally, with new techniques to measure mucoadhesion and a better understanding of the methodologies underlying the mucoadhesion phenomenon, more advanced and optimized drug delivery platforms can be developed.

10.11 KEY POINTS

- Mucoadhesion is an attraction between a mucus membrane and a polymer. Mucoadhesion is a complex process comprising two stages, contact and consolidation.
- Major benefits of mucoadhesive drug delivery systems are increased residence time, improved bioavailability, and controlled release.
- Challenges encountered in developing a successful mucoadhesive system are rate of mucin turnover, mucus–drug interactions, and mucus–polymer interactions.
- Polymer–mucus interactions play a key role in the mucoadhesive mechanism. They can be either covalent in nature or occur through weak physical interactions such as hydrogen bonding or van der Waal forces.

TABLE 10.4. Examples of Commercial Mucoadhesive Products

Tablet	Description	References
Aftach (triamcinolone acetonide); Teijin Limited Japan	Bilayer tablet applied to oral cavity, white adhesive layer containing drug and a colored layer for support. Used for treatment of aphthous stomatitis, the white layer of the tablet attaches to the application site; it contains hydroxypropyl cellulose and Carbopol 934 to improve mucoadhesion	96
Carafate (aluminum hydroxide and sucralfate); Axcan Scandipharm, Inc.	Applied to GI ulcers, it adheres to ulcer sites and provides protection from acids, bile salts, and enzymes; contains sucrose octasulfate for mucoadhesion	97
Susadrin (Nitroglycerin); Marion Merrells-Dows	Applied buccally, the tablet prepared using Synchrons of Forest Laboratories, provides up to 6 h of controlled release; contains Synchron (modified HPMC) for mucoadhesion	98
Buccastem (prochlorperazine maleate); Alliance Pharmaceutical Inc.	Applied buccally, the tablet is placed under upper lip and top gum, usually taken once or twice daily; contains Ceronia, xanthan gum for mucoadhesion	99
Fentora (fentanyl citrate); Cephalon	Applied to the oral cavity, it employs OraVescent® drug delivery technology. When the tablet comes into contact with saliva, a reaction takes place with the release of carbon dioxide. Applied to the buccal cavity, above a rear molar, between upper cheek and gum; contains sodium starch glycolate and mannitol for mucoadhesion	100
Suscard (glyceryl trinitrate); Forest laboratories	Applied buccally between the upper lip and the gum; contains hypromellose for mucoadhesion	101
Striant SR (Testosterone); Columbia Pharmaceuticals	The white or off-white tablet applied buccally to the upper gum just above the incisor tooth on either side with flat surface facing cheek mucosa; contains Carbopol 934P and hypromellose for mucoadhesion	102
Gum		
Nicotinell (Nicotine); Novartis Consumer	Applied to the oral cavity, the Nicotinell lozenges are used as part of NRT; contains polyacrylate 30% dispersion and xanthan gum for mucoadhesion	103

(continued)

335

TABLE 10.4. (Continued)

Tablet	Description	References
Lozenge		
Actiq (fentanyl citrate); Cephalon	Applied to the oral cavity, placed in the mouth between the cheek and lower gum, with help of the handle the matrix is moved from one side to another; contains modified food starch (edible glue) for mucoadhesion	104
Film		
Onsolis (fentanyl citrate); Meda Pharmaceutical, Inc.	Applied buccally, Onsolis uses rapidly dissolving BEMA™ bioerodible mucoadhesive technology from BioDelivery Sciences. The drug delivery system consists of two layers; the first layer contains drug and is bioadhesive in nature, while the second layer is protective and prevents the bioadhesive layer to interact with saliva; contains carboxymethyl cellulose, hydroxyethyl cellulose, and hydroxypropyl cellulose for mucoadhesion	105
Powder		
Rhinocort nasal spray (Budesonide); Astrazeneca, US	Applied nasally, used in the treatment of nasal symptoms of perennial rhinitis; a metered dose manual pump spray, with micronized budesonide suspended in aqueous medium, contains microcrystalline cellulose and carboxymethyl cellulose sodium for mucoadhesion	106
Ophthalmic solution/suspension		
Azasite ophthalmic solution (Azithromycin); Inspire Pharmaceuticals, Inc., USA.	Contains 1% of azithromycin. Used for treatment of topical eye infections. Uses Durasite drug delivery technology in the formulation. Polycarbophil is the bioadhesive polymer used in the Durasite technology.	107
Besivance ophthalmic suspension (Besifloxacin); Bausch & Lomb, FL, USA.	Besivance suspension containing 0.6% besifloxacin and is used to treat bacterial conjunctivitis. Utilizes Durasite drug delivery technology in the formulation.	108

NRT, nicotine replacement therapy.

- Hydrophilic high molecular weight anionic polymers are traditionally used for achieving mucoadhesion, whereas second-generation mucoadhesives offer enhanced site specific adhesion.
- Common tests carried out to measure mucoadhesion are tensile strength, shear strength, and rheology.

10.12 HOMEWORK QUESTIONS

1. Explain how drink and food habits may affect the efficacy of a mucoadhesive-based delivery system in enhancing drug bioavailability.
2. Mucoadhesive drug delivery is utilized to prolong retention of drugs with a narrow absorption window, that is, those with primary absorption sites in the upper intestines and stomach. Explain what factors you should consider in formulating a mucoadhesive platform for such application.
3. Mucoadhesive approach is utilized in buccal delivery systems. Explain the biopharmaceutical factors that might affect the efficacy of such delivery systems.
4. Explain the behavior of a pH-dependent mucoadhesive dosage form across the GI tract.

REFERENCES

1. Scrivener CA, Schantz CW. Penicillin; new methods for its use in dentistry. J Am Dent Assoc 1947;35(9):644–647.
2. Khutoryanskiy VV. Advances in mucoadhesion and mucoadhesive polymers. Macromol Biosci 2011;11(6):748–764.
3. Ahuja A, Khar RK, Ali J. Mucoadhesive drug delivery systems. Drug Dev Ind Pharm 1997;23(5):489–515.
4. Smart JD, Keegan G. *Buccal drug delivery systems*. In: Wen H, Park K, editors. Oral Controlled Release Formulation Design and Drug Delivery: Theory to Practice. Hoboken: John Wiley & Sons, Inc.; 2010. p 169–184.
5. Omidian H, Park K. *Oral targeted drug delivery systems: Gastric retention devices*. In: Wen H, Park K, editors. Oral Controlled Release Formulation Design and Drug Delivery: Theory to Practice. Hoboken: John Wiley & Sons, Inc; 2010. p 185–203.
6. Rathbone MJ, Hadgraft J. Absorption of drugs from the human oral cavity. Int J Pharm 1991;74(1):9–24.
7. Birudaraj R et al. Advances in buccal drug delivery. Crit Rev Ther Drug Carrier Syst 2005;22(3):295–330.
8. Kharenko E, Larionova N, Demina N. Mucoadhesive drug delivery systems. Pharm Chem J 2009;43(4):200–208.
9. Peppas NA, Sahlin JJ. Hydrogels as mucoadhesive and bioadhesive materials: a review. Biomaterials 1996;17(16):1553–1561.
10. Jimenezcastellanos MR, Zia H, Rhodes CT. Mucoadhesive drug delivery systems. Drug Dev Ind Pharm 1993;19(1–2):143–194.

11. Ponchel G, Irache JM. Specific and non-specific bioadhesive particulate systems for oral delivery to the gastrointestinal tract. Adv Drug Deliv Rev 1998;34(2–3):191–219.

12. MacAdam A. The effect of gastro-intestinal mucus on drug absorption. Adv Drug Deliv Rev 1993;11(3):201–220.

13. Konietzko N. Mucus transport and inflammation. Eur J Respir Dis Suppl 1986;147:72–79.

14. Duchene D, Touchard F, Peppas NA. Pharmaceutical and medical aspects of bioadhesive systems for drug administration. Drug Dev Ind Pharm 1988;14(2–3):283–318.

15. Gurny R, Meyer JM, Peppas NA. Bioadhesive intraoral release systems: design, testing and analysis. Biomaterials 1984;5(6):336–340.

16. Bremecker KD et al. Formulation and clinical test of a novel mucosal adhesive ointment. Arzneimittelforschung 1983;33(4):591–594.

17. Ch'ng HS et al. Bioadhesive polymers as platforms for oral controlled drug delivery II: synthesis and evaluation of some swelling, water-insoluble bioadhesive polymers. J Pharm Sci 1985;74(4):399–405.

18. Lee JW, Park JH, Robinson JR. Bioadhesive-based dosage forms: the next generation. J Pharm Sci 2000;89(7):850–866.

19. Smart JD. The basics and underlying mechanisms of mucoadhesion. Adv Drug Deliv Rev 2005;57(11):1556–1568.

20. Huang Y et al. Molecular aspects of muco- and bioadhesion: tethered structures and site-specific surfaces. J Control Release 2000;65(1–2):63–71.

21. Hagerstrom H, Edsman K, Stromme M. Low-frequency dielectric spectroscopy as a tool for studying the compatibility between pharmaceutical gels and mucous tissue. J Pharm Sci 2003;92(9):1869–1881.

22. Carvalho FC et al. Mucoadhesive drug delivery systems. Brazilian J Pharm Sci 2010;46:1–17.

23. Asane GS et al. Polymers for mucoadhesive drug delivery system: a current status. Drug Dev Ind Pharm 2008;34(11):1246–1266.

24. Salamat-Miller N, Chittchang M, Johnston TP. The use of mucoadhesive polymers in buccal drug delivery. Adv Drug Deliv Rev 2005;57(11):1666–1691.

25. Woodley J. Bioadhesion: New possibilities for drug administration? Clin Pharmacokinet 2001;40(2):77–84.

26. Lin HR, Sung KC. Carbopol/pluronic phase change solutions for ophthalmic drug delivery. J Control Release 2000;69(3):379–388.

27. Nikonenko NA, Bushnak IA, Keddie JL. Spectroscopic ellipsometry of mucin layers on an amphiphilic diblock copolymer surface. Appl spectrosc 2009;63(8):889–898.

28. Park H, Robinson JR. Mechanisms of mucoadhesion of poly(acrylic acid) hydrogels. Pharm Res 1987;4(6):457–464.

29. Kumar V, Banker GS. Chemically-modified cellulosic polymers. Drug Dev Ind Pharm 1993;19(1–2):1–31.

30. Ali J et al. Buccoadhesive erodible disk for treatment of oro-dental infections: design and characterisation. Int J Pharm 2002;238(1–2):93–103.

31. Felt O, Buri P, Gurny R. Chitosan: a unique polysaccharide for drug delivery. Drug Dev Ind Pharm 1998;24(11):979–993.

32. Rekha MR, Sharma CP. Synthesis and evaluation of lauryl succinyl chitosan particles towards oral insulin delivery and absorption. J Control Release 2009;135(2):144–151.

33. Bogataj M et al. The correlation between zeta potential and mucoadhesion strength on pig vesical mucosa. Biol Pharm Bull 2003;26(5):743–746.

34. Ludwig A. The use of mucoadhesive polymers in ocular drug delivery. Adv Drug Deliv Rev 2005;57(11):1595–1639.

35. Jain S et al. Sustained release drug delivery system. Bangalore, India: Bioplus Life Sciences Pvt. Ltd; 2009. p 1–27.

36. Donovan S. Botulinum toxin formulations for oral administration. Irvine, CA: Allergen Inc; 2004.

37. Altaf MA, Sreedharan, Charyulu N. Ionic gelation controlled drug delivery systems for gastric mucoadhesive microparticles of captopril. Indian J Pharm Sci 2008;70(5):655–658.

38. Thorat YS, Modi VS, Dhavale SC. Use of carbomers to design mucoadhesive microspheres for anti h-pyroli drug, clarithromycin. Int J of pharmTech Research 2009;1(4):1421–1428.

39. Longer MA, Ch'ng HS, Robinson JR. Bioadhesive polymers as platforms for oral controlled drug delivery III: oral delivery of chlorothiazide using a bioadhesive polymer. J Pharm Sci 1985;74(4):406–11.

40. Arya RKK, Ripudam S, Vijay J. Mucoadhesive microspheres of famotidine: preparation, characterization and invitro evaluation. International Journal of Engineering Science and Technology 2010;2(6):1575–1580.

41. Mohana Raghava Srivalli K, Lakshmi PK, Balasubhramaniam J. Design of a novel bilayered gastric mucoadhesive system for localized and unidirectional release of lamotrigine. Saudi Pharm J 2013;21(1):45–52.

42. David AE, Zhang R, Yoon JP, Yang AJ-M, Yang VC. Mucoadhesive Nanocomposite Delivery System. Newyork, US: Jones Day; 2009.

43. Shaikh AA, Pawar YD, Kumbhar ST. An in-vitro study for mucoadhesion and control release properties of guar gum and chitosan in itraconazole mucoadhesive tablets. Int J Pharm Sci Res 2012;3(5):1411–1414.

44. Wang J, Tauchi Y, Deguchi Y, Morimoto K, Tabata Y, Ikada Y. Positively Charged Gelatin Microspheres as Gastric Mucoadhesive Drug Delivery System for Eradication of H. pylori. Drug Deliv 2000;7(4):237–243.

45. Akiyama Y, Nagahara N. *Novel formulation approaches to oral mucoadhesive drug delivery systems.* In: Mathiowitz E, Chickering DE, Lehr CM, editors. Bioadhesive Drug Delivery Systems Fundamentals, Novel Approaches, and Development. New York: Marcel Dekker; 1999. p 477–505.

46. Geary RS, Schlameus HW. Vancomycin and Insulin used as models for oral delivery of peptides. J Control Release 1993;23:65–74.

47. Dhaval JP, Jayvadan KP. Mucoadhesive effect of polyethylene oxide on famotidine nanosuspension prepared by solvent evaporation method. Int J Pharm Pharm Sci 2010;2(2): 122–127.

48. Bernkop-Schnurch A. Thiomers: a new generation of mucoadhesive polymers. Adv Drug Deliv Rev 2005;57(11):1569–82.

49. Grabovac V, Guggi D, Bernkop-Schnurch A. Comparison of the mucoadhesive properties of various polymers. Adv Drug Deliv Rev 2005;57(11):1713–23.

50. Lehr CM. Lectin-mediated drug delivery: the second generation of bioadhesives. J Control Release 2000;65(1–2):19–29.

51. Haas J, Lehr CM. Developments in the area of bioadhesive drug delivery systems. Expert Opin Biol Ther 2002;2(3):287–98.

52. Chowdary KP, Rao YS. Mucoadhesive microspheres for controlled drug delivery. Biol Pharm Bull 2004;27(11):1717–24.

53. Bernkop-Schnürch A et al. An adhesive drug delivery system based on K99-fimbriae. Eur J Pharm Sci 1995;3:293–299.

54. Haltner E, Easson JH, Lehr CM. Lectins and Bacterial invasion factors for controlled endo- and transcytosis of bioadhesive drug carrier systems. Eur J Pharm Biopharm 1997;44:3–13.

55. Davidovich-Pinhas M, Bianco-Peled H. Novel mucoadhesive system based on sulfhydryl-acrylate interactions. J Mater Sci Mater Med 2010;21(7):2027–34.

56. Ladmiral V, Melia E, Haddleton DM. Synthetic glycopolymers: an overview. Eur Polym J 2004;40(3):431–449.

57. Rathi RC et al. N-(2-Hydroxypropyl) methacrylamide copolymers containing pendant saccharide moieties - synthesis and bioadhesive properties. J Polym Sci A Polym Chem 1991;29(13):1895–1902.

58. Vandamme TF, Brobeck L. Poly(amidoamine) dendrimers as ophthalmic vehicles for ocular delivery of pilocarpine nitrate and tropicamide. J Control Release 2005;102(1):23–38.

59. Ivanov AE et al. Boronate-containing polymers form affinity complexes with mucin and enable tight and reversible occlusion of mucosal lumen by poly(vinyl alcohol) gel. Int J Pharm 2008;358(1–2):36–43.

60. Smart JD, Kellaway IW, Worthington HE. An in-vitro investigation of mucosa-adhesive materials for use in controlled drug delivery. J Pharm Pharmacol 1984;36(5):295–299.

61. Teng CLC, Ho NFH. Mechanistic studies in the simultaneous flow and adsorption of polymer coated latex particles on intestinal mucus. I . Methods and physical model development. J Control Release 1987;6(1):133–149.

62. Nielson LS, Schubert L, Hansen J. Bioadhesive drug delivery systems. I. Characterization of mucoadhesive properties of systems based on glyceryl mono-oleate and glyceryl monolinoleate. Eur J Pharm Sci 1998;6(3):231–239.

63. Hassan EE, Gallo JM. A simple rheological method for the in vitro assessment of mucin-polymer bioadhesive bond strength. Pharm Res 1990;7(5):491–495.

64. Park K. A new approach to study mucoadhesion: colloidal gold staining. Int J Pharm 1989;53(3):209–217.

65. Kerr LJ, IWK , Rowlands C, Parr GD. The influence of poly acrylic acids on the rheology of glycoprotein gels. Proc Int Symp Control Rel Bioact Mater 1990;17:122.

66. Mortazavi SA, Carpenter BG, Smart JD. An Investigation of the rheological behavior of the mucoadhesive mucosal interface. Int J Pharm 1992;83(1–3):221–225.

67. Park K, Robinson JR. Bioadhesive polymers as platforms for oral controlled drug delivery: Method to study bioadhesion. Int J Pharm 1984;19(1):107–127.

68. Mikos AG, Peppas NA. *Scaling concepts and molecular theories of adhesion of synthetic polymers to glycoprotenic networks.* In: Lenaerts V, Gurny R, editors. Bioadhesive Drug Delivery Systems. Boca Raton, FL: CRC press; 1990. p 25.

69. Smart JD, Kellaway IW. In-vitro techniques for measuring mucoadhesion. J Pharm Pharmacol 1982;34:70.

70. Kamath KR, Park K. *Mucosal adhesive preparations.* In: Swarbrick J, Boylan JC, editors. Encyclopedia of Pharmaceutical Technology. New york: Marcel Dekker; 1994. p 133.

71. Sakkinen M et al. Are chitosan formulations mucoadhesive in the human small intestine? An evaluation based on gamma scintigraphy. Int J Pharm 2006;307(2):285–91.

72. Singh AK, Bhardwaj N, Bhatnagar A. Pharmacoscintigraphy: An unexplored modality in India. Ind J Pharm Sci 2004;66(1):18–25.

73. Chary RB, Vani G, Rao YM. In vitro and in vivo adhesion testing of mucoadhesive drug delivery systems. Drug Dev Ind Pharm 1999;25(5):685–90.

74. Petelin M et al. In vivo study of different ointments for drug delivery into oral mucosa by EPR oximetry. Int J Pharm 2004;270(1–2):83–91.

75. Ahmed MG, Satish Kumar BP, Kiran Kumar GB. Formulation and evaluation of gastric mucoadhesive drug delivery systems of captopril. J Curr Pharm Res 2010;2(1):26–32.

76. Krishna SS. Formulation and evaluation of mucoadhesive dosage form containing rosiglitazone maleate. Pak J Pharm Sci 2006;19(3):208–213.

77. Vasir JK, Garg KTS. Mucoadhesive tablets as a controlled drug delivery system. Int J Pharm 2003;255:13–32.

78. Decrosta, M.T., N.B. Jain, and E.M. Rudnic, Controlled release formulation, US Patent 4,666,705A, Published May 19, 1987.

79. Duchene DPG. Principle and investigation of the bioadhesion mechanism of solid dosage forms. Biomaterials 1992;13:709–714.

80. Arora S et al. Floating drug delivery systems: a review. AAPS PharmSciTech 2005;6(3): E372–90.

81. Nagahara N et al. Mucoadhesive microspheres containing amoxicillin for clearance of Helicobacter pylori. Antimicrob Agents Chemother 1998;42(10):2492–4.

82. Han H-K, Shin H-J, Ha DH. Improved oral bioavailability of alendronate via the mucoadhesive liposomal delivery system. Eur J Pharm Sci 2012;46(5):500–507.

83. Choi H-G, Oh Y-K, Kim C-K. In situ gelling and mucoadhesive liquid suppository containing acetaminophen: enhanced bioavailability. Int J Pharm 1998;165(1):23–32.

84. Cao Q-R et al. Enhanced oral bioavailability of novel mucoadhesive pellets containing valsartan prepared by a dry powder-coating technique. Int J Pharm 2012;434(1–2):325–333.

85. Durrani AM et al. Pilocarpine bioavailability from a mucoadhesive liposomal ophthalmic drug delivery system. Int J Pharm 1992;88(1–3):409–415.

86. Lim ST et al. In vivo evaluation of novel hyaluronan/chitosan microparticulate delivery systems for the nasal delivery of gentamicin in rabbits. Int J Pharm 2002;231(1):73–82.

87. Jacobs C, Kayser O, Müller RH. Production and characterisation of mucoadhesive nanosuspensions for the formulation of bupravaquone. Int J Pharm 2001;214(1–2):3–7.

88. Luessen HL et al. Mucoadhesive polymers in peroral peptide drug delivery. VI. Carbomer and chitosan improve the intestinal absorption of the peptide drug buserelin in vivo. Pharm Res 1996;13(11):1668–1672.

89. Tao Y et al. Development of mucoadhesive microspheres of acyclovir with enhanced bioavailability. Int J Pharm 2009;378(1–2):30–36.

90. Moro DG, Callahan H, Nowotnik D. Mucoadhesive Erodible Drug Delivery Device for Controlled Administration of Pharmaceuticals and Other Active Compounds. Dallas, US: Access Pharmaceutical Inc; 2003.

91. Bromet NE. Heterofunctional Mucoadhesive Pharmaceutical Dosage Composition. Orleans Cedex 2, France: Biotec Centre S.A; 1999.

92. Dobrozsi DJ. Oral Liquid Mucoadhesive Compositions. Ohio, US: The Procter & Gamble Company; 2003.

93. Putteman P, Francois MKJ, Snoeckx ECL. Mucoadhesive Emulsion Containing Cyclodextrins. Belgium: Janssen Pharmaceutica, N.V.; 1998.

94. Santus, G., G. Bottoni, and C. Lazzarini, Controlled- release mucoadhesive pharmaceutical composition for the oral administration of furosemide. 1996, Recordati S.A., Chemical and Pharmaceutical Company, Chiasso, Switzerland.

95. Dettmar PW et al. Mucoadhesive Granules of Carbomer Suitable for Oral Administration of Drugs. GB: Reckitt Benckiser Healthcare UK Ltd; 2001.

96. Teijin Limited Japan. Patient information leaflet: AFTACH 2003; Available at http://www.angelinipharma.com/public/schedepharma/aftach.htm. Accessed 2012 May 12.

97. Axcan Pharma US Inc. Carafate® (sucralfate) tablets US package insert. 2008; Available at http://www.aptalispharma.com/pdf/Car_Tablets_PI.pdf. Accessed 2012 April 12.

98. Schor JM et al. Susadrin transmucosal tablets (Nitroglycerin in Synchron® controlled-release base). Drug Dev Ind Pharm 1983;9(7):1359–1377.

99. Alliance Pharmaceutical Inc. Buccastem 3mg tablets: Patient information leaflet. 2009; Available at http://www.alliancepharma.co.uk/alliance/en/products/productsearch?prodsearch=Buccastem. Accessed 2012 April 14.

100. Cephalon Inc. Presciption information: Fentora. 2011; Available at http://www.fentora.com/pdfs/pdf100_prescribing_info.pdf. Accessed 2012 March 25.

101. Forest Laboratories. Package leaflet: Information for the user, Suscard 2 mg, 3mg or 5mg buccal tablets, glyceryl trinitrate. 2011; Available at http://www.forest-labs.co.uk/products/prescription/suscard_buccal_tablets/#. Accessed 2012 April 29.

102. Columbia Laboratories Inc. Package Insert & Patient Package Insert: Striant (testosterone buccal system mucoadhesive). 2003; Available at http://www.accessdata.fda.gov/drugsatfda_docs/label/2004/21543s002lbl.pdf. Accessed 2012 March 21.

103. Novartis Consumer Inc. Patient information leaflet: Nicotinell. 2009; Available at http://www.novartis.com.ph/products/over_counter.html. Accessed 2012 March 22.

104. Cephalon Inc. Actiq ACT-011 Prescribing information. 2011; Available at http://www.actiq.com/pdf/actiq_package_insert_4_5_07.pdf. Accessed 2012 April 09.

105. Meda Pharmaceuticals Inc. Onsolis: Patient information. 2011; Available at http://www.onsolis.com/pdf/onsolis_pi.pdf. Accessed 2012 May 05.

106. AstraZeneca Inc. Rhinocort Aqua: Patient information. 2010; Available at http://www1.astrazeneca-us.com/pi/Rhinocort_Aqua.pdf. Accessed 2012 May 07.

107. http://www.merck.com/product/usa/pi_circulars/a/azasite/azasite_pi.pdf. Accessed 2013 July 19.

108. Bausch and Lomb http://www.bausch.com/en/Our-Products/Rx-Pharmaceutical/Besivance. Accessed 2013 July 19.

11

ENHANCED ORAL DRUG DELIVERY THROUGH METABOLIC PATHWAYS

Gregory Russell-Jones

Mentor Pharmaceutical Consulting Pty Ltd, Middle Cove, Australia

11.1 INTRODUCTION

By far the most convenient method of drug delivery is via the oral route of administration. Within the gut, a single cell layer of intestinal epithelial cells (enterocytes) provides a barrier to the uptake of viruses, bacteria, and protozoa as well as the majority of ingested material, particularly water-soluble molecules. Even the uptake of water requires the presence of specific dedicated integral membrane proteins called *aquaporins* [1–5] to enable the transmembrane transport of water. The barrier properties of the enterocyte, whilst desirable as a defence mechanism against invasion, poses a problem for the body because most nutrients, such as amino acids, carbohydrates, and many vitamins, are highly water-soluble and must cross this barrier to gain access into the body. This chapter looks at how the body is able to overcome this barrier to allow the uptake of essential nutrients, and also describes how it is possible to use the natural nutrient uptake systems, particularly for water-soluble vitamins, to piggyback the uptake of other nondietary molecules, particularly whole peptides and proteins, from the intestine into the circulation.

Engineering Polymer Systems for Improved Drug Delivery, First Edition.
Edited by Rebecca A. Bader and David A. Putnam.
© 2014 John Wiley & Sons, Inc. Published 2014 by John Wiley & Sons, Inc.

11.2   UPTAKE OF NUTRIENTS FROM THE INTESTINE

As introduced in Chapter 2 and mentioned above, in order for the body to acquire ingested nutrients from the gut, these molecules must first cross the lipid bilayer, which constitutes the membrane that surrounds the intestinal epithelial cell, and then travel through the cell to be released from the basal side of the cell. This bilayer of lipids provides a barrier to the uptake of even very small molecules such as water, salts, as well as dietary amino acids and fats. In order to overcome this barrier, the body has devised a system of pores, receptors, and transporters, each of which shows some specificity for dietary compounds. Thus, very small molecules such as water require major intrinsic proteins (aquaporins) that form pores in the cell membrane, thereby allowing small hydrophilic molecules to pass through the hydrophobic medium, that is, the cell membrane [1–5]. Dietary sugars such as polysaccharides and disaccharides are digested into their component monosaccharides, and the resultant molecules, such as hexose, are transported into the cell by the sodium-glucose transporter SGLUT1, while fructose is taken up via the transporters GLUT2 and GLUT5.

For many years, it was thought that uptake of dietary fatty acids occurred by simple phase-partitioning of these molecules into the enterocyte membrane, followed by incorporation into lipoprotein complexes and/or chylomicrons. It is now known that, following the release of free fatty acids from triglycerides through the action of esterases and lipase secreted into the intestine, uptake and transport of these molecules into the enterocyte is via the fatty acid transporters FATP1, FATP2, and FATP4 [6] (Fig. 11.1). FATP4 is expressed in high amounts on the apical membrane surface of enterocytes [7].

There are also sodium-dependent monocarboxylate transporters (SMCT) expressed in the small intestine [8], which are responsible for transport of molecules such as γ-hydroxybutyrate, L-lactate, and pyruvate. Uptake of vitamin C has now been shown to be due to a sodium-dependent vitamin C transporter [9]. Dietary proteins are broken down in the intestine into small peptides and individual amino acids, which are then taken up via the peptide transporters PEPT1 and HPT1, and the amino acid transporters LAT3, PROT, CSNU1, CSNU3, 4F2HC, CT1, and ASCI

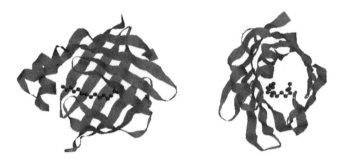

Figure 11.1. Fatty acid-binding protein (light gray) holding myristic acid (dark gray). Raswin representation of 21FB.PDB file.

[9–13]. DNA released from cells, or via digestion, is broken down into individual nucleosides, which in turn are taken up via the nucleoside transporters CNT2 and SBC2. Separate transporters have been found for organic cations (SFXN1, OCT5, OCTN2) [14], organic anions (NBC3, SDCT1, NADC1, NBC1), and bile acids (ASBT) [13, 15]. Uptake of drugs such as dopamine, serotonin, metformin, choline, cimetidine, verapamil, and ganciclovir is thought to occur via the organic cation transporter [14]. Separate transporters have also been identified for cholesterol, and these are now implicated in the uptake of fat-soluble vitamins such as vitamins D, E, A, and K, as well as carotenoids [16]. Additionally, small atoms such as copper have their own transporters [17].

One similarity with the uptake systems described above is that they all have relatively large capacities for uptake. Thus, at a single sitting, a human can ingest 10s to 100s of grams of carbohydrates, proteins, or fats, and still have the capacity to absorb the nutrients released by digestion. The absorptive area for uptake is very high and is increased by the structures of the intestine, including the finger-like projections (villi) (Fig. 11.2) and microvilli that are present on the surface of the enterocytes (Fig. 11.3).

Basically, there appears to be some sort of transporter for all small dietary molecules, but what about larger molecules such as the water-soluble vitamins and the various proteins and toxins that are known to be active after oral administration? The mechanism by which these molecules are taken up from the intestine will be discussed in later sections.

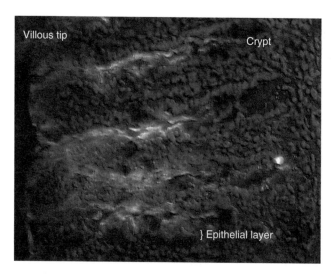

Figure 11.2. Structure of the small intestinal villous in a mouse. Each fingerlike projection is a whole villous. The lumen of the gut is on the left of the villous tip. The intestinal epithelium consists of a single cell layer. Cells divide in the base of the crypt (right) and gradually mature as they move up the villous to eventually be lost from the villous tip. Nuclei are dark gray, while the brush border layer at the tips of the enterocytes are light gray.

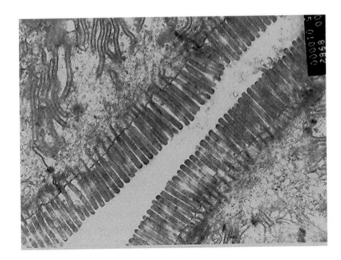

Figure 11.3. Electron micrograph of microvilli on the luminal surface of the enterocyte. Each microvilli is around 90 nm in diameter. The absorptive surface area of the intestine is greatly increased by the presence of microvilli on the apical surface of the enterocyte.

TABLE 11.1. Comparison of the Molecular Weight of Various Water-Soluble Molecules

Molecule	MW	Molecule	MW
Biotin	244	Folate	441
Nicotinic acid (niacin)	123	Riboflavin	376
Vitamin B_{12}	1356	Insulin	~6000
Epidermal growth factor	6045	Insulin-like growth factor	7649
Transferrin	~80,000	Lactoferrin	~80,000
Immunoglobulin G	~150,000	Secretory IgA	384,000

11.2.1 Uptake of Larger Molecules from the Intestine

From the description above, it would appear that the majority of nutrient molecules, be they hydrophobic, such as lipids, fats, and fat-soluble vitamins, or hydrophilic, such as water, amino acids, hexoses, and heptoses, are taken up from the gut via some sort of specific interaction with a membrane receptor (fats and fat-soluble vitamins) or via facilitated diffusion through some sort of pore (water, hexoses, heptoses, amino acids, etc.). These processes seem simple enough for such small, relatively low molecular weight compounds, but what about the uptake of larger molecules such as water-soluble vitamins, peptides, and proteins, whose molecular weights range from several hundreds up to many millions? Many of these molecules are highly water-soluble and as such are too big and hydrophilic to pass through small intramembranous pores. The molecular weight of some of these molecules is listed in Table 11.1.

11.2.2 Receptor-Mediated Endocytosis

There is one common process in the body that has the capacity to specifically take up small and large molecules from the gut. This process, called *receptor-mediated endocytosis* (RME), involves the binding of ligands to specific cell surface receptors. Following binding of the ligand to the receptor, a change occurs in the membrane structure, leading to the formation of a pit. This pit in turn becomes a vesicle, which internalizes the ligand and receptor. Depending upon the cell, the ligand, and the receptor, the internalized ligand can undergo intracellular sorting and, in polarized cells, such as enterocytes, the ligand can be transported from one side of the cell to the other, a process called *receptor-mediated transcytosis* (RMT). The advantage of this process for drug delivery is that very large peptides, proteins, viruses, and even nanoparticles can be taken up by the intestinal epithelial cells and transported across the single cell layer from the lumen of the intestine into the underlying interstitial space. Depending upon the ligand, it can then enter either the circulation or the draining lymphatics.

Three major factors are required for transcytosis across the enterocyte. First, there must be a receptor for the ligand that is to be transported, which is expressed on the apical/luminal side of the enterocyte. Second, binding of the ligand to the receptor must initiate endocytosis or internalization of the ligand, and, third, the ligand must be transported across the cell and released on the other side (the basal side) of the cell into the underlying interstitial space. Once the ligand has been released on the basal side of the cell, it can enter either the circulation via the hepatic portal vein or the draining lymphatics. If the ligand travels via the hepatic portal vein, its appearance in the serum will be quite rapid, but it will be subjected to removal by the liver, which is the first organ that it encounters, a process termed *hepatic first-pass metabolism*. On the other hand, if the ligand enters the draining lymphatic, it will first reach the mesenteric lymph node before traveling through the lymphatics to reach the superior vena cava. The majority of higher molecular weight ligands appear to travel via the lymphatics, the possible exception being IgG, which appears rapidly in serum following oral administration. The rapid appearance of IgG in serum is possibly due to transport via the neonatal Fc receptor FcRn, which has been shown to be expressed on vascular endothelium [18, 19] and is known to transport IgG from the interstitial space into the circulation.

11.2.2.1 RMT in the Embryo. As the embryo develops, be it in an egg or *in utero*, it must obtain its supply of nutrients and particularly vitamins from either the surrounding egg or via transplacental transfer. Particularly important in the development of vertebrate animals are vitamin B_{12} and folate (vitamin B_9), as deficiencies in these vitamins lead to problems in neural chord development [20]. There is a considerable amount of evidence to show that early in embryonic development the transport of vitamins and proteins into the developing embryo is dependent upon specific transporters. The earliest examples of these have come from the identification of various vitamin-binding proteins in the chicken egg yolk. These proteins are

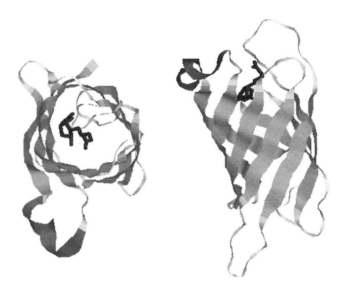

Figure 11.4. Chicken biotin-binding protein A (light gray ribbons) holding biotin (dark gray). Raswin representation of 2CIS.PDB.

generally found in association with their corresponding vitamin and have been postulated to be involved in the uptake of these vitamins into the developing embryo. Separate transporters have been identified that are required for the uptake of several B-group vitamins in the developing embryo, including biotin-binding proteins I and II (Fig. 11.4) [21–24], vitamin B_{12}-binding proteins, intrinsic factor (IF), and transcobalamin (TC) in human embryonic fluid [25]; folate-binding proteins [26–28], riboflavin-binding proteins [29–32], and also thiamine-binding proteins [31, 33–35].

11.2.2.2 RMT in the Neonate. During the growth of the fetus in the womb, one of the many changes that occur is the development of RMT in the intestine, which matures near the time of birth [35]. Evidence suggests that the offspring of many suckling mammals obtain maternal serum proteins, which are actively secreted into the colostrum and milk. Uptake of these proteins occurs via RMT of these proteins from ingested colostrum in the neonatal intestine. These colostrally derived proteins are found to accumulate in the serum of the neonate following suckling [25]. The implication of this is that the newborn mammal must have an active transcytotic mechanism in its intestine and also that the receptors involved in uptake of these macromolecules are also expressed on the luminal side of the small intestine of the neonate.

The major proteins identified in colostrum include immunoglobulins (Igs), particularly IgG, IgA, and IgM, the cytokines IL1, IL2, and IL6, iron-binding proteins such as lactoferrin and transferrin (Tf) [36], the oligonucleotidepeptide transfer factors [35], growth and maturation factors such as fibroblast growth factor, insulin-like growth factor (IGF)-I, IGF-II, erythropoietin (EPO), and somatostatin [37–39], trans-forming growth factors α and β (TGFα and TGFβ), insulin, platelet-derived growth factor (PDGF), and epithelial growth factor (EGF) [38, 39]. It has been shown that there are receptors for many of these factors distributed along the intestinal epithelium. The possibility exists that the neonate requires these factors for successful intestinal growth and development [38, 40]. Receptors for these molecules appear to be fairly ubiquitous among mammals, as orally administered bovine colostrum is effective in altering immune function in species as diverse as cattle, horses, pigs [41], sheep, cats, mice, rats, hamsters, and ferrets. In the human, apically expressed receptors involved in uptake of EGF, insulin, IGF-I, hepatocyte growth factor, glucagon-like polypeptide receptor, leptin [42], and IgG Fc have all been identified [37, 38]. Exper-iments in rats and mice have shown that many of the receptors present are active in RMT. Thus, suckling and weanling rats and mice have been found to transport cor-ticosterone, prostaglandins, insulin, prolactin, EGF, IGF, thyroid-releasing hormone (TRH), thyroid-stimulating hormone (TSH), and somatostatin from the intestine into the circulation [35].

11.2.2.3 ***RMT in the Adult.*** For many years, it was thought that the majority of intestinal receptors expressed in the neonate were those that were required during development. These were subsequently lost during maturation and as such were absent in the adult. This has now been found not to be the case, and many receptors involved in protein uptake in the gut of the neonate still show functional uptake in the adult. Of these, the nutrient transporters must obviously be retained, or a state of malnutrition would result.

In the rat, leptin is secreted by the Chief cells in the stomach; Cammisotto and coworkers [42] have found that in the adult rat leptin crosses the intestinal mucosa by transcytosis through enterocytes to reach blood circulation. It has also been found that two pancreatic enzymes, amylase and lipase, that are released into the intestine are "rescued" from the intestinal milieu by the process of RMT [43, 44].

11.3 NUTRIENT TRANSPORT IN THE INTESTINE

11.3.1 Iron

The recommended daily allowance for iron is around $18\,mg\,day^{-1}$ in adults. Iron is essential for oxygen transport around the body through porphryin complexation in hemoglobin and myoglobin and as iron enzymes in catalase, cytochromes, and peroxidases. Iron in the body exists in two major forms, Fe^{3+} and its reduced form Fe^{2+}. In the cytochrome system, iron is continually oxidized and reduced from Fe^{2+} to Fe^{3+} and back again. Until recently, it was postulated that Tf was the only major protein involved in the uptake and transport of iron (Fe^{3+}) from the intestine into the circulation and around the body [45–47]. However, it has now been found that there is also a receptor for the iron-binding protein in milk lactoferrin (see below). Iron transport into the fetus of placental mammals occurs via transplacental transfer following binding of Tf-bound Fe^{3+} to a Tf receptor on the placenta. In the suckling animal, Fe^{3+} bound by lactoferrin is bound to a lactoferrin receptor on the enterocyte, with resultant transcytosis of the iron [48–59]. Post weaning, Tf, produced in the liver is secreted into bile, which in turn is secreted into the small intestine. Intestinal Tf binds Fe^{3+} released from food, and the resulting $(Fe^{3+})_2$–Tf complex is bound either to TfR on the surface of the duodenal enterocyte, or, as suggested by Widera and coworkers [60], to cubulin, which has been shown to have receptor-binding activity for $(Fe^{3+})_2$–Tf complex. The complex is then internalized and transported across the enterocyte cell into the lymphatic system, appearing several hours later in the serum. More recently, it has been found that there is a separate transporter for the reduced form of iron, Fe^{2+}. This transporter, the divalent cation/metal ion transporter (DCT1), has been shown to transport the reduced form of iron Fe^{2+} from the intestine [61–63]. It has now been found that this transporter is also responsible for the cellular uptake of not only Fe^{2+} but also Zn^{2+}, Mn^{2+}, Cu^{2+}, Co^{2+}, Ni^{2+}, Pb^{2+}, and Cd^{2+} [61].

11.3.2   Vitamin B$_{12}$

Dietary vitamin B_{12} (VB$_{12}$) occurs as one of two naturally occurring cofactors in the body, namely 5′-deoxy-adenosylcobalamin (MW 1578) and methylcobalamin (MW 1344). These forms are quite different to the pro-vitamin form cyanocobalamin (MW 1355), which is normally found in dietary supplements. All three forms of the vitamin are variously water-soluble (25–100 mg ml^{-1}, depending upon the analog) and can only cross the intestinal cell membrane by receptor-mediated transcytosis. VB$_{12}$ is released from food by the action of acid in the stomach. The released vitamin B_{12} is then bound to haptocorrin in the stomach, which is subsequently degraded in the duodenum by intestinal proteases, thereby releasing the bound VB$_{12}$. The VB$_{12}$ is then transferred to IF. The resultant complex of VB$_{12}$ to IF is then bound by an IF receptor cubulin [64–66], which is located on the luminal surface of the enterocytes of the duodenum, jejunum, and ileum, with the largest concentration of receptors being found in the ileum [67–69] (Figs 11.5 and 11.6).

The daily requirement for vitamin B_{12} is quite low, only 1–2 μg VB$_{12}$ per feed in humans, approximately 30 ng in the mouse, and 100 ng in the rat (personal observations). This is reflected by the small number of receptors present on the enterocyte.

The binding of the VB$_{12}$–IF complex to cubulin triggers the endocytosis of the VB$_{12}$–IF–cubulin via a clathrin-coated pit [70, 74, 75]. Once inside the enterocyte, the IF is degraded and the vitamin B_{12} is then bound to the locally produced VB$_{12}$-binding protein TC II [70, 76, 77]. The resultant VB$_{12}$–TC II complex is secreted from the basal surface of the intestinal epithelial cell (see Fig. 11.5). There is no known basal to apical transport of TC II in the vascular epithelium, so the VB$_{12}$–TC II complex enters the draining lacteal lymph vessel in the villous and travels from there into the mesenteric lymph node [78]. Several hours after oral administration, vitamin B_{12} can be detected in the circulation, with levels peaking at 4–8 h following ingestion.

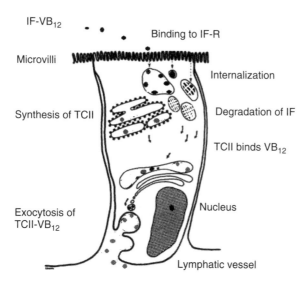

Figure 11.5. Receptor-mediated transcytosis of vitamin B_{12} across the intestinal epithelial cell. Ingested vitamin B_{12} (VB_{12}) binds to IF in the lumen of the small intestine. The $IF-VB_{12}$ complex in turn is bound by an IF receptor (IF-R; cubulin) located on the luminal/apical enterocyte membrane. Binding to the receptor initiates endocytosis (internalization) of the whole cubulin/$IF-VB_{12}$ complex into a clathrin-coated endocytotic vesicle [70]. The IF is cleaved by cathepsin L within the cell, and the released VB_{12} is then bound by locally produced TC II (TC-II). Sometime later, the TC $II-VB_{12}$ complex is released from the basal surface of the enterocyte.

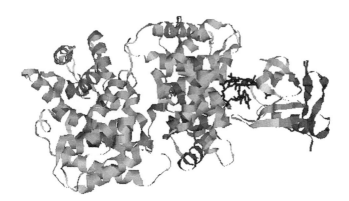

Figure 11.6. The structure of the vitamin B_{12}–IF complex. Cartoon showing the structure of human IF (represented by ribbons) with cyanocobalamin (dark gray stick shapes) shown (Structure modified from PDB file SPMV http://www.pdb.org/pdb/explore/explore.do?structureId=2PMV). Original structure from Mathews and coworkers (2007) following recombinant expression [71–73].

11.4   USE OF NUTRIENT TRANSPORTERS FOR DRUG DELIVERY

In the preceding sections, we have discussed the binding and uptake of a number of nutrient molecules via large proteins secreted into the small intestine. During this uptake and transport, these transporters are taken up into large vesicles that would allow the concomitant uptake of other molecules linked to the transporters. In the following sections, we will discuss the potential use of two of these nutrient transporters to cotransport various peptides, proteins, and even nanoparticles from the intestine into the circulation.

11.4.1   CoTransport Using Transferrin

The intestinal transport mechanism for iron involving the uptake of Fe^{3+} by Tf has been utilized by several workers as a means to achieve oral delivery of various proteins. Initial experiments concentrated on the covalent linkage of granulocyte colony-stimulating factor (GCSF) to Tf [36, 79], and conjugates have also been formed between insulin and Tf [80, 81]. Subsequent oral testing of the insulin–Tf conjugates in rats demonstrated that they were active in inducing blood glucose reduction in diabetic rats [81].

One of the problems encountered during the chemical linkage of GCSF or insulin to Tf is the need to avoid aggregation during conjugation and the often nonreproducible nature of such conjugates. For this reason, Shen and others [82–87] have produced genetically constructed fusion proteins between GCSF and Tf [82–86], and growth hormone (GH) and Tf [85, 87]. The GH–Tf fusion, when given orally, caused an increase in weight gain, although the effect correlated with an oral bioavailability of less than 6%. This could have been due to proteolysis of the GH, which is known to be susceptible to tryptic and chymotryptic cleavage [87]. Similarly, an oral bioavailability of around 5% was found for GCSF–Tf fusions [83].

Despite the successful formation of chemical conjugates between proteins and Tf, and the successful production of these conjugates via genetic techniques, there exists a very real potential for such conjugates/fusions to be immunogenic following repeated applications in humans. Additionally, such fusion technology is not always possible because of changes in the chemical structure of the fused proteins and also because such conjugates may show increased susceptibility to digestion by intestinal proteases. Furthermore, the technology is not generally applicable to all peptides and proteins, and as such a simpler technology is required for successful oral delivery of peptides and proteins using nutrient transporters.

11.5   CASE STUDY: THE USE OF THE VITAMIN B_{12} UPTAKE SYSTEM FOR DRUG DELIVERY

During the process of vitamin B_{12} absorption, vitamin B_{12} is first bound to IF, which is much larger than vitamin B_{12}, and the complex is subsequently taken into the enterocyte by receptor-mediated endocytosis. The endosome, which is formed around the VB$_{12}$–IF complex, can be rather large and is able to accommodate particles even as large as viruses up to 200 nm. For this reason, the possibility exists that relatively large molecules, such as peptides, proteins, or even nanoparticles, could be linked to the VB$_{12}$, which would then act as a transporter.

11.5.1   Conjugation to Vitamin B$_{12}$

In order to use vitamin B$_{12}$ as a transporter for the oral uptake of a drug, the drug to be delivered must first be covalently linked to the vitamin B$_{12}$. The following section will deal with where and how this is done.

11.5.1.1   Location of VB$_{12}$ in the Binding Site of IF.   During conjugation to vitamin B$_{12}$, it is important that the affinity for both IF and TC II is maintained.

It can be seen from the structure of IF with VB$_{12}$ that the axial group (the CN) (Fig. 11.7) sits on "top" of vitamin B$_{12}$ and is accessible to the "environment". Conjugation to generate the axial ligand leads to conjugates that have been found to be light sensitive and are easily hydrolyzed [88–90]. Acid hydrolysis of vitamin B$_{12}$ generates a mixture of carboxyl derivatives (b-, d-, and e-isomers). It can be seen from Fig. 11.7 that the side groups on the corin ring are "held" by IF during binding, thus modification of these groups was found to greatly reduce the affinity of IF for VB$_{12}$ in the complex [91–93]. One of the acid isomers, the e-isomer, did produce some conjugates that maintained relatively strong affinity for IF; however, the yield of this preferred derivative (the e-isomer) was only 5%. For this reason, an alternative site for modification has been exploited.

Russell-Jones and coworkers [93–99] have shown that it is possible to modify the 5′OH group on the "bottom" of the structure and the resultant products were formed in relatively high yield (over 70%) and with only a small reduction in the affinity for IF when compared to unconjugated CN-Cbl. Additionally, the affinity for non-IF VB$_{12}$-binding proteins was substantially maintained (111%) (Fig. 11.8) [93, 94].

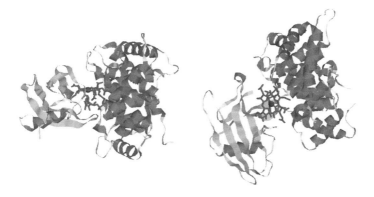

Figure 11.7. Orientation of B$_{12}$ in the IF binding site, seen from the side (left) and top view (right). The cartoon clearly shows the accessibility of the cobalt (dark gray, top view) and the ribose protein of the molecule.

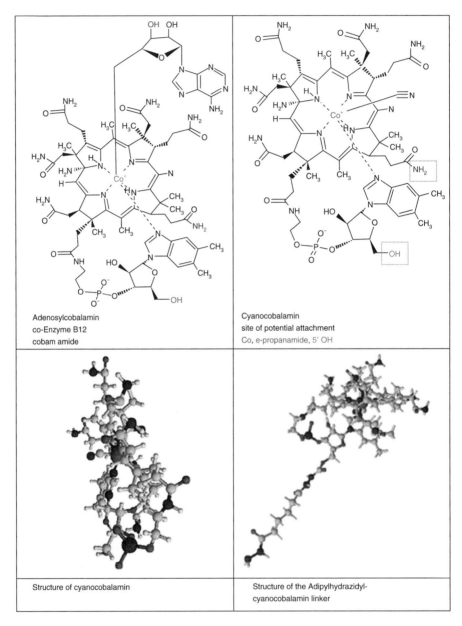

Adenosylcobalamin
co-Enzyme B12
cobam amide

Cyanocobalamin
site of potential attachment
Co, e-propanamide, 5′ OH

Structure of cyanocobalamin

Structure of the Adipylhydrazidyl-
cyanocobalamin linker

Figure 11.8. Structure of adenosyl cobalamin, cyanocobalamin, and an adipylhydrazidy-cyanocobalamin derivative. The relative binding affinity of the adipylhydrazidycyanocobal-amin for IF was 30% of native and for non-IF (haptocorrin) it was 111%.

Crystallization of the VB$_{12}$–IF complex by Matthews and coworkers [71] has demonstrated that there is an open "channel" in IF that allows access to the top and bottom of the VB$_{12}$ molecule. Russell-Jones and coworkers produced a variety of spacer molecules linked to both the e-VB$_{12}$ derivative and at the 5′OH position and these have been used to make conjugates to an assortment of peptides and proteins [91–99].

While linkage to small peptides generally produces single species in high yield, linkage of vitamin B$_{12}$ to proteins generally results in a heterogeneous mixture of products. Several of these conjugates are worthy of further discussion.

1. VB$_{12}$–D-Arg$_8$-vasopressin
   This was one of the earliest attempts at conjugation between VB$_{12}$ and a small peptide. The free amino terminal amine was chosen for conjugation. The conjugate was obtained in good yield; however, subsequent testing of antidiuretic activity in the standing dog model showed that the biological activity had been completely destroyed during conjugation. This is obviously one potential problem of conjugation to small molecules.

2. VB$_{12}$–SS–GCSF
   GCSF contains a single free thiol group on a free cysteine that is not involved in disulfide bond formation within the molecule. A covalently linked 1:1 conjugate between VB$_{12}$ and GCSF was made using thiol insertion chemistry, in which a long dithiopyridyl spacer ($NH(CH_2)_2NHCO(CH_2)_6CONH$-$(CH_2)_{12}NHCO(CH_2)_2SSPy$) was first linked to e-carboxy-VB$_{12}$ (Fig. 11.9). The free thiol on Cys$_{17}$ in GCSF was found to displace the pyridyl group from the extended linker, generating a 1:1 conjugate via a thiol cleavable bond. This linker was obtained in nearly 100% yield and maintained good affinity for IF (23%) and good bioactivity (66% relative to the parent molecule). A shorter spacer was found to have slightly lower yields (85%) and lower IF affinity (2.3%), but still retained good bioactivity (61%) [93].

3. VB$_{12}$–EPO
   The hydrophilic nature of many proteins, as well as the common occurrence of the alpha helix as part of their structure, often means that hydrophilic amino acids such as lysine, glutamic acid, and aspartic acid are located on the outer more water-exposed part of the molecule. This can be readily seen in the cartoon of the EPO structure (Fig. 11.10), where the aspartic acid (magenta), glutamic acid (yellow), and lysine (red) groups are shown. Experiments on amino acid modification of EPO established that functional activity was rapidly lost upon modification of the ϵ-amino groups on lysine. Therefore, in order to prepare conjugates between EPO and vitamin B$_{12}$, various hydrazidyl vitamin B$_{12}$ derivatives were made. These hydrazidyl–vitamin B$_{12}$ spacers were mixed with EPO and activated using water soluble 1-ethyl-3-(3-dimethylaminopropyl)carbodiimide (EDAC) and used to prepare VB$_{12}$–EPO conjugates at an acidic pH. This method has the dual advantage of high conjugate yield and avoidance of the formation of multimers of EPO which were often formed when amino derivatives of VB$_{12}$ were used [94–98].

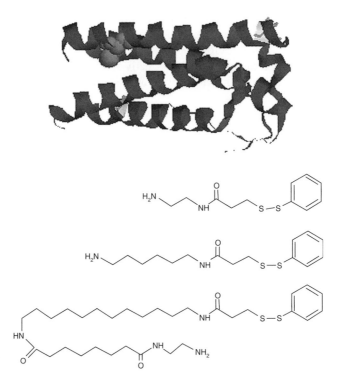

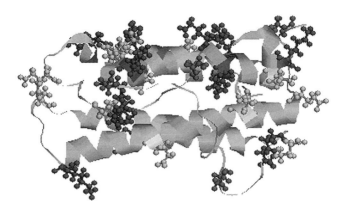

Figure 11.9. Structure of GCSF showing the Cys_{17} (medium gray) (top) and three of the spacers used to try to conjugate to the free thiol of the cysteine (bottom).

Figure 11.10. Cartoon of the structure of EPO showing lysine (dark gray), glutamic acid (light gray), and aspartic acid (medium gray).

11.5.2   Uptake Capacity of the VB$_{12}$ Uptake System

While some success was obtained with several high-potency peptides and proteins, such as leutenizing hormone releasing hormone (LHRH), EPO and GCSF, which are biologically effective in the picomolar range, many other biologics are much less effective and must be given at much higher doses [91–96]. Thus, insulin is normally administered in doses of 10–100 IU (26 IU mg^{-1}, 1 IU/38.8 µg), which is equivalent to 388–3880 µg of insulin. In molar terms, this is (388–3880 µg)/5808, or 66.8–688 nmoles, of insulin. The amount of vitamin B$_{12}$ taken up per feed is roughly 1 nmole in humans, which means that the uptake capacity would be approximately 1 nmole of conjugate. This is clearly a long way below the 66.8–688 nmoles per feed required for insulin. Similarly, the dose of monoclonal antibodies required per administration is around 25–50 mg per dose. IgG antibodies have a molecular weight of approximately 150,000, so the dose required is approximately 166–333 nmole per dose, which once again is considerably more than the uptake capacity for vitamin B$_{12}$.

11.5.2.1   Amplification of the Uptake Capacity of the VB$_{12}$ Transport System.   Apart from the limited uptake capacity of the vitamin B$_{12}$ oral delivery system, there are several other potential problems with the oral administration of 1:1 conjugates between vitamin B$_{12}$ and a peptide or protein.

1. There can be a loss of activity of the conjugated peptide or protein as a result of the conjugation (see discussion above).
2. Unless the conjugate between vitamin B$_{12}$ and the peptides or protein is fully biodegradable, the conjugate does produce a new chemical entity, the safety and efficacy of which must be established.
3. The conjugated peptide or protein is subject to the highly proteolytic environment within the intestine.

As a result of the problems outlined above, considerable work has been performed to try to encapsulate the peptide or protein within a nanoparticulate structure, then coat the nanoparticles with vitamin B$_{12}$, and determine if they are active orally.

Initially, these experiments were simply designed to determine whether the vitamin B$_{12}$ transport system is capable of transporting nanoparticles across intestinal epithelial cells. Preliminary experiments were performed with cells grown in tissue culture on semipermeable membranes. Two cell lines are available that have shown good IF-mediated uptake and transcytosis of VB$_{12}$. One of these, the opossum kidney (OK) cell line, shows polarized transport of vitamin B$_{12}$ when grown on semipermeable membranes; however, the cell line does not express microvilli on its surface [99–101]. For some reason, these cells also make IF, haptocorrin, and TC II [100], which presumably explains some of the VB$_{12}$–nanoparticle transport that was seen with these cells in the absence of IF [101]. The advantage of this cell line for transport studies is, however, that it shows similar levels of transport regardless of cell passage number. A second commonly used but more highly variable cell line for studying VB$_{12}$ transcytosis is the human colon cancer cell line Caco-2 [100, 102–106]. This cell line has a morphology similar to that of intestinal epithelial cells

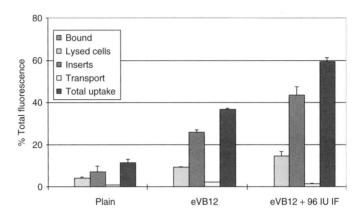

Figure 11.11. Enhanced binding, uptake, and transport of 50 nm fluorescent latex nanoparticles following surface coating with e-VB$_{12}$ and addition of IF. Data is represented as the mean and standard deviation of triplicate well cultures.

and possesses surface microvilli. Initial studies on particle uptake utilized commercial fluorescently tagged latex nanoparticles of defined sizes (Fluoresbrite™ Polysciences). In both Caco-2 cell cultures and OK cell models, it was found that particles as large as 500 nm could be taken up into the cells via IF-mediated RMT [101] (Fig. 11.11). Uptake increased as the surface density of VB$_{12}$ was increased, with greatest uptake seen with 200 and 400 nm particles [101]. Similar IF-mediated uptake has also been observed for polymeric micelles [107], Gantrez nanoparticles [97], and poly(acrylic acid)–cysteine nanoparticles [108].

The ability for VB$_{12}$ to promote uptake of nanoparticles has been confirmed in intestinal loops surgically instilled in anesthetized mice, rats, dogs, and pigs. Uptake is maximal at 100–200 nm particle size, with particles larger than 400 nm appearing to be physically excluded from reaching the enterocytes because of the mucous layer covering the tips of the villi (Fig. 11.12). Vitamin B$_{12}$-coated particle uptake was found to be quite rapid, with particle clearance from the loops occurring within 1 h of instillation into the loops. In contrast, over 90% of control uncoated particles were recoverable from the loops at 180 min (Fig. 11.13). Particles that were taken up were first found in the draining lacteal vessel that is located in the center of the villous "fingers". Particles were later found to accumulate in the mesenteric lymph nodes (Fig. 11.14).

The experiments described above utilized VB$_{12}$-coated latex nanoparticles containing a fluorophore. While they are useful to demonstrate particle uptake, they cannot be modified to deliver peptides or proteins. Several nanoparticle systems are available that allow peptide or protein incorporation into the nanoparticles while the nanoparticles are being formulated. Initially, isobutylcyanoacrylate nanoparticles were prepared containing ^{125}I-insulin [109, 110]. These were surface-coated with octadecyl–eVB$_{12}$ (C18–VB$_{12}$) and instilled into mouse intestine. It was found that the insulin was not really buried within the nanoparticle structure and that the majority of insulin was

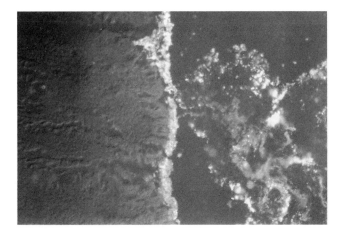

Figure 11.12. Exclusion by the gastrointestinal mucous layer of 500 nm latex particles. Particles can be seen aggregated in the lumen of the intestine and crowded among the mucous lining, but no particles were seen to penetrate into the entocytes, or between the villi. Data is presented for 120 min after administration into gastrointestinal loops instilled in anesthetized mice.

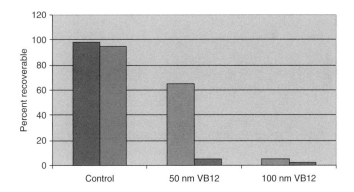

Figure 11.13. Recovery of 50 and 100 nm fluorescent Polysciences latex nanoparticles from intestinal loops instilled in anesthetized dogs. Particles were injected into separate loops, and at 60 min (left bar) and 180 min (right bar) the dogs were euthanized and the contents of the loops recovered following saline washout. Particles were surface-modified with adipylhydrazidyl–e–VB$_{12}$ following activation with EDAC/NHS and were subsequently blocked with ethanolamine. Because of the cost, animal ethics requirements, and technical feasibility of these experiments, they were performed as single dog experiments, which were repeated three times. Data is presented for one representative experiment.

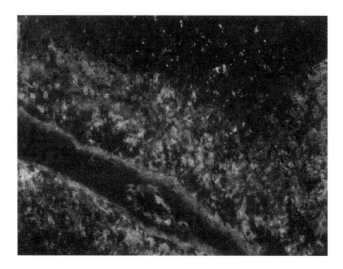

Figure 11.14. Presence of Vitamin B_{12}-coated 100 nm Polysciences nanoparticles (light gray) in the mesenteric lymph node of pigs (T240 min).

located on or near the surface and so was quickly degraded by intestinal proteases. A surface cross-linking agent was devised that contained an esterase-cleavable cross-linker, 2-aminoethyl-2-amino-2-benzyl-ethanoate (AEABE), and particles were once again fed to conscious mice (Fig. 11.15) [78, 111]. The stability of these particles was established by incubating the particles at 37 °C in the small intestinal fluid obtained from mice. Increasing the level of the cross-linking agent was found to greatly improve the stability of the insulin against degradation (Fig. 11.16) [78, 111]. Particles coated with various $C18-VB_{12}$ derivatives were prepared, and the bioavailability was compared to that of noncoated particles. Uptake of nontargeted particles was found to be rather low (2% of total amount fed). A significant increase in bioavailability was seen for each of the VB_{12} isomer conjugates, with bioavailability increasing from

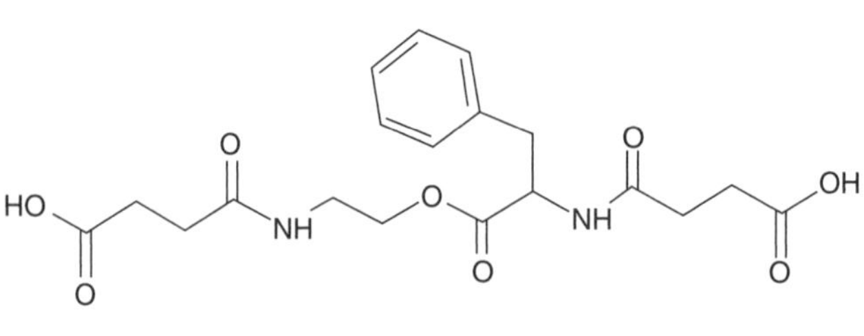

Figure 11.15. Esterase-cleavable cross-linker. One of several cross-linkers produced containing a hindered ester bond that was slowly cleaved in serum, but not in the intestine. Cross-linking was achieved following activation of the terminal COOH groups with EDAC/NHS. Such cross-linkers can be used on insulin-loaded IBCA nanoparticles, with the extent of cross-linking controlling the rate of release of insulin.

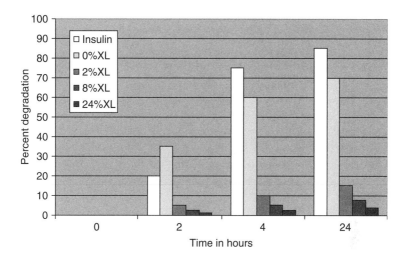

Figure 11.16. Resistance of ^{125}I-labeled insulin to enzymatic degradation following incorporation into IBCA nanoparticles and surface cross-linking with esterase-cleavable cross-linkers. ^{125}I-insulin containing IBCA nanoparticles were surface cross-linked with increasing amounts of an esterase-cleavable dipeptide. Percentage cross-linking refers to the weight percent of cross-linker that was activated. The nanoparticles were then washed, were placed in a dialysis bag (10,000 molecular weight cut-off), and were incubated with mouse small intestinal washout at 37 °C. At various times, samples of the dialysate were removed and the percentage of released insulin was determined.

2% of total with uncoated particles to 15% of total administered with C18–5'OH –VB_{12}-coated nanoparticles ($P < 0.05\%$) (Fig. 11.17).

The positive results from the VB_{12}-coated latex particles instilled into gut loops, combined with the evidence of significant levels of uptake of VB_{12}-coated isobutyl-cyanoacrylate (IBCA) nanoparticles, was very encouraging because it established the feasibility of using the VB_{12} transport system to transport protein-loaded nanoparticles from the intestine into the circulation. Despite this, work with IBCA nanoparticles was discontinued because of the potential modification of the entrapped protein during the surface cross-linking of the particles and so an alternative nanoparticle system was required.

Several attempts have been made to produce protein-loaded nanoparticles that are capable of trapping proteins within the particle and which can be pretargeted with vitamin B_{12}. Thus, Chalasani and coworkers [112–115] produced drug-loadable "cross-linked dextran nanosponges," which could be pretargeted with vitamin B_{12} and used to soak up solutions of proteins such as insulin or IgG. Cross-linking of the dextran was achieved using epichlorohydrin, while the size was controlled by homogenization of an oil/surfactant/water mix. Once cross-linked, the nanosponges were surface-activated with succinic anhydride, which was subsequently substituted with aminohexyl–VB_{12} using a suitable carbodiimide and N-hydroxysuccinimide. Once the excess reagents were removed by positive-pressure dialysis, the dried particles were

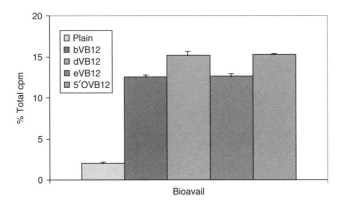

Figure 11.17. Comparison of the bioavailability of ^{125}I-insulin following oral administration of surface cross-linked VB$_{12}$-modified IBCA nanoparticles. Various C18-derivatives of vitamin B$_{12}$ were used to coat the nanoparticles. These were prepared from reacting the "b", "d", and "e" carboxylic acid isomers with octadecylamine using EDAC, as well as through the carbonyldiimidazole (CDI) activation of the 5'-OH group followed by conjugation to octadecylamine. Total counts recovered in the liver, heart, lung, spleen, blood, skin, muscles, kidney, and thyroid were summed and presented as the percentage of the total counts fed to the conscious mice. Counts still present in the stomach, small intestine, and colon have been omitted from bioavailability measurements.

swollen in the presence of the protein solution. Vitamin B$_{12}$-targeted insulin-loaded nanosponges when fed to diabetic rats caused a significant reduction in serum glucose levels, thus demonstrating the feasibility of this approach [78, 112–115]. Reduced serum glucose levels were observed for several hours, which returned to pretreatment levels after 12–16 h (Fig. 11.18). The nanosponges were well tolerated, and similar

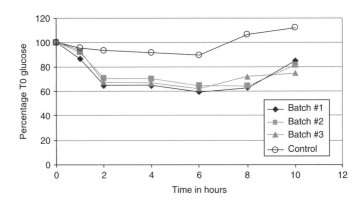

Figure 11.18. Comparison of the glucose-lowering activity in diabetic rats of three batches of vitamin B$_{12}$-targeted insulin-loaded dextran nanosponges. Blood glucose levels were determined at T0, and these were used as a reference level for subsequent bloods. Data represents the blood glucose level over time following oral feeding.

glucose reductions were seen on five successive days of feeding. Interestingly, the rats also reduced their water intake, as would be expected from the lowered glucose levels, and also reduced their food intake. Although good progress was made with these particles in again demonstrating the proof of concept, it was found that the ester linkage of the succinate group slowly hydrolyzed upon storage, and so the targeting agent was gradually lost.

Salman and associates [97] prepared vitamin B$_{12}$-coated Gantrez nanoparticles containing ovalbumen (OVA), which were found to elicit higher anti-OVA titres than either subcutaneously injected antigen or nontargeted OVA-containing Gantrez nanoparticles [97]

As mentioned above, although it was possible to prepare targeted nanoparticles containing protein pharmaceuticals and demonstrate that they were taken up from the intestine in relatively good amounts, these particles were hard to produce at scale, and so an alternative scaleable nanoparticle system was developed. A novel nanolattice particle system was formulated by chelating the carboxyl group on carboxymethyl dextran (CMD) with zinc ions (Zn^{2+}) [116] to form "nanolattices." In essence, CMD was dissolved in water and dispersed in an oil/surfactant mix to form a water-in-oil microemulsion (W/O ME). Proteins to be incorporated within the lattices were also dispersed in a W/O emulsion and were allowed to associate with the CMD. Zinc chloride at various concentrations was added to cross-link the CMD and entrap the protein within the structure. The nanolattices were readily isolated by precipitation from ethanol. Targeting agents such as lysyl–vitamin B$_{12}$ or lysyl–biotin were added to the surface of the particles either immediately after cross-linking or following isolation from ethanol (Fig. 11.19). The size of the nanolattices was altered by changing

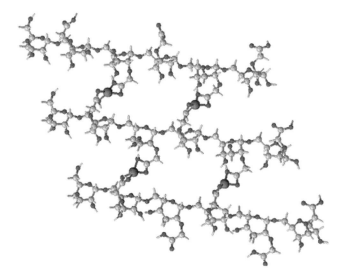

Figure 11.19. Structure of zinc-chelated carboxymethyl dextran. Zinc (dark gray), carbon (light gray), oxygen (medium gray).

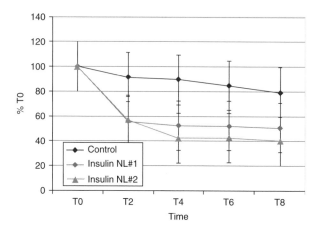

Figure 11.20. Reduction in serum glucose levels following oral administration of insulin-loaded, vitamin B_{12}-targeted dextran nanolattices to diabetic rats. The data is represented as the mean glucose level ($n = 4$), expressed as a percentage of values at T0 over the period of 2, 4, 6, and 8 h. Data is presented for two separate nanolattice preparations.

the amount of water in the W/O ME. Nanolattices were readily isolated following freeze-drying, and vitamin B_{12}-targeted nanolattices containing insulin or IgG have been found to be stable for periods of over 9 months at room temperature.

Carboxymethyl–dextran nanolattices containing human insulin were formulated as described previously using lysyl–5′OH –VB_{12} as the targeting agent. These particles were fed to diabetic rats and their serum glucose levels monitored over time. Glucose levels were reduced by around 40% of the control levels and were maintained at this level for more than 8 h (Fig. 11.20).

Several features of the above experiment are notable. First, the delay in appearance of a glucose-lowering effect is typical of the vitamin B_{12} uptake system. Second, the peak in uptake at around 4 h and the extended time of glucose lowering are also features of the vitamin B_{12} uptake system and were seen in all studies carried out using either the vitamin B_{12} transport system as a targeting agent [78, 91–93, 95, 97, 100, 112–115] or Tf [80–82].

Because of the many developments in the use of the vitamin B_{12} uptake system as a transport mechanism for orally administered peptides, proteins, nanoparticles, and protein-loaded nanolattices, most of hurdles that have prevented successful oral delivery of peptides and proteins have been overcome. Successful oral delivery via the transport system has now been achieved by many workers [78, 91–93, 95, 97, 100, 112–115], and so there is every reason to believe that the delivery system will find its way into clinical trials in the near future. The author wishes all who take the system forward good luck in the future, and hopes that needle-free oral delivery will soon become a reality, thereby giving vast relief to those patients, such as those with diabetes, who must inject themselves with medications on a daily basis.

11.6   KEY POINTS

- There are many nutrient transporters that have been identified in the gastrointestinal tract of mammals.
- Transport of several of these nutrients occurs via receptor-mediated transcytosis.
- The processes involved in the transport of these nutrients allow the cotransport of peptides, proteins, and nanoparticles with the nutrients.
- Successful cotransport of peptides, proteins, and nanoparticles via the vitamin B_{12} transport system has been achieved.
- The possibility exists that the transport processes for nutrients other than vitamin B_{12} can also be hijacked for drug delivery.

11.7   WORKED EXAMPLE

As mentioned in the text, the vitamin B_{12} uptake capacity in the mouse is approximately 30 ng (Um), in the rat 100 ng (Ur), and in humans approximately 1.36 µg (Uh). The molecular weight of VB_{12} is approximately 1360. Assuming that one is able to conjugate one VB_{12} molecule to insulin (MW ~6000) or IgG (MW 150,000), calculate the amount of insulin and IgG that can be taken up with a single feed in each animal species.

$$Uh = 1.36 \ \mu g$$

$$= 1360 \ ng/1360(MW) = 1 \ nmole$$

Therefore, 1 nmole insulin or 1 nmole IgG can be taken up.

$$1 \ nmole \ insulin = 6000 \ MW \times 1 \ ng$$

$$= 6000 \ ng = 6 \ \mu g$$

$$1 \ nMole \ IgG = 150,000 \ MW \times 1 \ nmole$$

$$= 150,000 \ ng = 150 \ \mu g$$

$$Um = 30 \ ng$$

$$= 30,000 \ pg/1360(MW) = 22 \ pmole$$

Therefore, 22 pmole insulin or 22 pmole IgG can be taken up.

$$22 \ pmole \ insulin = 6000 \ MW \times 22 \ pmole$$

$$= 132,000 \ pg = 132 \ \mu g$$

$$22 \text{ pmole IgG} = 150,000 \ MW \times 22 \text{ pmole}$$
$$= 3,300,000 \text{ pg} = 3.3 \ \mu g$$
$$Ur = 100 \ \text{ng}$$
$$= 100,000 \ \text{pg}/1360(MW) = 73 \text{ pMole}$$

Therefore 73 pmole insulin or 73 pmole IgG can be taken up.

$$73 \text{ pmole insulin} = 6000 \ MW \times 73 \text{ pmole}$$
$$= 438,000 \text{ pg} = 438 \text{ ng}$$
$$73 \text{ pmole IgG} = 150,000 \ MW \times 73 \text{ pmole}$$
$$= 10,950,000 \text{ pg} = 10.95 \ \mu g$$

Note: The dose of various IgG preparations given by injection to humans is around 25 mg. Thus, the uptake of only 150 μg via a VB_{12}:IgG 1:1 conjugate is far too low to be of therapeutic benefit to humans.

11.8 HOMEWORK PROBLEMS

1. A researcher has successfully conjugated vitamin B_{12} to a peptide of 3795 MW and now wants to test the efficacy of the peptide by orally feeding to a rat.
   a. What is the maximal dose of conjugated peptide that can be taken up in a single feed?
   b. Calculate the dose in picomoles and convert this value to picograms or nanograms.

2. A research scientist has successfully formed a conjugate between vitamin B_{12} and insulin. Upon testing the conjugate by subcutaneous injection, the scientist determines that he has managed to maintain full bioactivity of the insulin as judged by glucose reduction. The scientist then feeds 100 nmole of the VB_{12}–insulin conjugate (MW = 7388) to diabetic rats and measures the reduction in blood glucose. As a control, he would like to administer the VB_{12}–insulin conjugate with a 100,000-fold excess free vitamin B_{12}.
   a. Calculate the weight conjugate that has been administered.
   b. Calculate the weight of the excess vitamin B_{12} that has to be administered. Given that the maximum solubility of vitamin B_{12} is 25 mg ml^{-1}, is it possible to administer the conjugate plus excess vitamin B_{12} in a total volume of 1 ml.
   c. Compare the amount of conjugate administered to the uptake capacity for vitamin B_{12} in the rat. Is it an excess? If so, how much excess is it?

REFERENCES

1. Henin J, Tajkhorshid E, Schulten K, Chipot C. Diffusion of glycerol through *Escherichia coli* aquaglyceroporin GlpF. Biophys J 2008;94:832–839.

2. Wang Y, Schulten K, Tajkhorshid E. What makes an aquaporin a glycerol channel: a comparative study of AqpZ and GlpF. Structure 2005;13:1107–1118.

3. Wang Y, Cohen J, Boron WF, Schulten K, Tajkhorshid E. Exploring gas permeability of cellular membranes and membrane channels with molecular dynamics. J Struct Biol 2007;157:534–544.

4. Yu J, Yool AJ, Schulten K, Tajkhorshid E. Mechanism of gating and ion conductivity of a possible tetrameric pore in Aquaporin-1. Structure 2006;14:1411–1423.

5. Törnroth-Horsefield S, Wang Y, Hedfalk K, Johanson U, et al. Structural mechanism of plant aquaporin gating. Nature 2006;439:688–694.

6. Kaemmerer E, Plum P, Klaus C, Weiskerchen R, Liedtke C, Adolf M, Schippers A, Wagner N, Reinartz A, Gassler N. Fatty acid binding receptors in intestinal physiology and pathophysiology. World J Gastrointest Pathophysiol 2010;15:147–153.

7. Kim H-R, Park S-W, Cho H-J, Chae K-A, et al. Comparative gene expression profiles of intestinal transporters in mice, rats and humans. Pharm Res 2007;56:224–236.

8. Ganapathy V, Thangaraju M, Gopal E, Martin PM, et al. Sodium-coupled monocarboxylate transporters in normal tissues and in cancer. AAPS J 2008;10:193–199.

9. Luo S, Wang Z, Kansara V, Pal D, Mitra AK. Activity of a sodium-dependent vitamin C transporter (SVCT) in MDCK-MDR1 cells and mechanism of ascorbate uptake. Int J Pharm 2008;358:168–176.

10. Adibi SA. The oligopeptide transporter (PepT1) in human intestine: Biology and function. Gastroenterology 1997;113:332–340.

11. Adibi SA, Soleimanpour MR. Functional characterization of dipeptide transport system in human jejunum. J Clin Invest 1974;53:1368–1374.

12. Adibi SA, Morse EL, Masilamani SS, Amin PM. Evidence for two different modes of tripeptide disappearance in human intestine. Uptake by peptide carrier systems and hydrolysis by peptide hydrolases. J Clin Invest 1975;56:1355–1363.

13. Kramer W. Transporters, Trojan horses and therapeutics: suitability of bile acid and peptide transporters for drug delivery. Biol Chem 2011;392(1–2):77–94 Review.

14. Saborowski M, Kullak-Ublick GA, Eloranta JJ. The human organic cation transporter-1 gene is transactivated by hepatocyte nuclear factor-4alpha. J Pharm Exp Ther 2006;317:778–785.

15. Alrefai WA, Sarwar Z, Tyagi S, Saksena S, Dudeja PK, Gill RK. Cholesterol modulates human intestinal sodium dependent bile acid transporter. Am J Physiol Gastrointest Liver Physiol 2005;288:G978–G985.

16. Reboul E, Borel P. Proteins involved in uptake, intracellular transport and basolateral secretion of fat-soluble vitamins and carotenoids by mammalian enterocytes. Prog Lipid Res 2011;50:388–402.

17. Zimnicka AM, Maryon EB, Kaplan JH. Human copper transporter hCTR1 mediates basolateral uptake of copper into enterocytes: implications for copper homeostasis. J Biol Chem 2007;282(36):26471–26480.

18. Deane R, Sagare A, Hamme K, Parisi M, LaRue B, Guo H, Wu Z, Holtzman DM, Zlokovic BV. IgG-assisted age-dependent clearance of Alzheimer's amylois β –peptide by the blood–brain barrier neonatal Fc receptor. J Neurosci 2005;25(50):11495–11503.

19. Schlachetzki F, Chunn F, Pardridge WM. Expression of the neonatal Fc receptor (FcRn) at the blood brain barrier. J Neurochem 2002;81:203–206.

20. Stover PJ. Vitamin B12 and older adults. Curr Opin Clin Nutr Metab Care 2010;13:24–27.

21. Määttä JAE, Niskanen EA, Huuskonen J, Helttunen KJ, et al. Structure and characterization of a novel chicken biotin-binding. BMC Struct Biol 2007;7(8). DOI: 10.1186/1472-6807-7-8.

22. Hytönen VP et al. Structure and characterization of a novel chicken biotin-binding protein A (BBP-A). BMC Struct Biol 2007;7(8).

23. Murphy CV, Adiga PR. Purification of biotin-binding protein from chicken egg yolk and comparison with avidin. Biochim Biophys Acta 1984;786:222–230.

24. White HB, Dennison BA, Della Fera MA, Whitney CJ, McGuire JC, Meslar HW, Sammelwitz PH. Biotin-binding protein from chicken egg yolk. Assay and relationship to egg-white avidin. Biochem J 1976;157:395–400.

25. Aimone-Gastin I, Gueant JL, Plenat F, Muhale F, Maury F, Djalali M, Gerard P, Duprez A. Assimilation of [57Co]-labeled cobamin in human fetal gastrointestinal xenographts into nude mice. Pediatr Res 1999;45:860–866.

26. Vallet JL, Christenson RK, Klemcke HG. Purification and characterization of intrauterine folate-binding proteins from swine. Biol Reprod 1998;59(1):176–181.

27. Vallet JL, Klemcke HG, Christenson PK. Interrelationships among conceptus size, uterine protein secretion, fetal erythropoiesis, and uterine capacity. J Anim Sci 2002;80:729–737.

28. Shaw DT, Rozeboom DW, Hill GM, Booren AM, Link JE. Impact of vitamin and mineral supplement withdrawal and wheat middling inclusion on finishing pig growth performance, fecal mineral concentration, carcass characteristics, and the nutrient content and oxidative stability of pork. J Anim Sci 2002;80:2920–2930.

29. Zanette D, Monaco HL, Zanotti G, Spadon P. Crystallization of hen eggwhite riboflavin-binding protein. J Mol Biol 1984;180:1185–1187.

30. Monaco HL. Crystal structure of chicken riboflavin binding protein. Embo J 1997;16:1475–1483.

31. Adiga PR, Visweswariah SS, Karande A, Kuzhandkaivelu N. Biochemical and immunological characteristics of riboflavin carrier protein. J Biosci 1988;13:87–104.

32. Adiga PR, Subramanian S, Rao J, Kumar M. Prospects of riboflavin carrier protein (RCP) as an antifertility vaccine in male and female mammals. Hum Reprod Update 1997;3:325–334.

33. Muniyappa K, Adiga PR. Isolation and characterization of thiamin-binding protein from chicken egg white. Biochem J 1979;177:887–894.

34. Muniyappa K, Adiga PR. Nature of the thiamin binding protein from chicken egg yolk. Biochem J 1981;193:678–685.

35. Pácha J. Development of intestinal transport function in mammals. Physiol Rev 2000;80:1633–1667.

36. Widera A, Kim KJ, Crandall ED, Shen WC. Transcytosis of GCSF-transferrin across rat alveolar epithelial cell monolayers. Pharm Res 2003;20:1231–1238.

37. Matsuura M et al. Therapeutic effects of rectal administration of basic fibroblast growth factor on experimental murine colitis. Gastroenterology 2005;128:975–986.

38. Cummins AG, Thompson FM. Effect of breast milk and weaning on epithelial growth of the small intestine in humans. Gut 2002;51:748–754.

39. Taillon C, Andreasen A. Veterinary nutraceutical medicine. Can Vet J 2000;41:231–234.

40. Montaner B, Asbert M, Perez-Tomas R. Immunolocalization of transforming growth factor-2 and epidermal growth factor receptor in the rat gastroduodenal area. Dig Dis Sci 1999;44:1408–1416.

41. Stirling CMA, Charleston B, Takamatsu H, Claypool S, et al. Characterization of the porcine neonatal Fc receptor—potential use for trans-epithelial protein delivery. Immunology 2005;114:542–553.

42. Cammisotto PG, Gingras D, Bendayan M. Transcytosis of gastric leptin through the rat duodenal mucosa. Am J Physiol Gastrointest Liver Physiol 2007;293:G773–G779.

43. Bruneau N, Bendayan M, Gingras D, Ghitescu L, Levy E, Lombardo D. Circulating bile salt-dependent lipase originates from the pancreas via intestinal transcytosis. Gastroenterology 2003;124(2):470–480.

44. Cloutier M, Gingras D, Bendayan M. Internalization and transcytosis of pancreatic enzymes by the intestinal mucosa. J Histochem Cytochem 2006;54:781–794.

45. Wan J, Taub ME, Shah D, Shen WC. Brefeldin A enhances receptor-mediated transcytosis of transferrin in filter-grown Madin-Darby canine kidney cells. J Biol Chem 1992;267:13446–13450.

46. Shah D, Shen WC. The establishment of polarity and enhanced transcytosis of transferrin receptors in enterocyte-like caco-2 cells. J Drug Target 1994;2:93–99.

47. Shah D, Shen WC. Transepithelial delivery of an insulin-transferrin conjugate in enterocyte-like Caco-2 cells. J Pharm Sci 1996;85:1306–1311.

48. Jiang R, Lopez V, Kelleher SL, Lönnerdal B. Apo- and holo-lactoferrin are both internalized by lactoferrin receptor via clathrin-mediated endocytosis but differentially affect ERK-signaling and cell proliferation in Caco-2 cells. J Cell Physiol 2011;226(11):3022–3031. DOI: 10.1002/jcp.22650.

49. Liao Y, Lönnerdal B. miR-584 mediates post-transcriptional expression of lactoferrin receptor in Caco-2 cells and in mouse small intestine during the perinatal period. Int J Biochem Cell Biol 2010;42(8):1363–1369 Epub Aug 07, 2009.

50. Lönnerdal B. Lactoferrin binding to its intestinal receptor. Adv Exp Med Biol 1991;310:145–150.

51. Kawakami H, Lönnerdal B. Isolation and function of a receptor for human lactoferrin in human fetal intestinal brush-border membranes. Am J Physiol 1991;261(5 Pt 1):G841–G846.

52. Lönnerdal B. Lactoferrin receptors in intestinal brush border membranes. Adv Exp Med Biol 1994;357:171–175 Review.

53. Gíslason J, Iyer S, Douglas GC, Hutchens TW, Lönnerdal B. Binding of porcine milk lactoferrin to piglet intestinal lactoferrin receptor. Adv Exp Med Biol 1994;357:239–244.

54. Iyer S, Yip TT, Hutchens TW, Lonnerdal B. Lactoferrin-receptor interaction. Effect of surface exposed histidine residues. Adv Exp Med Biol 1994;357:245–252.

55. Suzuki YA, Lönnerdal B. Characterization of mammalian receptors for lactoferrin. Biochem Cell Biol 2002;80(1):75–80 Review.

56. Suzuki YA, Shin K, Lönnerdal B. Molecular cloning and functional expression of a human intestinal lactoferrin receptor. Biochemistry 2001;40(51):15771–15779.

57. Gíslason J, Douglas GC, Hutchens TW, Lönnerdal B. Receptor-mediated binding of milk lactoferrin to nursing piglet enterocytes: a model for studies on absorption of lactoferrin-bound iron. J Pediatr Gastroenterol Nutr 1995;21(1):37–43.

58. Suzuki YA, Lopez V, Lönnerdal B. Mammalian lactoferrin receptors: structure and function. Cell Mol Life Sci 2005;62(22):2560–2575 Review.

59. Ashida K, Sasaki H, Suzuki YA, Lönnerdal B. Cellular internalization of lactoferrin in intestinal epithelial cells. Biometals 2004;17(3):311–315.

60. Widera A, Norouziyan F, Shen WC. Mechanisms of TfR-mediated transcytosis and sorting in epithelial cells and applications toward drug delivery. Adv Drug Deliv Rev 2003;55:1439–1466.

61. Rolfs A, Hediger MA. Metal ion transporters in mammals: structure, function and pathological implications. J Physiol 1999;518(Pt 1):1–12.

62. Núñez MT, Tapia V, Rojas A, Aguirre P, Gómez F, Nualart F. Iron supply determines apical/basolateral membrane distribution of intestinal iron transporters DMT1 and ferroportin 1. Am J Physiol Cell Physiol 2010 Mar;298(3):C477–C485 Epub Dec 09, 2009.

63. Thompson K, Molina RM, Donaghey T, Brain JD, Wessling-Resnick M. Iron absorption by Belgrade rat pups during lactation. Am J Physiol Gastrointest Liver Physiol 2007 Sep;293(3):G640–G644 Epub July 19, 2007.

64. Katz M, Cooper BA. Solubilized receptor for intrinsic factor-vitamin B_{12} complex from guinea pig intestinal mucosa. J Clin Invest 1974;54:733–739.

65. Kozyraki R, Fyfe J, Kristiansen M, Gerdes C, et al. The intrinsic factor vitamin B_{12} receptor, cubilin, is a high affinity apolipoprotein A-1 receptor facilitating endocytosis of high-density lipoprotein. Nat Med 1999;5:656–661.

66. Kozyraki R, Kirstiansen M, Silahtarogly A, Hansen C, et al. The human intrinsic factor-vitamin B12 receptor, cubilin: molecular characterization and chromosomal mapping of the gene to 10p within the autosomal recessive megaloblastic anemia (MGA1) region. Blood 1998;91:3593–3600.

67. Andersen CBF, Madsen M, Storm T, Moestrup SK, Andersen GR. Structural basis for receptor recognition of vitamin B_{12}-intrinsic factor complexes. Nature 2010;464:445–4448.

68. Moestrup SK, Birn H, Fischer PB, Petersen CM, Verroust PJ, Sim RB, Christensen EI, Nexo E. Megalin-mediated endocytosis of TC–vitamin-B12 complexes suggests a role of the receptor in vitamin-B12 homeostasis. Proc Natl Acad Sci U S A 1996;93:8612–8617.

69. Christensen EI, Birn H. Megalin and cubilin: multifunctional endocytic receptors. Nat Rev Mol Cell Biol 2002;3:256–266.

70. Alpers DH, Russell-Jones GJ. Intrinsic factor and haptocorrin and their receptorsIn: Banerjee R, editor. Chemistry and Biochemistry of B12: Part II: Biochemistry of B12. New York: John Wiley & Sons, Inc.; 1999.

71. Wen J, Kinnear MB, Richardson MA, Willetts NS, Russell-Jones GJ, Gordon MM, Alpers DH. Functional expression in Pichia pastoris of human and rat intrinsic factor. Biochim Biophys Acta 2000;1490:43–53.

72. Gordon MM, Russell-Jones G, Alpers DH. Expression of functional intrinsic factor using recombinant baculovirus. Methods Enzymol 1997;281:255–261.

73. Mathews FS, Gordon MM, Chen Z, Rajashankar KR, Ealick SE, Alpers DH, Sukumar N. Crystal structure of human intrinsic factor: cobalamin complex at 2.6-A resolution. Proc Natl Acad Sci USA 2007;104(44):17311–17316 Epub Oct 22, 2007.

74. Gordon MM, Howard T, Becich MJ, Alpers DH. Cathepsin L mediates intracellular ileal digestion of gastric intrinsic factor. Am J Physiol 1995;268:G33–G40.

75. Ramasamy M, Alpers DH, Tiruppathi C, Seetharam B. Cobalamin release from intrinsic factor and transfer to transcobalamin II within the rat enterocyte. Am J Physiol 1989;257(5 Pt 1):G791–G797.

76. Quadros EV, Regec AL, Khan KM, Quadros E, Rothenberg SP. Transcobalamin II synthesized in the intestinal villi facilitates transfer of cobalamin to the portal blood. Am J Physiol 1999;277:G161–G166.

77. Moestrup SK, Kozyraki R, Kristiansen M, Kaysen JH, et al. The intrinsic factor-vitamin B12 receptor and target of teratogenic antibodies is a megalin-binding peripheral membrane protein with homology to developmental proteins. J Biol Chem 1998;273:5235–5242.

78. Russell-Jones GJ. Intestinal receptor targeting for peptide delivery: reasons for failure and new opportunitiesInvited Review. Ther Deliv 2011;2(12):1575–1593.

79. Widera A, Bai Y, Shen WC. The transepithelial transport of a G-CSF-transferrin conjugate in Caco-2 cells and its myelopoietic effect in BDF1 mice. Pharm Res 2004;21:278–284.

80. Wang J, Shen D, Shen WC. Oral delivery of an insulin-transferrin conjugate in streptozotocin-treated CF/1 mice. Pharm Res 1997;14 abstract in press.

81. Xia CQ, Wang J, Shen WC. Hypoglycemic effect of insulin-transferrin conjugate in streptozotocin-induced diabetic rats. J Pharmacol Exp Ther 2000;295:594–600.

82. Bai Y, Ann DK, Shen WC. Recombinant granulocyte colony-stimulating factor-transferrin fusion protein as an oral myelopoietic agent. Proc Natl Acad Sci USA 2005;102:7292–7296.

83. Bai Y, Shen WC. Improving the oral efficacy of recombinant granulocyte colony-stimulating factor and transferrin fusion protein by spacer optimization. Pharm Res 2006;23:2116–2121.

84. Chen X, Bai Y, Zaro JL, Shen WC. Design of an in vivo cleavable disulfide linker in recombinant fusion proteins. Biotechniques 2010;49:513–518.

85. Amet N, Lee HF, Shen WC. Insertion of the designed helical linker led to increased expression of Tf-based fusion proteins. Pharm Res 2009;26:523–528.

86. Lim CJ, Shen WC. Comparison of monomeric and oligomeric transferrin as potential carrier in oral delivery of protein drugs. J Control Release 2005;106:273–286.

87. Amet N, Wang W, Shen WC. Human growth hormone-transferrin fusion protein for oral delivery in hypophysectomized rats. J Control Release 2010;141:177–182.

88. McGreevy JM, Cannon MJ, Grissom CB. Minimally invasive lymphatic mapping using fluorescently labeled vitamin B12. J Surg Res 2003;111(1):38–44.

89. Smeltzer CC, Cannon MJ, Pinson PR, Munger JD Jr, West FG, Grissom CB. Synthesis and characterization of fluorescent cobalamin (CobalaFluor) derivatives for imaging. Org Lett 2001;3(6):799–801.

90. Howard WA Jr, Bayomi A, Natarajan E, Aziza MA, el-Ahmady O, Grissom CB, West FG. Sonolysis promotes indirect Co-C bond cleavage of alkylcob(III)alamin bioconjugates. Bioconjug Chem 1997;8(4):498–502.

91. Russell-Jones GJ. Oral delivery of therapeutic proteins and peptides by the vitamin B_{12} uptake system. In: Taylor M, Amidon G, editors. Peptide-based Drug Design: Controlling Transport and Metabolism. Washington, DC: ACS Publications; 1995. p 181–198.

92. Russell-Jones GJ. Utilisation of the natural mechanism for vitamin B_{12} uptake for the oral delivery of therapeutics. Eur J Pharm Biopharm 1996;42:241–249.

93. Russell-Jones GJ. Use of Vitamin B_{12} conjugates to deliver protein drugs by the oral route. Crit Rev Ther Drug Carrier Syst 1998;16:557–558(Review).

94. McEwan JF, Veitch HS, Russell-Jones GJ. Synthesis and biological activity of ribose-5'carbamate derivatives of vitamin B_{12}. Bioconjug Chem 1999;10:1131–1136.

95. Alsenz J, Russell-Jones GJ, Westwood S, Levet-Trafit B, de Smidt PC. 2000 Oral absorption of peptides through the cobalamin (vitamin B12) pathway in the rat intestine. Pharm Res 2000;17(7):825–832.

96. Russell-Jones GJ, Westwood SW, Habberfield A. Vitamin B12 mediated oral delivery systems for granulocyte colony stimulating factor and erythropoietin. Bioconjug Chem 1995;6:459–465.

97. Salman HH, Gamazo C, de Smidt PC, Russell-Jones G, Irache JM. Evaluation of bioadhesive capacity and immunoadjuvant properties of vitamin B12-Gantrez Nanoparticles. Pharm Res 2008;12:2859–2868.

98. Habberfield A, Jensen-Pippo K, Ralph L, Westwood SW, Russell-Jones GJ. Vitamin B_{12}-mediated uptake of erythropoietin and granulocyte colony stimulating factor in vitro and in vivo. Int J Pharm 1996;145:1–8.

99. Ramanujam KS, Seetharam S, Dahms NM, Seetharam B. Effect of processing inhibitors on cobalamin (vitamin B12) transcytosis in polarized opossum kidney cells. Arch Biochem Biophys 1994;315(1):8–15.

100. Brada N, Gordon MM, Shao JS, Wen J. Alpers DH Production of gastric intrinsic factor, transcobalamin, and haptocorrin in opossum kidney cells. Am J Physiol Renal Physiol 2000;279(6):F1006–F1013.

101. Russell-Jones GJ, Arthur L, Walker H. Vitamin B_{12}-mediated transport of nanoparticles across Caco-2 cells. Int J Pharm 1999;179:247–255.

102. Ramanujam KS, Seetharam S, Ramasamy M, Seetharam B. Expression of cobalamin transport proteins and cobalamin transcytosis by colon adenocarcinoma cells. Am J Physiol 1991;260(3 Pt 1):G416–G422.

103. Bose S, Kalra S, Yammani RR, Ahuja R, Seetharam B. Plasma membrane delivery, endocytosis and turnover of transcobalamin receptor in polarized human intestinal epithelial cells. J Physiol 2007;581(Pt 2):457–466 Epub March 08, 2007.

104. Pons L, Guy M, Lambert D, Hatier R, Guéant J. Transcytosis and coenzymatic conversion of [(57)Co]cobalamin bound to either endogenous transcobalamin II or exogenous intrinsic factor in caco-2 cells. Cell Physiol Biochem 2000;10(3):135–148.

105. Bose S, Seetharam S, Dahms NM, Seetharam B. Bipolar functional expression of transcobalamin II receptor in human intestinal epithelial Caco-2 cells. J Biol Chem 1997;272(6):3538–3543.

106. Dan N, Cutler DF. Transcytosis and processing of intrinsic factor-cobalamin in Caco-2 cells. J Biol Chem 1994;269(29):18849–18855.

107. Francis MF, Cristea M, Winnik FM. Exploiting the vitamin B12 pathway to enhance oral drug delivery via polymeric micelles. Biomacromolecules 2005;6:2462–2467.

108. Sarti F, Iqbal J, Müller C, Shahnaz G, Rahmat D, Bernkop-Schnürch A. Poly(acrylic acid)-cysteine for oral vitamin B12 delivery. Anal Biochem 2012;420(1):13–19 Epub Sep 10, 2011.

109. Damgé C, Michel C, Aprahamian M, Couvreur P, Devissaguet JP. Nanocapsules as carriers for oral peptide delivery. J Control Release 1990;13:233–239.

110. Damgé C, Michel C, Aprahamian M, Couvreur P. New approach for oral adminis-tration of insulin with polyalkylcyanoacrylate nanocapsules as drug carrier. Diabetes 1988;37:246–251.

111. Russell-Jones GJ, Starling S, McEwan JF. Surface cross-linked particles suitable for con-trolled delivery. PO8880/97 {29/9/97; FL 060042/0179 {28/9/98} US patent 6,221,397. 1997.

112. Chalasani KB, Russell-Jones GJ, Jain AK, Diwan PV, Jain SK. Effective oral delivery of insulin in animal models using vitamin B12-coated dextran nanoparticles. J Control Release 2007;122:141–150.

113. Chalasani KB, Russell-Jones GJ, Yandrapu SK, Diwan PV, Jain SK. A novel vitamin B12-nanosphere conjugate carrier system for peroral delivery of insulin. J Control Release 2007;117:421–429.

114. Chalsani KB, Diwan PV, Raghaven DV, Russell-Jones GJ, Jain SK. Novel vitamin B12-microparticulate conjugate carrier systems for peroral delivery of injectable drugs, therapeutic peptides/proteins and vaccines. US Patent 6,482,413. 2000.

115. Chalsani KB, Diwan V, Raghaven DV, Russell-Jones GJ, et al. Novel vitamin B12-biodegradable microparticulate conjugate carrier systems for peroral delivery of drugs, therapeutic peptides/proteins and vaccines. US Patent 2002, 0192235. 2000.

116. Russell-Jones GJ, Luke MR; 2006 Nanostructures suitable for delivery of agents. WO 2007/131286.

PART V

ADVANCED POLYMERIC DRUG DELIVERY

12

STIMULI-RESPONSIVE POLYMER DELIVERY SYSTEMS

Amy Van Hove, Zhanwu Cui, and Danielle S.W. Benoit

Department of Biomedical Engineering, University of Rochester, Rochester, NY, USA

12.1 INTRODUCTION

Stimuli-responsive polymers exhibit sharp changes in their physical properties upon exposure to specific stimuli. This change can be an alteration in conformation, solubility, or hydrophilic/hydrophobic balance, and can be employed to trigger the release of drugs. For use clinically, stimuli-responsive polymers must exhibit their stimuli response within the context of physiological conditions: a $37\,^{\circ}C$ aqueous environment with high salt concentration and pH $\sim$7.4 (with noted exceptions listed herein). There is a large repertoire of stimuli that have been exploited for drug delivery purposes. These stimuli include temperature, pH, electric field, magnetic field, light, redox state, as well as concentration or presence of enzymes, glucose, and other physiological compounds [1]. This chapter focuses on temperature, pH, redox, and enzymatically responsive drug delivery systems, as these are the stimuli most predominantly employed to trigger drug release. Figure 12.1 is a schematic of some hypothetical uses of polymers responding to a variety of stimuli within different drug delivery devices.

Engineering Polymer Systems for Improved Drug Delivery, First Edition.
Edited by Rebecca A. Bader and David A. Putnam.
© 2014 John Wiley & Sons, Inc. Published 2014 by John Wiley & Sons, Inc.

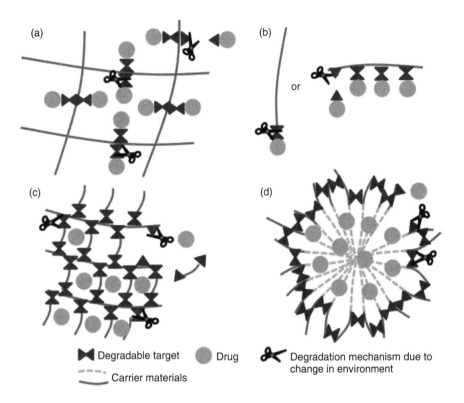

◗◖ Degradable target   ● Drug   ✂ Degradation mechanism due to change in environment

‑‑‑‑ Carrier materials

Figure 12.1. Stimuli-responsive drug delivery systems. (a, b) The drug is conjugated to the carrier via a degradable target (tether). When the environmental conditions change, the tether is cleaved, allowing drug to diffuse into nearby tissue. (a) The carrier is a bulk material. (b) The carrier is a soluble conjugate. (c, d) The drug is encapsulated within a network which contains environmentally responsive degradable targets (linkers). When the environmental conditions change, the linker is cleaved, degrading the network. This allows the drug to diffuse into nearby tissue. (c) The carrier is a bulk material. (d) The carrier is a micelle or nanoparticle.

12.2 TEMPERATURE-RESPONSIVE POLYMERS FOR DRUG DELIVERY

The most well-studied responsive polymers are those that respond to changes in temperature. For physiologically relevant drug delivery systems, however, temperature-responsive drug delivery is somewhat limited, as the body temperature does not deviate much from 37 °C, with rare exceptions of hypo- or hyperthermia; therefore, temperature can be feasibly altered only externally. However, several studies have illustrated that temperature-responsive polymers can be introduced into the body, where they undergo a solution-to-gel (sol-to-gel) transition as a result of the change from ambient to physiological temperature, creating localized drug delivery depots. In addition, there are a multitude of approaches that can be used to externally modulate body temperature to trigger drug delivery (e.g., in the form of ultrasound-mediated heating of gold nanoparticles or subdermal implants). We will first describe the fundamental concepts that govern temperature-responsive polymers, and then introduce specific temperature-responsive polymers and how they have been utilized in drug delivery *in vitro* and *in vivo*.

12.2.1 Fundamental Characteristics of Temperature-Responsive Polymers

To fully understand the mechanism of temperature-responsive polymers for drug delivery applications, it is important to understand the phase transition behavior of these polymers.

12.2.1.1 Lower Critical Solution Temperature and Upper Critical Solution Temperature.
Temperature-responsive polymers exhibit phase transitions at specific temperatures, which cause a sudden change in their solvated state and their overall volume. This temperature is known as either the lower critical solution temperature (LCST) or the upper critical solution temperature (UCST). The LCST and UCST are defined as the minimum or maximum temperature, respectively, in the phase diagram of polymer/solvent mixtures exhibiting both a one-phase and a two-phase region (Fig. 12.2). For polymers with an LCST, the polymer is soluble below the LCST and undergoes a phase transition to become insoluble when the solution is above the LCST. For polymers with a UCST, the polymer behaves in the opposite fashion: it is soluble above the UCST but insoluble below the UCST. LCST or UCST behavior is completely reversible and is dependent upon several factors. These factors

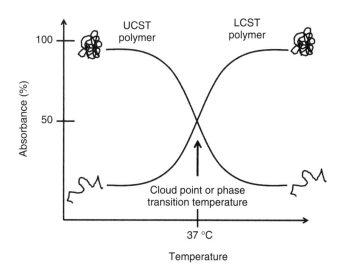

Figure 12.2. Phase behavior of representative LCST and UCST temperature-responsive polymers.

include polymer composition, molecular weight, concentration, and the presence of cosolvent or other additives.

Phase transition behaviors such as UCST and LCST are governed by the thermodynamics of polymer solvation/desolvation. Typically, temperature-responsive polymers are comprised of amphiphilic monomers in which the common hydrophilic groups include amides, carbonyls, or secondary, tertiary, or quaternary amines, and hydrophobic moieties include methyl, ethyl, or propyl groups. These polymers exhibit interesting temperature-dependent phase behavior because of their amphiphilic nature. Although LCST and UCST behavior is not limited to aqueous environments, only aqueous systems are relevant for drug delivery applications; thus, here we assume the solvent is water. Many theories have been proposed to explain the behavior of LCST and UCST polymers. The most commonly cited and well-supported theory is that posed by Schild [2]. Recall from thermodynamics that $\Delta G_{mix} = \Delta H_{mix} - T \Delta S_{mix}$, where G is the Gibbs free energy, H is the enthalpy, T is the temperature (K), and S is the entropy. For mixing (solvation) to occur, the Gibbs free energy of mixing (ΔG_{mix}) must be negative. Therefore, a negative ΔG_{mix} favors solvation and a positive ΔG_{mix} favors desolvation (gel formation). Solvation of polymers requires hydrogen bonding between water and polymer chains. Below the LCST or above the UCST, solvation is an exothermic reaction primarily due to enthalpic contributions ($-\Delta H_{mix}$) associated with hydrogen bonding with only modest increases in entropy (ΔS_{mix}), resulting in an overall negative free energy of mixing ($-\Delta G_{mix}$).

As the temperature changes (an increase for LCST or a decrease for UCST behavior), the hydrophilic–hydrophobic balance of the polymer chain is altered, resulting in more hydrophobic characteristics. As the polymer chain becomes more hydrophobic, water molecules must reorient and become highly organized around the newly revealed hydrophobic regions of the polymer. As the water molecules organize, they no longer form hydrogen bonds with the polymer, resulting in a change to a positive ΔH_{mix}. In addition to these unfavorable enthalpic changes, the entropy of the system decreases ($-\Delta S_{mix}$) because water becomes more organized as it arranges itself around the hydrophobic polymer interface, a phenomenon known as the hydrophobic effect. These two factors combine to make the overall free energy change (ΔG_{mix}) positive, making desolvation and phase separation an energetically favorable process. This desolvation behavior is shown in Fig. 12.3 for the LCST polymer, poly(N-isopropylacrylamide) (PNIPAM).

LCST or UCST behavior can be characterized with a variety of methods, including differential scanning calorimetry, static and dynamic light scattering, and turbidity (optical density at 350 nm) measurements. As an example, Fig. 12.3 highlights typical turbidity behavior of temperature-responsive polymers. A polymer solution at low concentration (e.g., 0.5 wt%) is introduced into a spectrophotometer (wavelength of 350 nm) and the transition temperature, also known as the cloud point temperature, is determined when the absorbance of the polymer solution decreases (UCST) or increases (LCST) to 50% of its maximum absorbance. The turbidity of PNIPAM is shown as a function of temperature in Fig. 12.3.

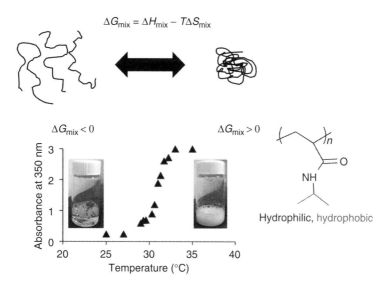

$$\Delta G_{mix} = \Delta H_{mix} - T\Delta S_{mix}$$

$\Delta G_{mix} < 0$ $\Delta G_{mix} > 0$

Hydrophilic, hydrophobic

Figure 12.3. Illustration of thermodynamics of temperature-responsive polymers and representative turbidity test of PNIPAM.

12.2.2 Temperature-Responsive Polymers and Their Applications in Drug Delivery

A number of temperature-responsive polymers have been discovered and developed for drug delivery applications (see Fig. 12.4 for chemical structures and transition temperatures (T_{tr})). Polymers with LCST behaviors include poly(N-alkylacrylamides) such as PNIPAM and poly(N,N-diethylacrylamide), poly(methyl vinyl ether), poly(N-vinyl caprolactam), poly(2-ethyl-2-oxazoline), and the pseudo-natural polymer, elastin-like polypeptide (ELP) poly(GVGVP). The most common polymers with UCST behavior are interpenetrating networks of poly(alkylacrylamides) and poly(acrylic acid).

All the polymers identified in Fig. 12.4 have transition temperatures of interest for biomedical applications (approximately 37 °C). One exception is poly(2-oxazoline) (POx), whose transition temperature is 62 °C. To exploit this and other temperature-responsive polymers, the transition temperature can be altered through incorporation of hydrophilic or hydrophobic comonomers, or by incorporating additives after polymerization. For example, the LCST of PNIPAM can be decreased through copolymerization with hydrophobic comonomers and increased through copolymerization with hydrophilic comonomers [5, 6]. This is due to a change in the temperature at which point polymer amphiphilic behavior switches to hydrophobic behavior caused by changes in hydrogen bonding. Three additives that can similarly be used to change transition temperatures are salts, surfactants, and cosolvents. These additives are conducive to the use of these polymers for drug delivery, as they are states of common drug molecules (salt) or drug formulations (surfactants, cosolvents) and are also commonly found within the body. The additives' effects on transition temperatures are

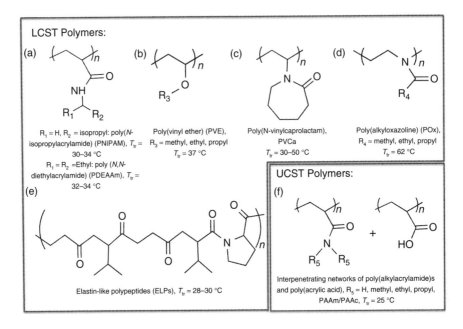

Figure 12.4. Chemical structures and transition temperatures of selected LCST (a–e) and UCST (f) polymers [2–4, 151–154].

varied and must be examined on a case-by-case basis. Surfactants, in particular, can be problematic for temperature-responsive drug delivery, as they can substantially alter the polymer's hydrophilic/hydrophobic balance. Incorporation of surfactants, therefore, can shift the transition temperature to a large extent, or can even remove the transition behavior altogether. Two LCST polymers, PNIPAM and poly(N-vinylcaprolactam) (PVCa), have been shown to exhibit large increases in transition temperature as a result of addition of surfactants [3, 7].

12.2.2.1 LCST Polymers.

POLY(*N*-ALKYL ACRYLAMIDE)S. The most common group of polymers showing LCST behavior is the poly(*N*-substituted acrylamide) family (Fig. 12.4a). Of all the temperature-responsive polymers, PNIPAM is the most investigated, exhibiting an LCST close to body temperature. Related polymers, such as poly(*N*,*N*-diethyl acrylamide) (PDEAAM, Fig. 12.4a), exhibit an LCST in the range 26–35 °C, and among the poly(*N*-alkylacrylamides), PDEAAM has drawn the most attention recently because of its favorable biocompatibility [8, 9].

POLY(VINYL ETHER). Poly(vinyl ether) based materials (PVE, Fig. 12.4b) represent another group of temperature-responsive materials with LCST behavior. The living cationic polymerization of PVE-based polymers leads to well-controlled molecular weight, polydispersity, and polymer architectures, which provide control over drug delivery [10–13]. Although both PVE based random copolymers and block copolymers have been synthesized, random copolymers generally do not exhibit a sharp thermoresponsive behavior [10–13]. Another unique characteristics of PVE is that end-group modification affects the temperature-responsive behavior quite extensively, where hydrophilic end groups increase the transition temperature, and hydrophobic end groups decrease the transition temperature or eliminate phase transition behavior altogether [11].

POLY(*N*-VINYL CAPROLACTAM). PVCa (Fig. 12.4c) polymers possess LCSTs in the range of 30–50 °C, with a strong dependence upon concentration and molecular weight [14–17], making them unique amongst all known LCST polymers. PVCa does not produce toxic low molecular-weight amines during degradation, which is a huge advantage for drug delivery applications [14].

POLY(OXAZOLINE)S. POxs (Fig. 12.4d) with ethyl, isopropyl, or *n*-propyl side chains are water soluble and show LCST behavior in water [18–21]. The cloud point of POx increases with increasing hydrophobicity, but it also depends on the degree of polymerization (DP) and concentration. Poly(2-ethyl-2-oxazoline) shows a transition temperature only when the DP is above 100 because the smaller polymer chains are soluble up to 100 °C. Poly(2-isopropyl-2-oxazoline) has a cloud point close to body temperature, making it advantageous in drug delivery applications. However, its thermoresponsiveness is irreversible after annealing above the LCST because of its semicrystallinity [18]. Recently, control of the LCST of POx was demonstrated over a broad range of temperatures by gradient or random copolymerization between 2-*n*-propyl-2-oxazolin (nProX) and either 2-isopropyl-2-oxazoline (iPrOx) or 2-ethyl-2-oxazoline (EtOx) [20].

ELASTIN-LIKE POLYPEPTIDES. Polypeptides such as ELPs (Fig. 12.4c) can also show LCST behavior. Tropoelastin is the soluble precursor to elastin, the main elastic protein found in mammals. Tropoelastin is known to undergo a phase transition *in vivo* as the first step of assembly into elastin. This phase transition process is known as coacervation and can be mimicked by ELPs. *In vivo*, coacervation can be triggered through changes in temperature, pH, and ionic strength. Similarly, a protein that contains the pentapeptide mimic of elastin GVGVP as a repeating unit, exhibits a phase transition temperature of 30 °C. However, the peptide's primary structure can be easily altered using recombinant DNA techniques to modulate the phase transition behavior. This pentapeptide can then be used to exploit the subtle alterations in physiological temperature that occur within diseased tissues. For example, a responsive doxorubicin–polypeptide conjugate was developed to improve the efficacy of doxorubicin's chemotherapeutic effect. This conjugate accumulated in tumor tissue because of its large size and enhanced tumor permeation and retention. As the LCST behavior of these polymers were designed to undergo phase transition at the slightly elevated temperatures of the tumor tissue, the drug conjugate became insoluble in or near tumors, allowing doxorubicin to be released by hydrolysis of drug–polymer linkers [22].

12.2.2.2 UCST Polymers.
SEMI-INTERPENETRATING POLYMER NETWORKS CONSISTING OF A POLY(ALKYL ACRYLAMIDE) AND POLY(ACRYLIC ACID). Semi-interpenetrating polymer networks (IPNs) consisting of a poly(alkyl acrylamide) and poly(acrylic acid) (PAAm/PAAc, Fig. 12.4f) have been developed as UCST polymers [4, 23]. The complex between poly(N,N'-dimethylacrylamide) (PDMAAm) and PAAc forms through hydrogen bonding, with PDMAAm acting as the hydrogen-bond acceptor and PAAc as the hydrogen-bond donor. Generally, transition temperature of these networks is broad (5–10 °C) and can be shifted to higher values by increasing the PDMAAm content.

12.2.2.3 Examples of Temperature-Responsive Polymers for Drug Delivery Applications.
Temperature-responsive polymers have been used in many devices to control the delivery of a variety of drugs. Some interesting applications are compiled in Table 12.1 and will be reviewed briefly here.

Temperature-responsive polymers have been formed into nanoparticles, microgels, microparticles, liposomes, micelles, and hydrogels [26–28, 31–35] with all or part of the polymer acting as the drug delivery device. As an example, ABA triblock copolymers of the poly(2-oxazoline)s (POx), specifically poly(2-methyl-2-oxazoline) (A)-block-(2-isopropyl-2-oxazoline-co-2-butyl-2-oxazoline   (B)-block-2-methyl-2-oxazoline (A) (hydrophilic, hydrophobic and thermoresponsive, hydrophilic blocks, respectively), were synthesized and formed micelles within narrow temperature ranges [36], enabling temperature dependent loading and release of hydrophobic drugs. In fact, these micelles have shown unprecedentedly high solubilization capacity for drugs, such as the chemotherapeutic paclitaxel, the antifungal drug amphotericin B, and the immunosuppressant cyclosporin A. In addition, paclitaxel remained fully active when delivered *in vitro* and *in vivo* using this micelle carrier [29].

Many other drugs have been delivered using temperature-responsive devices, including bovine serum albumin (a model for protein-based therapeutics), doxorubicin, etc. In designing temperature-responsive delivery systems, one must be cognizant of possible drug–polymer interactions that may alter drug release and activity. For example, studies on the potential interactions between model drugs (benzoates, diltiazem, cyanocobalamin, dextrans) and thermoresponsive PNIPAM hydrogels [37] showed that there are hydrophobic interactions between PNIPAM and the aromatic ring/ester side chain of the unionized benzoate at relatively low drug concentrations (<0.01 M). This interaction affects the equilibrium swelling ratio of the hydrogel, leading to alterations in drug release kinetics [38].

More hydrophilic drugs (nadolol) lead to lower nanoparticle swelling compared to hydrophobic drugs (propranolol and tacrine). Both nadolol and propranolol exhibit slowed release with increasing temperature because of enhanced polymer–drug interactions through hydrophobic bonding. Loading with the slightly hydrophobic beta-blocker nadolol in temperature-responsive nanoparticles composed of pNVCa resulted in lower swelling ratios as compared with the very hydrophobic beta-blocker propranolol and Alzheimer's medication tacrine. Loading with either propranolol or tacrine caused the nanoparticles to swell considerably, whereas reduced swelling was

TABLE 12.1. Examples of Drug Delivery Applications for Temperature-Responsive Polymers

Class	Polymer composition	Drug delivered	Drug utilized	Discussion	References
LCST	poly(N,N-diethylacrylamide)	Insulin	Hydrogels	Insulin release reaches 80% within the first 10 h, very different from poly(N-isopropylacrylamide) gels which have biphasic release	9
	poly(N,N-diethylacrylamide)	Paclitaxel	Nanoparticles	Good colloidal stability in physiologically relevant buffers may support long circulation time *in vivo*. Initial burst release over the first 10 h with much greater release rate at 43 °C versus 37 °C	24
	poly(N-isopropylacrylamide)	Hydrophobic and hydrophilic drugs	Hydrogels	Above the LCST the hydrogel is in a dehydrated state and hydrophobic drug–polymer interactions dictate whether or not the drug is released, while the rate of release is dictated by steric interactions between hydrophilic drugs and the hydrogel network	25
	poly(2-(2-ethoxy)ethoxyethyl vinyl ether (EOEOVE))	Doxorubicin	Liposomes (block copolymers with octadecyl vinyl ether)	Liposomes were stable below physiological temperature but exhibited significant release of drug above 40 °C, releasing doxorubicin entirely within 1 min at 45 °C. Long circulation times *in vivo* and biodistribution similar to other liposomal formulations were observed. Tumor growth was suppressed after systemic treatment of drug-loaded liposomes combined with tumor site heating to 45 °C for 10 min at 6 and 12 h after injection	26
	Poly(N-vinylcaprolactam)	Nadolol, Propranolol, Tacrine	Nanoparticles	More hydrophilic drugs (Nadolol) lead to lower nanoparticle swelling versus hydrophobic drugs (Propranolol and Tacrine). Both Nadolol and Propranolol exhibit slowed release with increasing temperature due to enhanced polymer-drug interactions (hydrophobic effect)	27

(continued)

385

TABLE 12.1. (*Continued*)

Class	Polymer composition	Drug delivered	Drug utilized	Discussion	References
LCST	Poly(*N*-vinylcaprolactam)	Hypothetical	Micelles (block copolymers with poly(ethylene glycol))	Have prolonged stability in physiologically relevant buffer systems and have been modified with folic acid to target tumors which overexpress the folate receptor	28
	Poly(2-oxazolines)	Paclitaxel, Amphotericin B, Cyclosporin A	Micelles	Hydrophilic, thermoresponsive, hydrophilic ABA polyoxazoline diblock copolymers form micelles in a temperature-responsive manner. These micelles have been demonstrated to have high loading of hydrophobic drugs (Paclitaxel, Amphotericin B, Cyclosporin A) without loss of activity	29
	Elastin-like polypeptides	Doxorubicin	Drug conjugates	Drug-conjugated ELPs are endocytosed by squamous cell carcinoma cells and result in near equivalent *in vitro* cytotoxicity to free doxorubicin. Phase transition temperature was 40 °C. Upon combination of ELP delivery and hyperthermia, cytotoxicity of the drug conjugate was increased 20-fold	22
UCST	poly(acrylamide)/ poly(acrylic acid) interpenetrating networks	Ibuprofen	Hydrogels	Drug was released faster at 37 °C than at 25 °C	30

observed for the less hydrophobic nadolol. Nadolol incorporation decreased the transition temperature of the pNVCa nanoparticles, while the more hydrophobic propranolol and tacrine did not. However, hydrophobicity alone is not sufficient to determine the effect that a drug will have on the behavior of the delivery system: attenuated release of nadolol and propranolol indicated that these drugs bind more favorably to the polymer chains within the particles than tacrine [27].

12.3 pH-RESPONSIVE POLYMERS FOR DRUG DELIVERY

Although physiological pH is typically between 7.35 and 7.45 (the normal pH of blood), a variety of tissues, cellular compartments, and pathological states exhibit pH values that deviate from this range. Table 12.2 lists examples of pH values found in different types of normal tissues and pathological conditions. Because these alterations in pH are localized to specific tissues or pathological states, the use of pH has significant potential as a stimulus for responsive drug delivery systems. In particular,

TABLE 12.2. Examples of Tissues and Conditions Resulting in Deviation from Physiological pH[a]

	System	pH
Normal	Blood	7.35–7.45
	Stomach	1.0–3.0
	Duodenum	4.8–8.2
	Skin [39]	5.2–5.9
	Small intestine [40]	6–7.4
	Large intestine [40]	5.7–6.7
	Vagina [41, 42]	4.0–5.0
	Muscle (lower limb)	
	Before exercise [43]	7.2
	After a 30-s sprint [43]	6.6
	Intracellular compartments	
	Early endosome	6.0–6.5
	Late endosome	5.0–6.0
	Lysosome	4.5–5.0
	Golgi	6.4
Pathologic	Ischemic tissue, extracellular	
	Ischemic myocardium, aortic clamp [44–46]	6.0–7.0
	Ischemic hindlimb, tourniquet model [47]	6.3–7.1
	Ischemic brain tissue [48]	6.0–6.6
	Sites of wound healing/inflammation	
	Acute wounds [49]	5.2–6.2
	Chronic wounds [49]	7.3–8.9
	Tumors, extracellular	6.5–7.2

[a] Adapted from Reference 50 unless otherwise noted.

pH-responsive drug delivery may allow drug targeting to regions of local acidosis, including sites of inflammation, neoplasia, or ischemia, or could be used to protect the drug from the harsh environment of the stomach, ensuring downstream drug delivery.

12.3.1 Fundamental Characteristics of pH-Responsive Smart Polymers

To better understand the mechanism of pH-responsive polymers for drug delivery applications, it is important to review the basics of acid–base equilibrium.

12.3.1.1 Acid–Base Equilibrium. pH-responsive polymers are composed of functional groups capable of accepting or donating protons, making them weak acids or bases. A weak acid (HA) is a proton (H^+) donor and its conjugate base (A^-) is a proton acceptor. The equilibrium between the donor and acceptor is dependent on the local pH and the strength of the acid involved in the equilibrium reaction.

$$HA \rightleftharpoons H^+ + A^- \tag{12.1}$$

When in solution, equilibrium is obtained between the protonated and deprotonated form of the acid. This equilibrium is quantified by the acid dissociation constant, K_a:

$$K_a = \frac{[A^-][H^+]}{[HA]} \tag{12.2}$$

where [HA] is the concentration of the protonated acid, $[A^-]$ is the concentration of the conjugate base, and $[H^+]$ is the concentration of free protons in solution. Depending on the relative strength of the acid and the solvent used, this value can vary over many orders of magnitude. To facilitate comparison of the highly variable range of K_a values, the logarithmic form pK_a is used:

$$pK_a = -\log_{10} K_a = -\log_{10} \frac{[A^-][H^+]}{[HA]} \tag{12.3}$$

On the basis of this convention, strong acids have a lower pK_a (less than -2) and weak acids have a higher pK_a (-2 to 12).

For bases that serve as proton acceptors, a similar relationship exists. When a base (B) accepts a proton from water, it becomes protonated (BH^+) while simultaneously converting the water molecule into a hydroxide anion (OH^-):

$$B + H_2O \rightleftharpoons BH^+ + OH^- \tag{12.4}$$

The equilibrium between the protonated and deprotonated forms is expressed by an analogous set of equations to characterize the degree of basicity:

$$K_b = \frac{[BH^+][OH^-]}{[B]} \tag{12.5}$$

where $[BH^+]$ is the concentration of the protonated base, $[B]$ is the concentration of the deprotonated base, and $[OH^-]$ is the concentration of hydroxide anions in solution. Similar to the acids previously discussed, the log form of K_b is often used.

$$pK_b = -\log_{10} K_b = -\log_{10} \frac{[BH^+][OH^-]}{[B]} \tag{12.6}$$

Similar to strong acids, strong bases have low values of pK_b.

Derived from Eqs. 12.1–12.6, the Henderson–Hasselbalch equation describes pH and pOH of a solution as follows:

$$pH = pK_a + \log \frac{[A^-]}{[HA]} \tag{12.7a}$$

$$pOH = pK_b + \log \frac{[BH^+]}{[B]} \tag{12.7b}$$

When the environmental pH is equal to pK_a, $\log \frac{[A^-]}{[HA]}$ is equal to 0. So, $[A^-]/[HA]=1$, meaning that the concentration of protonated acid $[HA]$ is equal of that of deprotonated acid $[A^-]$. If the environmental pH is below pK_a, the protonated form of the acid is favored; similarly for bases, if the environmental pOH is below pK_b, the deprotonated form of the acid is favored.

12.3.2 pH-Responsive Polymer Compositions and their Applications in Drug Delivery

pH-responsive polymers are typically polyelectrolytes that bear weak acidic or basic groups. These polyelectrolytes are capable of accepting or donating protons in response to the environmental pH. Generally, alterations in the protonated state result in changes of polymer solubility, conformation, size, and so on. For example, upon protonation of an amine-containing polymer, a charge is generated along the polymer and electrostatic repulsion results in an increase in hydrodynamic volume [51]. Polyelectrolytes that contain carboxylic acids or secondary, tertiary, and/or quaternary amines have both been employed for pH-responsive drug delivery applications (Fig. 12.5); thus, polyelectrolytes can be subdivided into carboxylic and amine-containing architectures. pH can also be utilized to trigger drug release through enhanced degradation of polymer cross-links or tethers. These linkages can be composed of ester, hydrazone, anhydride, or orthoester bonds (Fig. 12.6). While these linkers typically degrade hydrolytically, the kinetics of degradation are greatly accelerated in the presence of elevated hydronium (H_3O^+) concentrations. A variety of polymers have been developed that respond to the altered pH of different tissues.

12.3.2.1 Anionic pH-Responsive Polymers.
Anionic polymers formed from carboxylic acid-containing monomers are commonly used as pH-responsive polymers. As the pH drops below the pK_a of the carboxyl groups in the polymer,

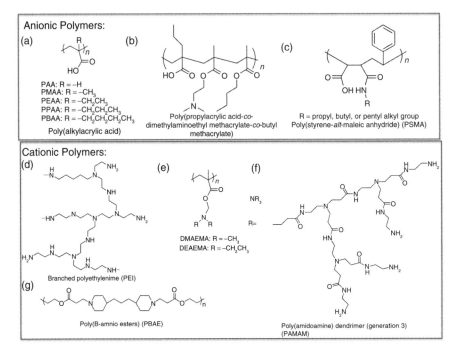

Figure 12.5. Structures of pH-responsive polymers useful in drug delivery applications.

protonation of the carboxylate anions results, which increases the overall polymer hydrophobicity. This causes the polymer to switch from a soluble, extended state to a less soluble, compact, globular morphology. Importantly, this transition can be tuned to occur at physiologically relevant pH by modifying carboxylic acid-containing monomers with aliphatic groups (see Fig. 12.5). In the absence of aliphatic groups, the typical pK_a of carboxylic acids is approximately 10–11. Anionic pH-responsive polymers have been utilized to deliver a variety of drugs including peptides, proteins, DNA, siRNA, and small-molecule drugs (Table 12.3). Anionic polymers have also been shown to enhance drug circulation times and are well-suited for *in vivo* delivery because of their cytocompatibility [52].

POLY(ALKYLACRYLIC ACID)S. The most prominent pH-responsive polymers utilized for drug delivery are the poly(alkylacrylic acid)s (PAAAs) (Fig. 12.5a). The pH-responsive behavior of PAAA polymers was first described for poly(ethylacrylic acid) (PEAA). PEAA was found to change from an ionized, expanded conformation into a collapsed, hydrophobic globular coil in acidic conditions with a transition mid-point at approximately pH = 6.2 [60]. Since this pioneering work, PAAA polymers, including PAAc, poly(methacrylic acid) (PMAA), PEAA, poly(propylacrylic acid) (PPAA), and poly(butylacrylic acid) (PBAA) (Fig. 12.5a) have been extensively studied. The systematic increase in the length of the hydrophobic alkyl group with the methylene group (CH_2) results in an increase in the polymer's pK_a value, consequently affecting the pH at which the polymer transitions from a hydrophilic to a hydrophobic conformation. This is evident by the increase in the polymer's pK_a from 6.3 for PEAA to 6.7 for PPAA and 7.4 (physiological) for PBAA. Because of its physiologically relevant pK_a and hydrophobic, membrane-interactive characteristics at normal pH, PBAA is not utilized as a pH-responsive polymer. As the pH-responsive behavior of PAAAs is intimately tied to the alkyl chain and can be tuned over physiologically relevant pH, this family of pH-responsive polymers has been extensively used in a variety of drug delivery applications. We will discuss PMAA and PPAA specifically in depth below, and offer more examples of the drug delivery applications of these important polymers in Table 12.3.

POLY(METHACRYLIC ACID)S. Anionic pH-responsive PMAA containing polymers have primarily been used for oral delivery of biotherapeutics (Fig. 12.5a, $R=CH_3$) because of their low pK_a (5.4). Thus, PMAA collapses in the highly acidic stomach environment (pH $= 1-3$), making it useful as a protective barrier for oral delivery of drugs that would otherwise be destroyed by the pH and proteolytic enzymes present in the stomach. For example, nanosized poly(methacrylic acid-g-ethylene glycol) (P(MAA-g-EG)) hydrogels were developed for oral delivery of insulin [61]. In the acidic stomach, the gels remain collapsed as a result of the low pH and protonation of the methacrylic acid moieties. Under these acidic conditions, the mesh size of the nanogels was as low as 70 Å, and insulin remained entrapped and protected from proteolytic degradation. However, once the carriers passed into the neutral pH of the intestine, the polymer chains elongated with a resulting network mesh size of 210 Å, resulting in rapid hydrogel swelling and release of insulin. These carriers were effective *in vivo*; within 2 h of oral administration to either healthy or diabetic rats, dose-dependent hypoglycemic effects were observed, with blood sugar control lasting for up to 8 h after administration [62].

POLY(PROPYLACRYLIC ACID) (PPAA). PPAA (Fig. 12.5a) has shown great utility for intracellular delivery of macromolecular drugs (e.g., proteins, peptides, and nucleic acids) because of its pH-responsive behavior. The pK_a of PPAA is just below physiological, making it ideal for use to modulate drug escape from intracellular endosomal trafficking. Generally, cells uptake macromolecular drugs via endocytosis. Once within the endosome, molecules are gradually transported to lysosomes in a process known as endosomal trafficking. During trafficking, there is a gradual reduction of endosomal pH from 7.4 to 5.0. Once a molecule reaches the lysosome, pH and lysosomal enzymes degrade the endocytosed cargo. Drug molecules must escape this trafficking before reaching the lysosome to avoid degradation and act intracellularly. At pH ranges occurring during endosomal–lysosomal trafficking, PPAA becomes protonated and hydrophobic, mediating endosomal membrane disruption through hydrophobic interactions with the lipid bilayer and enabling release of cargo into the cytoplasm. For example, PPAA was conjugated to a model antigen, ovalbumin. PPAA–ovalbumin was delivered to macrophages *in vitro* as a first step toward a polymeric vaccine delivery

TABLE 12.3. Examples of Drug Delivery Applications for pH-Responsive Polymers

Class	Polymer composition	Drug delivered	Drug utilized	Discussion	References
Anionic	Poly (propylacrylic acid)	Fibroblast growth factor, vascular endothelial growth factor	Hydrogel	pH-dependent release of growth factors was observed.	53
	Poly(styrene-alt-maleic anhydride) (PSMA)	siRNA, doxorubicin	Micelles	Pentyl amine modified PSMA complexed with cationic micelles were capable of loading doxorubicin. This system was non-cytotoxic and mediated efficient cell uptake of siRNA ($>70\%$) through endosomal release in ovarian cell lines.	54
Cationic	Polyethyleneimine (PEI)	Diltiazem	Nanoparticles	PEI-modified nanoparticles modulated drug release, with slower release at pH 1.2 than at 6.8.	55
	Poly(amidoamine)	DNA	Nanosized poly-electrolyte	Showed high buffering capacity between pH 5–7 and excellent DNA binding ability. Comparable or higher transfection efficiency than PEI observed through 'proton sponge' effects.	56
	DMAEMA	Protamine and insulin	Hydrogel	Release of drugs from hydrogels was Fickian in nature. As pH of the release media decreased from 7.3 to 4.0, the rate of release of both biomolecules increased due to the protonation of DMAEMA and increased mesh size of the hydrogel.	57
Degradable	'Encrypted polymer' linked through acetal groups	Oligonucleotides	Drug conjugates	PEG was grafted to pH sensitive backbone through acid-degradable acetal linkages. The carrier directed uptake and endosomal release of oligonucleotides in hepatocytes.	58
	Acid-cleavable carriers	DNA	Drug conjugates	pH sensitive PEG lipids bearing acid-cleavable acetal linkage and short PEG chains were synthesized. The pH these lipids were susceptible to degradation at depends on lipid structures, and varies from 3.0 to 5.5 at 37 °C.	59

system. This treatment resulted in antigen presentation which required cytosolic delivery of antigen and proved useful in vaccination of mice *in vivo* [63].

Block copolymers have also been synthesized bearing propylacrylic acid (PAA) to exploit its pH-responsive, endosomal-escape properties. Typically, diblock copolymers have been designed with a dual delivery mechanism—for example, increased circulation times or drug complexation and protection in addition to endosomal escape. One copolymer designed specifically for siRNA delivery is a block copolymer consisting of poly(dimethylaminoethyl methacrylate)-*b*-Poly(propylacrylic acid-co-dimethylaminoethyl methacrylate-co-butyl methacrylate) (pDMAEMA-*b*-p(PAA-*co*-DMAEMA-*co*-BMA)) [64]. This diblock copolymer was designed to complex with, and protect, negatively charged siRNA while also providing a mechanism for endosomal escape. Therefore, a cationic first block to condense and protect siRNA as well as a terpolymer second block containing PAA for endosomal escape (see Fig. 12.5b) was synthesized. Delivery of siRNA using the diblock copolymer resulted in gene knockdown of up to 80% compared to untreated cells and resulted in no detectable cytotoxicity [64].

Similarly, the polymer poly(*N*-(2-hydroxypropylmethacrylamide))-*b*-poly(propylacrylic acid-*co*-butyl methacrylate-*co*-dimethylaminoethyl methacrylate) (pHPMA-*b*-p(PAA-*co*-BMA-*co*-DMAEMA)) was utilized to confer long circulation times (pHPMA block) and endosomal escape (PAA containing terpolymer block) to an intracellular-acting pro-apoptotic peptide [65]. These peptide—polymer conjugates increased HeLa cervical carcinoma cell apoptotic activity over free peptide and resulted in 50% tumor cell death in cultures after 6 h of treatment [65]. Data gathered using these polymer delivery systems indicate that cytosolic delivery is enhanced using PAA functionalities, even when incorporated into a diblock copolymer—opening up new and exciting avenues for delivery systems requiring multiple functionalities.

POLY(STYRENE-*alt*-MALEIC ANHYDRIDE). Another class of anionic, pH-responsive polymers are copolymers of styrene and maleic anhydride (poly(styrene-*alt*-maleic anhydride), PSMA, Fig. 12.5c). Styrene and maleic anhydride are known to produce alternating copolymers that have been used in a variety of applications [66]. PSMA has many desirable attributes for use as a polymer therapeutic. It enhances drug circulation half-life and lipid solubility and binds noncovalently with albumin during systemic circulation, thereby reducing polymer clearance [67]. In the initial use of PSMA aimed to exploit these properties, Maeda and coworkers used low molecular-weight PSMA copolymers (<6 kDa) clinically to deliver an antitumor protein, neocarzinostatin (NCS) [68–70]. The polymer—protein conjugate styrene-alt-maleic anhydride-NCS (SMANCS) [68–70] significantly improved the pharmacological properties of NCS and has been clinically effective in treating liver cancer. Similar to that of PAAAs, the pH-responsive behavior of PSMA can be extensively modified depending for the intended application. The pK_a of PSMA was altered by modification of the maleic anhydride segment with alkyl chains (Fig. 12.6c) [71]. By varying the length of alkyl chain used, the percent modification, and the overall molecular weight of PSMA, the pK_a of these derivatives was varied from 5.0 to 7.5. The pH-dependent activity of PSMA has been utilized to mediate the endosomal escape required for efficient delivery of macromolecular drugs including siRNA [54].

12.3.2.2 Cationic pH-Responsive Polymers. Cationic pH-responsive polymers consist of functional groups that are weak acids, typically secondary, tertiary, or quaternary amines. Unlike anionic polymers, which exhibit pK_as around pH 4–7, amine-containing polymers undergo hydrophobic to hydrophilic transitions at or above pH = 8. These polymers also include poly(β-amino esters) (PBAE) and poly(amidoamine) dendrimers (PAMAM) (Fig. 12.6 d–f). Two polymers whose pK_a s are not above 8 are dimethylaminoethyl methacrylate (DMAEMA, pK_a = 7.5) and diethylaminoethyl methacrylate (DEAEMA, pK_a = 7.3) (Fig. 12.5e). The pK_a of these polymers was decreased by increasing the length of the alkyl chains conjugated to the tertiary amine from methyl groups to ethyl groups, which is the opposite trend of pK_a and hydrophobicity observed for anionic polymers. Beyond DMAEMA and DEAEMA, several other cationic polymers have been modified to reduce their pK_a values for use in drug delivery applications. Cationic polymers have also shown great utility for extracellular drug delivery, as well as for intracellular macromolecular drug delivery via the "proton sponge effect." We will explore these classes of amine-containing cationic polymers both below and within Table 12.3.

CATIONIC POLYMERS FOR EXTRACELLULAR DRUG DELIVERY. Poly(β-amino esters) (Fig. 12.5g) are an example of cationic polymers that have been used for pH-dependent drug delivery. For example, micelles composed of poly(ethylene glycol)-b-poly(β-amino esters) (PEG–PBAE) were examined as pH-responsive micelles for a chemotherapeutic delivery vehicle [72]. The diblock pK_a was approximately 6.5, causing the PBAE block to become deprotonated and hydrophobic at physiological pH, where it assembled into the interior of micelles able to load hydrophobic drugs. As the pH decreased, amine protonation increased polymer solubility and induced a sharp demicellization behavior at pH $\sim$ 6.4–6.8. As the pH of many pathological conditions is between 6.0 and 7.0 (Table 12.3), this demicellization behavior may allow precise targeting of drug to target tissues.

Similarly, poly(amidoamine) dendrimers (Fig. 12.6f) were capable of self-assembly into nanoparticles at physiological pH. Upon reduction of the pH below 6, drug was released as a resullt of protonation of the amines of the dendrimers and dissolution of the nanoparticles [73]. pH-sensitive nanoparticle hydrogels comprised of crosslinked DMAEMA and 2-hydroxyethyl methacrylate (HEMA) have also been investigated for pH-responsive drug delivery applications [57, 74]. Upon exposure to a low pH environment (e.g., a tumor [75]), the nanoparticles swelled, resulting in release of paclitaxel, while little to no release was observed at physiological pH [74].

CATIONIC POLYMERS FOR INTRACELLULAR DRUG DELIVERY. Intracellular drug delivery presents a unique challenge, as the drug has to pass through the protective outer cell membrane and escape endosomal–lysosomal degradation. Cationic polymers currently used for intracellular delivery were initially investigated because of their ability to complex with negatively charged nucleic acid drugs such as DNA and siRNA, where they could mediate cellular uptake through electrostatic interactions with the negatively charged lipid bilayer. In addition to mediating complexation and uptake of negatively charged drugs, cationic polymers containing proton-accepting amine groups were found to facilitate endosomal release by osmotic disruption through the "proton sponge" effect. After endocytosis, acidification of endosomes occurs. By accepting protons, cationic polymers neutralize endosomes and inhibit the typical reduction in pH, resulting in a continued influx of protons and their counter ions (typically Cl^-). This causes the osmotic pressure inside the vesicle to increase, resulting in greater water influx, causing swelling and disruption of the endosomal membrane, and finally resulting in the release of endocytosed cargo. There are many examples of amine-containing "proton sponge" polymers, including poly(DMAEMA), poly(DEAEMA) (Fig. 12.5e), poly(ethylenenimine) (PEI, Fig. 12.5d), and PAMAM (Fig. 12.5f). These polymers generally contain a plethora of proton-accepting groups, including primary, secondary, and tertiary amines, to mediate the "proton sponge" activity.

PEI "proton sponge" polymers have been used to effectively deliver oligonu-cleotides [76, 77], plasmid DNA (pDNA) [78–80], Epstein–Barr virus-based plasmid vectors [81–85], as well as RNA, siRNA [86, 87], and intact ribozymes [88], both *in vitro* and *in vivo*. While the amine-rich structure of PEI generates its endoso-molytic activity, they are also exploited for electrostatically condensing drug cargo (nucleic acids or anionic proteins) and enhancing drug uptake. More recent work has also exploited PEI's primary amines to conjugate macromolecular drugs [89] and/or molecules that enhance endosomal escape or enable tissue-specific targeting [90–95].

Poly(amidoamine) (PAMAM) dendrimers (Fig. 12.5f) are particularly potent weak bases and proton sponges. Haensler and Szoka originally reported the use of PAMAM dendrimers for gene delivery [96]. Because of its relatively high gene delivery effi-ciency, PAMAM dendrimers have recently been used in several *in vivo* gene delivery studies [97–100]. Although they are remarkably potent with respect to intracellu-lar drug delivery both *in vitro* and *in vivo*, "proton sponge" polymers suffer from high levels of cytotoxicity, which has limited their translation into clinical use. See Table 12.3 for additional applications of these polymers.

12.3.2.3 pH-Responsive Linkers for Drug Delivery.
Another way to exploit pH for tissue-specific drug delivery is based on the use of acid-degradable chemical linkages. These linkages can control drug delivery in two ways. They can couple drug into cross-linked networks or to polymer chains, where degradation results in released drug; or they can used as part of cross-linkers within networks entrapping drug, and as the cross-links are degraded, drug is released, as depicted in Fig. 12.1. Many chemistries have been used for these applications, including ester, hydrazone, anhydride, acetal/ketal linkage, and orthoester linkages, as shown in Fig. 12.6. Generally, the rates of degradation of these linkers follows the order: anhydride > hydrazone > ketal > orthoester > acetal > ester [101, 102]. However, the degradation rate is also greatly impacted by the overall chemistry of the R-groups, depicted in Fig. 12.6

Polyesters are a great example of R-group-dependent degradation behavior. Ring-opening polymerization of cyclic lactones produces poly(ε-caprolactone), poly(lactic

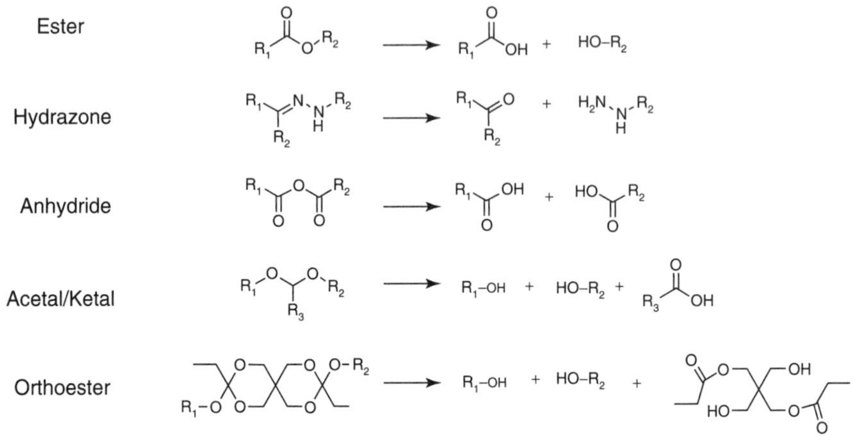

Figure 12.6. Acid-labile chemistries employed for pH-responsive drug delivery.

acid) (PLA), and poly(glycolic acid), commonly used biomedical materials. These polymers contain ester bonds. The degradation rate of the ester bond is highly dependent on the hydrophobicity of the R-group. As the hydrophobicity of the R-group increases, the rate of degradation of the ester dramatically decreases. For example, decreasing the hydrophobicity of R_1 from C_6H_{12} (caprolactone) to CH_2CH_3 (lactide) and even further to CH_2 (glycolide) causes an increase in the degradation rate and an associated decrease in the total degradation time. Typical times for complete degradation of poly(ε-caprolactone), PLA, and poly(glycolic acid) polymers are 2 years, 1 year, and 0.5 years, respectively [103]. These linkers are degradable at physiological pH. However, in environments that are more acidic, degradation rates increase dramatically. For example, the rate of hydrolysis of acetals is first-order relative to the concentration of the hydronium ion, and, therefore, per unit decrease in pH, the rate of hydrolysis increases by a factor of 10. The rate of hydrolysis also can be changed by modifying the structure of the acetal [104], which can be useful for controlling the point at which physiological hydrolysis occurs. Similarly, the rate of hydrolysis of orthoesters also increases with the hydronium ion concentration, but the relationship is not first-order with respect to time and is, therefore, more difficult to predict.

There are numerous examples of degradation as pH-responsive mechanisms for drug release. We will highlight a few here, and urge the reader to explore Table 12.3 and the literature described therein for more information. For example, nanoparticles were formulated with camptothecin, a chemotherapeutic drug, conjugated to short PEG chains via an ester bond. Camptothecin release was rapid at pH <5 or in the presence of an esterase, and was nonexistent over the same time period at physiological pH [105]. Likewise, a series of orthoester-containing model compounds were synthesized and observed to have different hydrolysis rates at pH s between 4.5 and 7.4 [106]. Drug–polymer conjugated nanoparticles containing the chemotherapeutic drug cisplatin were formed using hydrazone as a cross-linker to achieve low pH drug release. Cisplatin release occurred at pH <6 as a result of hydrazone hydrolysis.

Cisplatin release enhanced cellular cytotoxicity compared to the free drug because of more favorable uptake and intracellular degradation kinetics. A ketal-based pH-responsive drug delivery vehicle was developed, which was based on the polymer poly(1,4-phenyleneacetone dimethylene ketal) (PPADK). PPADK contains ketal linkages allowing acid-catalyzed hydrolysis of the polymer into low molecular-weight hydrophilic compounds. The release of drugs encapsulated into these cross-linked networks was highly dependent on environmental conditions, with acidic conditions greatly accelerating drug release [107].

12.4 REDUCTION/OXIDATION (REDOX)-RESPONSIVE POLYMERS

Redox reactions are characterized by the transfer of electrons between chemical species. As electrons are responsible for the formation of covalent bonds, this transfer of electrons simultaneously breaks existing bonds while generating new ones. Different regions of the body, and even different intracellular compartments, have different redox states. These properties of redox reactions make them an ideal target for a stimuli-responsive drug delivery system. For example, if a redox-responsive chemical group is utilized as a tether for a drug, it will be stable when the redox state is neutral, preventing premature release of drug. By choosing a linker that is sensitive to cleavage in the particular redox state in target tissue, drug release can be localized to that tissue.

12.4.1 Fundamentals of Redox-Responsive Drug Delivery

Before we delve into the specifics of redox responsive drug delivery, we will review the basics of redox reactions, explain how redox states are defined in biological systems, and discuss physiologically unique redox conditions that can be exploited for drug delivery.

12.4.1.1 Reduction–Oxidation (Redox) Reactions. Redox reactions occur when there is a transfer of electrons between atoms, ions, or molecules [108]. These reactions are split into two half-reactions: an oxidation and a reduction reaction. Oxidative reactions are characterized by the loss of electrons and an increase in charge and oxidative state of the atom, ion, or molecule. Reductive reactions, on the other hand, are characterized by the gain of electrons and a decrease in charge and oxidative state of the atom, ion, or molecule. For redox reactions to occur, the exchange of electrons between the two half-reactions must be conserved. Together, these two half-reactions are called a "redox pair."

Redox reactions can be simple, such as the reaction of hydrogen and fluorine:

$$H_2 + F_2 \rightarrow 2HF \tag{12.8}$$

$$H_2 \rightarrow 2H^+ + 2e^- \text{ Oxidative } 1/2 \text{ reaction} \tag{12.8a}$$

$$F_2 + 2e^- \rightarrow 2F^- \text{ Reductive } 1/2 \text{ reaction} \tag{12.8b}$$

Or they can be incredibly complex, requiring multiple series of electron-transfer reactions to reach completion, such as the oxidation of glucose in the human body:

$$C_6H_{12}O_6 + 6O_2 \rightarrow 6CO_2 + 6H_2O \tag{12.9}$$

$$C_6H_{12}O_6 + 3O_2 \rightarrow 6CO_2 + 6H_2O \text{ Oxidative 1/2 reaction} \tag{12.9a}$$

$$6H_2 + 3O_2 \rightarrow 6H_2O \text{ Reductive 1/2 reaction} \tag{12.9b}$$

12.4.1.2 Redox State in Biology. Biologically, redox state is used to describe the ratio of oxidized and reduced forms of redox pairs, such as NAD^+/NADH (the oxidized and reduced form of nicotinamide adenine dinucleotide, respectively) in biological reactions, as well as the state of an intracellular or extracellular environment [109]. The overall redox environment in biological fluids, organelles, cells, and tissues is the summation of the products of the reduction potential and reducing capacity of the linked redox couples of the redox pairs present in that biological environment:

$$\text{Overall Redox Environment} = \sum_{i=1}^{N} E_i \times [S]_i \tag{12.10}$$

where E_i is the half-cell reduction potential for pair i, $[S]_i$ is the concentration of reduced species in pair i, and N is the total number of pairs. Reduction potential is defined such that E_i is positive for oxidative agents and negative for reductive agents. Therefore, an overall redox environment that is positive will induce oxidation of the drug delivery system, and an overall redox environment that is negative will induce reduction of the drug delivery system.

12.4.1.3 Physiologically Unique Redox Conditions. Among the many physiological redox couples, glutathione (γ-glutamyl–cysteinyl–glycine; GSH) is most commonly exploited to trigger drug delivery. In this case, GSH/glutathione disulfide (GSSG) is the major redox couple. Glutathione concentration in cells is 50–10,000 μM and most of the cellular GSH (85–90%) exists in the cytosol with the rest present in organelles, such as the nucleus and mitochondria. Conveniently, extracellular concentrations of GSH are relatively low, between 2 and 20 μM. Because of its cysteine residue, GSH is easily oxidized by free radicals and reactive oxygen/nitrogen species, and is converted into GSSG. GSSG is then removed from cells by efflux pumps, resulting in a net loss of intracellular GSH. The ratio of GSH to GSSG is often used to indicate the cellular redox state and is typically greater than 10 under normal physiological conditions but can be as high as 1000 in cancer cells. This causes an overall reduced intracellular environment, which can be exploited for drug delivery. Although GSH/GSSG is the major redox couple determining the redox state of cells, the intracellular level of GSH is also dependent on other redox couples within cells, including $NADH/NAD^+$, $NADPH/NADP^+$, etc. [110, 111].

Oxidative environments are commonly associated with inflammation. Inflammation is a common comorbidity in pathological processes such as cancer, rheumatoid arthritis, and atherosclerosis. Inflammation is mediated through cellular increase in peroxide and nitric oxide, as well as through the production of reactive oxygen and nitrogen species that are released extracellularly and produce a locally oxidative environment. Many inflammatory cells including neutrophils, dendritic cells, macrophages, eosinophils, and mast cells produce these reactive species.

12.4.2 Redox-Responsive Polymers and their Applications in Drug Delivery

A number of redox-responsive polymers have been developed for drug delivery applications (see Fig. 12.7). These compositions can be divided into oxidative-responsive and reductive-responsive polymer categories. Redox-responsive polymers have been used in many devices to control the delivery of a huge variety of drugs. Some interesting applications are compiled in Table 12.4 and a few will be reviewed here.

12.4.2.1 Oxidative-Responsive Drug Delivery Mechanisms and Applications. For oxidative-responsive drug delivery, limited chemistries have been

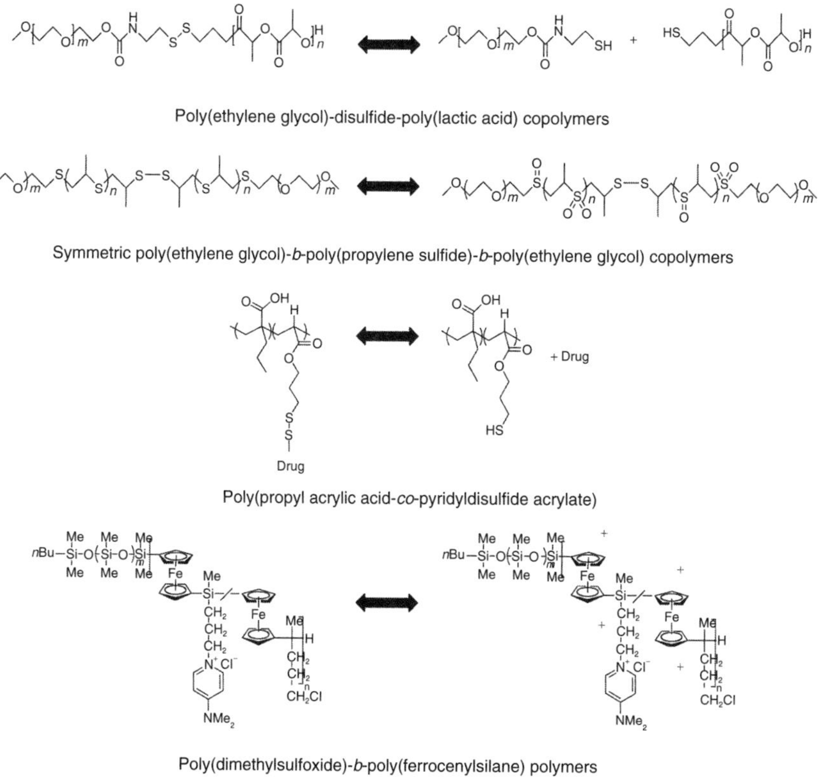

Poly(ethylene glycol)-disulfide-poly(lactic acid) copolymers

Symmetric poly(ethylene glycol)-b-poly(propylene sulfide)-b-poly(ethylene glycol) copolymers

Poly(propyl acrylic acid-co-pyridyldisulfide acrylate)

Poly(dimethylsulfoxide)-b-poly(ferrocenylsilane) polymers

Figure 12.7. Selected redox-responsive polymers for drug delivery

TABLE 12.4. Examples of Applications of Redox-Responsive Polymers in Drug delivery

Class	Polymer composition	Drug delivered	Device utilized	Discussion	References
Oxidative responsive polymers	Poly(ethylene glycol)-*b*-poly(propylene sulfide)-*b*-poly(ethylene glycol)	Hypothetical	Vesicles	Block copolymers self-assemble into unilamellar vesicles. Under oxidative conditions, poly(porpylene sulfide) is converted to poly(propylene sulfonoxide) and ultimately poly(propylene sulfone). This was the first example of polymer carriers that destabilize due to an oxidative environment	112–114
	Poly(ethylene glycol)-*b*-poly(propylene sulfide)-*b*-poly(ethyleneimine)	Plasmid DNA	Micelles	Carriers successfully transfected melanoma cells *in vitro* and when delivering a plasmid coding for an antigen, tumor growth was reduced *in vivo*	115
	Poly(ethylene glycol)-*co*-poly(propylene sulfide) block copolymers	Cyclosporin A	Micelles	Drug solubility was increased up to 2 mg ml^{-1}, with loading levels up to 19% w/w achieved. Release was burst-free and sustained for 9–12 days	116
	Poly(dimethylsiloxane-*b*-ferrocenylsilane)	Hypothetical	Vesicles	The diblock copolymer formed nanoscale vesicular aggregates upon direct dissolution in water. These structures can be reversibly opened and reformed by sequential oxidation and reduction of the ferrocene units, thus vesicles may provide access to aggregate structures with redox-tunable drug encapsulation properties	117
Reductive responsive polymers	Poly(ethylene glycol)-SS-poly(lactic acid)	Paclitaxel (PTX)	Nanoparticles	Loading of PTX and formation of nanoparticles was performed using an O/W emulsion/solvent evaporation technique. PTX release from nanoparticles was sensitive to glutathione concentrations. Moreover, cancer cell lines were demonstrated to uptake the carriers, resulting in uniform intracellular distributions	118

Material	Payload	Form	Description	Ref.
poly(ethylene glycol acrylate)	siRNA	Drug conjugates	A straightforward synthetic method to prepare pyridyl disulfide end functionalized poly(PEG acrylate) by RAFT polymerization for efficient and reversible conjugation to siRNA was developed	119
Disulfide-linked peptide + poly(hydroxypropyl methacrylamide)-pH-responsive polymers	Pro-apoptotic peptide	Drug conjugates	Thiol-disulfide exchange reactions efficiently produced reversible polymer conjugates. Microscopy showed that peptide delivered via polymer conjugates significantly enhanced the apoptotic activity of peptide alone	65
Disulfide-linked protein with poly(propylacrylic acid-*co*-pyridyldisulfide acrylate)	Ovalbumin (model antigen)	Drug conjugates	Disulfide reduction resulted in cytosolic ovalbumin release from the polymer through GSH action. This occurred after endosomal escape via poly(propylacrylic acid) pH-responsive action, resulting in enhanced major histocompatibility complex-1 presentation. In a follow-up study, vaccine efficacy of this approach was demonstrated *in vivo*	63, 120
Poly(ethylene glycol)-modified thiolated gelatin	Plasmid DNA	Nanoparticles	Intracellular DNA delivery in response to glutathione concentration mediates enhanced gene transfection in breast cancer cells in an *in vivo* tumor model	121
Hyperbranched multiarm copolyphosphates (HPHSEP-star-PEPx)	Doxorubicin	Micelles	Disulfide linked dendrimers consisting of polyphosphates were self-assembled into doxorubicin-loaded spherical micelles. Upon treatment with the micelles, cervical carcinoma cell proliferation was inhibited. This effect was diminished upon pretreatment with a drug that abolishes the reducing environment of the cells	122

explored. The most prominent examples are polymers containing poly(propylene sulfide) (PPS). This chemistry, pioneered by Hubbell and coworkers [112, 115, 123–125], incorporates sulfide groups into a polymer backbone (Fig. 12.7). When these polymers encounter an oxidative environment, the sulfide becomes oxidized, first to a sulfonoxide and then further to a sulfone group. As this reaction progresses, the polymer undergoes a hydrophobic to hydrophilic transition similar to the phase transition behavior of temperature-responsive polymers (see Section 12.2.1). PPS segments of block copolymers are commonly utilized as the interior region of vesicles, micelles, or nanoparticles. Their reactive chemistry allows the drug carrier to be oxidized, resulting in carrier disintegration and release of the encapsulated drug. This behavior can be modified through changes in PPS molecular weight, copolymer incorporation, and hydrophilic corona composition.

PPS carriers have been used to deliver a variety of drugs including proteins and small-molecule drugs [112, 123, 124]. For example, cationic micelles formed from poly(ethylene glycol)-*b*-PPS-*b*-poly(ethyleneimine) (PEG–PPS–PEI) and from mixed micelle structures composed of mixtures PEG-*b*-PPS and PEG–PPS–PEI were explored as nonviral vectors for pDNA. Both formulations effectively transfected melanoma cells *in vitro*. To test efficacy *in vivo*, tumors were transfected with a gene that would result in tumor cell death mediated through host immune responses. A reduction in tumor growth, increase in intratumoral infiltration of cytotoxic T lymphocytes, and accumulation of inflammatory cytokines indicated that both micelle formulations mediated high pDNA delivery compared with naked pDNA. Moreover, these carriers were noncytotoxic [115]. Using similar formulations, drug encapsulation was explored in AB block copolymers PEG-*b*-PPS, using the immunosuppressive drug cyclosporin A (CsA) as an example of a highly hydrophobic drug. Block copolymers with a DP of 44 on the PEG and of 10, 20, and 40 on the PPS, respectively (abbreviated as PEG44-b-PPS10, PEG44-b-PPS20, PEG44-b-PPS40) were synthesized and characterized. Drug-loaded polymeric micelles were obtained by the cosolvent displacement method, with drug solubility up to 2 mg ml^{-1} and loading levels up to 19% w/w achieved. Release was burst-free and sustained over periods of 9–12 days [125].

Recently, another polymer chemistry, which exploits the oxidation of ferrocene groups, has emerged. This development is based on previous work [126], where ferrocene-based surfactants were observed to be reversibly opened and reformed by sequential oxidation and reduction of ferrocene units. Poly(dimethylsulfoxide)-*b*-poly(ferrocenylsilane) (PFS) polymers [117, 127] (Fig. 12.7) were synthesized. These polymers were formed into vesicles and examined for their ability to respond to oxidative environments. Reversible oxidation of the ferrocene units in the PFS block was demonstrated, highlighting their possible use for oxidation-controlled drug delivery. However, no specific drug delivery applications for this new class of polymers have been reported.

12.4.2.2 *Reductive-Responsive Drug Delivery Mechanisms and Applications.* Reductive-responsive drug delivery polymers typically respond to intracellularly elevated glutathione levels through reduction of disulfide linkages.

There are a number of ways to exploit this responsive behavior: the release of drugs conjugated to polymer carries via disulfide tethers, the release of drug via disruption of disulfide linkages acting as hydrogel cross-linkers, or the disruption of micelle or nanoparticle stabilizing disulfide bonds to release encapsulated drug. These generalized approaches are highlighted in Fig. 12.1.

As detailed in Table 12.4 [63, 118–122, 128], a variety of drugs have been delivered using disulfide reduction mechanisms including plasmid DNA, siRNA, peptides, proteins, and small-molecule drugs. Interestingly, many of these applications incorporate an additional type of responsive chemistry into the system. This second responsive chemistry is often used to mediate delivery. Chemistries that mediate endosomal escape, for example, are often integrated, as the carriers are primarily taken into cells via endosomes because of their molecular weight and size. Incorporation of this second chemistry ensures that the delivery system will reach the cytosol where the reductive environment will mediate release of the drug. For example, polymers composed of PEG and PLA linked with disulfides were synthesized. Loading of paclitaxel (PTX) and formation of nanoparticles was achieved using an oil/water (O/W) emulsion/solvent evaporation technique. At extracellular GSH concentrations or in the absence of GSH altogether, PTX release was only 40% but increased to almost 90% over 4 days when GSH was increased to typical cytosolic concentrations. *In vitro* cellular uptake and intracellular distribution of PTX-loaded nanoparticles was shown to be homogeneous within three different cancer cell lines [118].

Therapeutic, intracellular delivery of proapoptotic peptides has also been achieved using glutathione-responsive polymers. These applications have additional delivery system requirements, namely enhanced solubility and ability to escape endosomal trafficking. In one example, polymers were composed of an *N*-(2-hydroxypropyl) methacrylamide (HPMA) first block which was intended to enhance water solubility. The second polymer block, consisting of equimolar quantities of DMAEMA, PAA, and butyl methacrylate (BMA), was a pH-responsive composition designed to enhance endosomal escape. The polymer contained a pyridyl disulfide end-functionalization, allowing easy incorporation of the proapoptotic peptide, which was designed to include both a cysteine (the amino acid that bears a thiol R-group) and a cell-internalization peptide sequence. Microscopy studies showed that peptide delivered via polymer conjugates effectively escaped endosomes and achieved diffusion into the cytosol. Peptide–polymer conjugates also produced significantly increased apoptotic activity over peptide alone in HeLa cervical carcinoma cells, highlighting the intracellular delivery and efficacy of the proapoptotic peptide [65].

12.5 ENZYMATICALLY RESPONSIVE DRUG DELIVERY

Enzymes are proteins that catalyze biochemical reactions, including reactions occurring within the body. Enzymes convert substrates into products by reducing the activation energy (E_a) required for the chemical reaction to proceed. By lowering E_a, enzymes increase the likelihood that a reaction will occur, increasing the reaction rate and overall conversion of reactant to products. Enzymes are highly specific in their action, often interacting with only one or a few substrates to mediate very specific reactions. Moreover, enzymes are not consumed by reactions, so they may continue to act upon substrates if the proper conditions exist. These properties make their use as a drug delivery/drug release mechanism highly desirable. Imagine using an enzyme-sensitive linker to tether a drug to a stable carrier material. The linker will be stable when the enzyme is absent, preventing premature release of the drug; and by choosing a linker that is sensitive to an enzyme overexpressed, or only expressed, in target tissue, drug release can be localized specifically to that tissue. Before we delve into the specifics of enzymatically responsive drug delivery, let us first review enzyme kinetics and discuss some enzymes commonly found in the body [129].

12.5.1   Fundamentals of Enzyme Kinetics

In order to fully understand how enzyme–substrate interactions can be manipulated for controlled drug delivery, we must first understand the basics of enzyme kinetics. In order for an enzyme (E) to convert a substrate (S) into a product (P), the enzyme and substrate must bind; the substrate is then converted to product by the enzyme; and finally, the product is released by the enzyme, as illustrated in Fig. 12.8.

Figure 12.8 also illustrates the mechanism by which enzyme specificity occurs: the "lock and key" mechanism. Each enzyme has an active site (lock) to which substrates of proper conformation (key) must bind to in order to undergo a change in chemical structure. This helps to maintain specificity of the enzymes: only specific substrates with the proper conformation will be able to bind to the lock and undergo enzymatic conversion into product. In Fig. 12.8, for example, a circular substrate would not be converted to product, as it would not properly fit in the triangular lock.

In enzyme kinetics, the Michaelis–Menten model assumes that, after being released from the enzyme, the product rarely rebinds with the enzyme, as it is very atypical for an enzyme to catalyze both forward and reverse biological reactions.

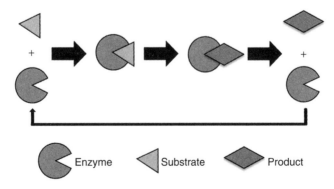

Figure 12.8. Lock and key mechanism of enzyme reactions.

This allows this process to be described as:

$$E + S \underset{k_{-1}}{\overset{k_1}{\rightleftharpoons}} ES \xrightarrow{k_{cat}} E + P \tag{12.11}$$

where k_1, k_{-1}, and k_{cat} are the rate constants for the formation of the ES complex from E and S, the breakdown of the ES complex into separate E and S, and the formation of E and P from the ES complex, respectively. The reaction velocity and rate of product formation, V, is therefore determined by:

$$V = k_{cat}[ES] \tag{12.12}$$

where [ES] is the concentration of the enzyme–substrate complex. By using the Briggs–Haldane assumption that at steady state the change in [ES] with respect to time is zero, the Michaelis–Menten equation can be derived as

$$V = \frac{V_{max}[S]}{K_m + [S]} \tag{12.13}$$

where [S] is the concentration of the substrate, V_{max} is the maximum velocity of the reaction, and K_m is the Michaelis constant. In terms of the previously used variables and the initial enzyme concentration $[E_0]$:

$$V_{max} = k_{cat}[E_0] \tag{12.14}$$

$$K_m = \frac{k_{-1} + k_{cat}}{k_1} \tag{12.15}$$

These equations are commonly used to describe the kinetics of enzyme–substrate interactions and provide valuable insight into these reactions.

A typical Michaelis–Menten plot of enzyme kinetics is shown in Fig. 12.9. Let us pause for a minute and check that this equation makes sense with our theoretical understanding of enzyme reactions. At low concentrations of substrate, when excess enzyme is present, we would expect the reaction speed to be largely dependent on substrate concentration. At low concentrations of S, K_m dominates the denominator, and the equation reduces to $V = \frac{V_{max}}{K_m}[S]$, which is linearly dependent on [S]. When there is an excessive amount of substrate present, we expect the reaction to proceed very quickly, where the speed would depend on the amount of enzyme present. For high values of [S], [S] dominates the denominator, and the Michaelis–Menten equation reduces to $V = V_{max} = k_{cat}[E_0]$, consistent with our expectations.

In order to compare the efficiencies of different enzymes, the specificity constant $\frac{K_{cat}}{K_m}$ is often used. The specificity constant is the rate constant for the conversion of E + S to E + P, and higher values indicate a more efficient enzyme. The upper limit for $\frac{K_{cat}}{K_m}$ values is between 10^8 and 10^9 M^{-1} s^{-1}, the rate at which substrate can diffuse toward and product can diffuse away from the enzyme. In designing an enzyme-responsive drug delivery system, controlling the specificity constant is one

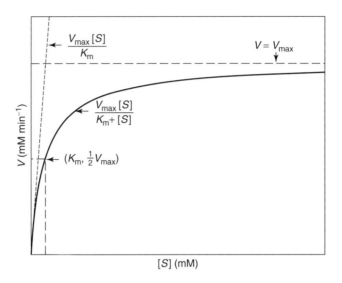

Figure 12.9. Michaelis–Menten plot of enzyme kinetics

aspect of the system that can be manipulated in order to achieve ideal drug delivery profiles and concentrations [129, 130].

12.5.2   Common Enzymes

A multitude of enzymes are produced by the body and each has a specific function. To identify the thousands of enzymes that are currently known, an international standard exists, which classifies them on the basis of the reaction they catalyze. This classification system is provided in Table 12.5, and the reader is directed to standard biochemistry text books, such as Reference 130, for additional information. While a complex system for numerically identifying enzymes exists, many enzymes are best known by their common names, which often give information regarding their function. Collagenase, for example, is an enzyme responsible for the hydrolytic cleavage of collagen, the main component of the human body's extracellular matrix. The substrate this enzyme acts on (collagen) is indicated, while the suffix "-ase" indicates it is an enzyme. However, other common names do not illustrate the enzyme's function. Renin, for example, is responsible for the hydrolytic cleavage of angiotensinogen, a hormone involved in blood pressure regulation.

As each enzyme has a specific chemical reaction it catalyzes, it is understandable that many enzymes are found performing specific functions within particular tissues. This can be exploited for the design of enzymatically responsive drug delivery systems: by choosing a drug tether that is degraded by an enzyme most highly concentrated in the target tissue, drug release can be localized to that tissue, reducing wasted drug and undesirable off-target side effects.

TABLE 12.5. International Enzyme Classification System

Class number	Class name	Reaction catalyzed
1	Oxioreductase	Catalyze reactions where one molecule is oxidized while another is reduced
2	Transferase	Catalyze the transfer of a functional group from one molecule to another
3	Hydrolase	Catalyze hydrolytic cleavage of a molecule
4	Lyase	Catalyze reactions either adding functional groups to double bonds, or forming new double bonds by removing functional groups
5	Isomerase	Catalyze the rearrangement of bonds within a single molecule
6	Ligase	Catalyze the joining of two molecules by forming a new bond

As listed in Table 12.6, there are numerous enzymes present in the body. This table is by no means complete; a diverse population of enzymes is present in the body, and a full list of these enzymes is well beyond the scope of this chapter. When designing an enzymatically responsive drug delivery system, it is important to remember that one organ/tissue will have multiple enzymes present in it at any given time. Additionally, as is illustrated with the case of procarboxypeptidases A and B, enzymes are often present in multiple locations within the body. Therefore, the relative amount of the enzyme in both the target tissue and nontarget areas of the body is of critical importance when choosing an enzyme to mediate drug release.

Enzyme levels are also dependent upon tissue homeostasis. Enzyme presence and/or activity is often altered during disease progression; enzymes typically present in a tissue can be over- or underexpressed. For example, while cathespin K is involved in healthy bone remodeling, its expression is drastically increased in osteoclastomas (bone cancer) [135]. Additionally, enzymes not usually expressed in the tissue can become highly expressed in diseased tissue. For example, enzymes produced in the pancreas, such as amylase, are usually not converted into their active form until they have been transported to the small intestine. In pancreatitis, however, pancreatic enzymes are prematurely activated, causing pain and inflammation [136]. This provides a unique opportunity to specifically target diseased areas of an organ/tissue. Table 12.7 illustrates this principle. As with Table 12.6, this is by no means an exhaustive list and mainly focuses on diseases that are associated with increases in enzymatic activity, as increases (rather than decreases) in local enzyme levels hold the key to enzymatically responsive drug delivery.

As can be seen in Table 12.7, matrix metalloproteinases (MMPs) are involved in numerous diseases, and are particularly important in cancer progression. These enzymes are responsible for degrading the components of the extracellular matrix, and are critically important in tumor invasion and cancer metastases. As is illustrated in Table 12.7, an increase in enzymatic activity is not always restricted to the location

TABLE 12.6. Examples of Tissue-Specific Enzymes in the Body

Organ system	Local enzyme
Mouth	Lingual lipase: Hydrolyzes triglycerides into diglycerides and free fatty acids
	Salivary amylase: Hydrolyzes carbohydrate chains [131]
Stomach	Pepsin: Hydrolytically cleaves peptides at bonds on the amino side of phenylalanine, tryptophan, and tyrosine amino acids
	Trypsin: Hydrolytically cleaves peptides on the carboxy side of lysine and arginine amino acids
	Chymotrypsin: Hydrolytically cleaves peptides on the carboxy side of phenylalanine, tryptophan and tyrosine amino acids [130, 132]
Small Intestine	Procarboxypeptidase A: Removes amino acids from the carboxy end of a peptide
	Procarboxypeptidase B: Removes arginine or lysine amino acids from the carboxy end of a peptide [132, 133]
Colon	Dextranase: Hydrolytically degrade glucosidic linkages in dexetran
	Glycosidase: Hydrolytically degrade glycosidic linkages in sugars [134]
Liver	L-glutamate dehydrogenase: Removes an amine group from an amino acid by an oxidative reaction
	Alkaline phosphatase: Hydrolytically dephosphorylates nucleotides, proteins, and alkaloids [132]
Pancreas	Trypsin: Hydrolytically cleaves peptides on the carboxy side of lysine and arginine amino acids
	Chymotrypsin: Hydrolytically cleaves peptides on the carboxy side of phenylalanine, tryptophan and tyrosine amino acids
	Elastase: Cleaves peptides after alanine, glycine and serine amino acids
	Procarboxypeptidase A: Removes amino acids from the carboxy end of a peptide
	Procarbozypeptidase B: Removes arginine or lysine amino acids from the carboxy end of a peptide
	Pancreatic lipase: A variety of lipases are produced by the pancreas; all hydrolyze fat
	Pancreatic α-amylase: Hydrolytically cleaves starches at interior glucose linkages [134]
Bone	Alkaline phosphatase: Hydrolytically dephosphorylates nucleotides, proteins and alkaloids
	Cathepsin K: Hydrolytically cleaves peptide bonds in extracellular matrix molecules such as collagen and elastin [135]

of the diseased tissue. While pancreatitis is a disease characterized by localized inflammation of the pancreas, the increase in enzymatic activity is not exclusively localized to the pancreas. Enzyme levels in the blood are often also increased as a side effect of increased enzyme production in the diseased tissue. This table also illustrates another complicating factor in the use of enzymatically responsive drug delivery: enzymes are not always increased to the same extent for the full duration of the disease. Consider

TABLE 12.7. Changes in Enzymatic Activity in Specific Disease States

Disease state	Change in enzyme levels
Cancer	
Bone	Cathespin K levels are significantly increased in osteoclastomas [135]
Breast	Blood levels of amylase are increased. MT-MMP levels are increased at the tumor site [136, 137]
Colon	Blood levels of amylase are increased. MMP-2 levels are increased at the tumor site [136]
Leukemia	Blood levels of alkaline phosphatase are increased [138]
Liver	Blood levels of lipase are increased [136]
Lung	Blood levels of amylase are increased. MT-MMP levels are increased at the tumor site [136, 137]
Ovarian	Blood levels of amylase are increased [136]
Wound healing	A variety of MMPs are involved in wound healing. Collagenase (MMP-1) expression peaks 1 day after wounding, while gelatinase levels peak 5–7 days after wounding [139]
Ischemia	Gelatinases (MMP-2 and 9) are increased 3–14 days after onset of ischemic conditions, and MT1-MMP expression is increased for 30 days after onset of ischemia [140]
Pancreatitis	A blockage in the pancreatic secretion pathway causes enzymes produced in the pancreas to accumulate and activate. Amylase and lipase levels are elevated more than threefold both in the pancreas and in the blood [136]
Diabetic ketoacidosis	In addition to the typical increase in blood glucose levels seen with diabetes, this disease also exhibits increases in blood lipase and amylase levels [136]

the increase in MMP activity in ischemic tissue, resulting from reduced oxygen supply. MMP-2 and -9 both are overexpressed in response to ischemia. This increase in expression is highest 3 days after the initiation of ischemia and slowly decreases over the next 11 days. MT1-MMP expression, however, is increased at relatively constant levels for a full 30 days after onset of ischemia [140]. It is important to consider both the spatial and temporal changes in enzyme expression when designing an enzymatically responsive drug delivery system: if the drug-releasing enzyme is present in the target tissue at low levels only for a short period, the drug will be released from the carrier at low levels only for a short period of time.

12.5.3 Design Considerations and Applications Within Drug Delivery

The unique behavior of enzymes and their spatial distribution in the body, especially in response to various disease states, have been exploited in a variety of enzyme-responsive drug delivery applications. We will discuss factors that should be considered in the design of such responsive drug delivery systems and will apply these design considerations to real-life applications by discussing five enzymatically responsive drug delivery systems. These systems are summarized in Table 12.8.

12.5.3.1 Enzyme Specificity.

12.5.3.1 Enzyme Specificity. The enzyme should be localized to the target tissue, with no (or significantly reduced) expression in other off-target tissues. There should be an appreciable concentration of the enzyme in the tissue, and it should be expressed for a therapeutically relevant duration. For example, targeting drugs specifically to the colon is useful both to treat colon diseases (Crohn's disease, colon cancer, etc.) and to maintain stability of the drug as it passes through the digestive system. Hovgaard et al. [144] developed an enzymatically responsive material to deliver drugs to the colon using a dextran carrier (Table 12.8). As dextranase is present in the colon, but not in previous stages of the digestive system, the dextran network remains stable and the drug remains protected as it passes through the stomach and small intestine. Once the network reaches the colon, dextranase cleaves the dextran molecules, releasing the encapsulated anti-inflammatory drug hydrocortisone specifically into colon tissue.

12.5.3.2 Enzyme Accessibility.

12.5.3.2 Enzyme Accessibility. The accessibility of the enzyme also needs to be considered: if the enzyme is expressed only within the cytosol, but the delivery vehicle is not able to be internalized by the cell, the drug will never be released from the vehicle because the enzyme will never interact with the target. Sakiyama-Elbert et al. [123] incorporated β-nerve growth factor (β-NGF) into fibrin matrices via a plasmin-sensitive tether to generate tissue-engineered constructs for peripheral nerve regeneration. This tether was chosen because plasmin is secreted by neural cells as they invade the fibrin-based tissue-engineered matrix, causing a cell/enzyme-dictated release of the conjugated growth factor [143].

12.5.3.3 Enzyme Classification.

12.5.3.3 Enzyme Classification. The type/classification of enzyme should also be considered (Table 12.5). It would be inadvisable, for example, to try and use a ligase (class 6) to release drug from a network: ligases catalyze the joining of two molecules into a single molecule and would not be effective at cleaving a bond to mediate drug release. Generally, hydrolases and lyases are the most common choice of enzyme type/classification to mediate drug release.

12.5.3.4 Ease of Synthesis.

12.5.3.4 Ease of Synthesis. Practical considerations regarding synthesis of the enzymatically degradable drug conjugate are also important. As is implied by the information presented in Table 12.6, enzymes are able to react with a variety of different targets, including proteins/peptides, sugars, extracellular matrix molecules, single-stranded DNA, and even specific chemical groups. Thus, there can be many options for degradable target chemistries depending upon the enzyme chosen to mediate drug release. To implement the drug delivery system, the drug and degradable target must be simply and efficiently incorporated with the carrier material. While the specific chemistry required to incorporate each tether is unique, "click" chemistries are a popular choice in generating this linkage. Click chemistry does not refer to any

TABLE 12.8. Enzymatically Responsive Drug Delivery Systems. ↓ Indicates the Site of Cleavage, if Specified

Enzyme to trigger release	Enzymatically degradable substrate	Release mechanism	Carrier	Drug	Tissue targeted/disease	References
α-chymotrypsin	GG peptide	Tether	N-(2-hydroxypropyl) methacrylamide copolymer	Procainamide	Postmyocardial infarction cardiac tissue/Arrhythmia	141
Human neutrophil elastase	YAPPG↓VGCG peptide	Tether	PEG–hydrogel	Theoretical	Any/Inflammation and wound healing	142
Plasmin	NIL↓MKP peptide	Tether	Fibrin	β-nerve growth factor	Peripheral nerve/Peripheral nerve damage	143
Dextranase	Glucosidic linkages	Linker	Dextran	Hydrocortisone	Colon/Chron's and other inflammatory diseases	144
α-amylase	Cyclodextrin	Linker (Cap)	Silica nanoparticle	Calcein	Pancreas/Acute pancreatitis	145
Cathepsin B	GFLG and GLG	Tether and Linker	PEG–hydrogel	Doxorubicin	Tumor site/Cancer	146

specific reaction, rather it refers to a reaction that is stereospecific, produces a stable product, results in high yield, produces biocompatible side products, has large driving forces, and can be easily used in numerous applications. One such chemistry is the reaction between alkyne groups and azide derivatives [147]; another is the reaction between alkene groups and thiol functionalities [148]. Choosing an enzymatically degradable target that can efficiently be integrated with the carrier material is critical for the ultimate success of the drug delivery system.

12.5.3.5 Target Specificity.
Many substrates are responsive to multiple enzymes, with varying efficiencies for each enzyme. Design of a target sequence that is responsive to multiple enzymes in the target tissue will result in an increased release rate, which may or may not be desirable depending on the application. However, this will also decrease the specificity with which the drug is released.

12.5.3.6 Enzyme Kinetics.
Reaction efficiencies can be compared by looking at the specificity constant for the enzyme–substrate system. Controlling the efficiency of this interaction is one method to modulate the release profile of a drug. Often, the substrate (the linker chemistry) can be modified slightly to control the rate at which it is cleaved by an enzyme. Aimetti et al. [142] developed a PEG-based enzymatically responsive drug delivery system to treat inflammation. A human neutrophil elastase (HNE) sensitive peptide tether was used, as HNE is overexpressed by neutrophils in an inflammatory environment, making the cleavage of the tether specific to disease or injury. While no drug was released in this study, the authors showed that the rate of tether cleavage could be controlled by modifying the amino acids immediately adjacent to the cleavage site, illustrating the highly tunable nature of enzymatically responsive delivery systems.

12.5.3.7 Drug Release Mechanisms.
There are two release mechanisms used in enzymatically responsive drug delivery: drug conjugation (Fig. 12.1a and b) where drug is tethered to a carrier by a responsive linker; and drug encapsulation, where drugs are trapped within an enzymatically degradable carrier (Fig. 12.1c and d).

In this first mechanism (Fig. 12.1 a and b), the drug is physically conjugated to a carrier by a degradable tether. This carrier can be one of the many drug delivery vehicles discussed throughout this book, including hydrogels, nanoparticles, linear or branched/dendrimer polymers, micelles, etc. When the drug–carrier complex comes into contact with the enzyme, the enzyme interacts with the tether and cleaves the drug from the carrier. This allows the drug to diffuse away from the carrier into nearby tissue. In the bulk material version of this delivery system (Fig. 12.1a), it is critical that the enzyme be able to reach all areas of the carrier that contain drug. This is ensured by coating the surface of the carrier with tethered drug, or by choosing a carrier that has sufficient porosity so that the enzyme is able to enter the carrier and release the internally bound drug. It is important to remember that, except in the cases of very specific chemistries, there will be a residual part of the tether remaining on the drug. The amino acid sequence IPVS↓LRSG, for example, is cleaved by MMP-2 at the "↓" between the serine (S) and leucine (L) [149]. If this amino acid sequence were used to create a MMP-2-degradable tether to release a peptide drug from a hydrogel network, the drug would have four additional amino acids on the end after release (either LRSG-Drug or Drug-IPVS). The presence of these residual amino acids may have an impact on the bioactivity of the drug, and should be considered when designing the release system.

For the second mechanism (Fig. 12.1c and d), the drug is entrapped within a three-dimensional carrier which can be degraded by the enzyme. Again, the carrier can be a hydrogel, nanoparticle, micelle, etc., but in this mechanism the drug is not tethered to the network but is instead physically entrapped. When the drug–carrier network comes into contact with the enzyme, the enzyme interacts with the linker and degrades the biomaterial. This releases the drug from the carrier network. In this delivery system, the relative sizes of the encapsulated drug and the enzyme are important. The encapsulated drug must be large enough so that the porosity of the carrier network does not allow it to freely diffuse out, bypassing the responsive aspect of the system entirely. If the enzyme is large compared to the network mesh size, the material will undergo surface degradation, as the enzyme will not be able to penetrate the network. However, if the enzyme is sufficiently small, and is able to diffuse freely through the network, bulk degradation of the network will occur. The drug release profile achieved depends on whether the network undergoes surface or bulk degradation; therefore, this is of critical importance when designing the system. Compared to the tethered delivery system, the drug in this second configuration is released in its original form, with no residual tether affecting its efficacy.

An interesting variation on this second release mechanism was developed by Park et al. [145]. They developed silica nanoparticles with porous channels which could be loaded with a "guest molecule" (drug). The porous channels are capped with a cyclodextrin gatekeeper, which prevents release of the guest molecule until the cyclodextrin is hydrolyzed by α-amylase. While the 2009 study released calcein (a fluorescent molecule) as a model of drug release, the delivery system could easily be adapted to deliver similarly sized therapeutic molecules.

Pechar et al. [146] developed a particularly interesting enzymatically responsive drug delivery system which integrates both drug conjugation and degradation of the carrier material. They used a carrier in which PEG molecules were linked by enzymatically degradable GLG peptide linkers. They then tethered the anticancer drug doxorubicin to the carrier via an enzymatically degradable GFLG linker. Both linkers are susceptible to nonspecific hydrolysis by enzymes such as cathepsin B, but the differences in their length and amino acid sequence cause them to have different enzyme kinetics. As the cleavage of the drug from the PEG carrier occurs at a significantly faster rate than the cleavage of the inter-PEG linkers, the drug is released from the carrier before the carrier molecule is degraded and becomes small enough to be cleared by the kidney.

12.5.3.8 Carrier Choice.
The final aspect of enzyme-responsive drug delivery systems that must be taken into account is the choice of carrier itself. As previously mentioned, many of the traditional drug delivery systems can be modified for use as an enzymatically responsive delivery system. These systems can be composed of a variety

of polymers, both synthetic and natural, in a variety of formats including hydrogels, nanoparticles, micelles, and soluble structures. The choice of the appropriate carrier material should be carefully considered. Refer to previous chapters regarding the benefits, draw backs, and design considerations for possible carrier materials.

12.5.4 Example Problem: Enzymatically Responsive Drug Delivery

You are investigating the use of the peptide sequence GPQG↓IWGQ as a degradable tether for a new drug delivery system. You suspect that it is degradable to MMP-1, but are unsure about its efficiency. Using a constant concentration of MMP-1 (1 mM), you vary the concentration of peptide in solution and measure the velocity with which the enzyme cleaves the peptide sequence. Determine the K_m, K_{cat}, and the specificity constant for the peptide sequence and MMP-1.

[S], mM	V, mM s^{-1}
1000	5.00
100	4.00
20	2.85
10	2.38
5	1.82
3	1.00
2	0.70

While one could determine the values of V_{max} and K_m by using the regular Michaelis–Menten equation (Eq. 12.13), it is much easier to determine these experimentally relevant values from a Lineweaver–Burke plot. This plot is a double-reciprocal plot of the Michaelis–Menten equation, and is defined by the Lineweaver–Burke equation:

$$\frac{1}{V} = \frac{K_m}{V_{max}[S]} + \frac{1}{V_{max}} \tag{12.16}$$

By plotting $\frac{1}{V}$ versus $\frac{1}{[S]}$ a linear graph is obtained which has a slope of $\frac{K_m}{V_{max}}$, a y-intercept of $\frac{1}{V_{max}}$, and an x-intercept of $-\frac{1}{K_m}$. This allows the experimentally relevant values of V_{max} and K_m to be determined without performing complicated nonlinear regression, as would be required with the standard Michaelis–Menten form of the equation. Additionally, the value of V_{max} obtained from the Lineweaver–Burke plot is significantly more accurate, because in the Michaelis–Menten plot this value has to be estimated on the basis of the apparent asymptote of the data trend, and therefore can only be approximated. For our data, we can generate the plot shown in Fig. 12.10. As is shown by our best-fit line and Eq. 12.16, $\frac{K_m}{V_{max}} = 2.40$ $secs$ and $\frac{1}{V_{max}} = 0.19$ s mM^{-1}. Therefore, we can calculate $V_{max} = \frac{1}{0.19 \text{ s mM}^{-1}} = 5.26$ mM s^{-1} and

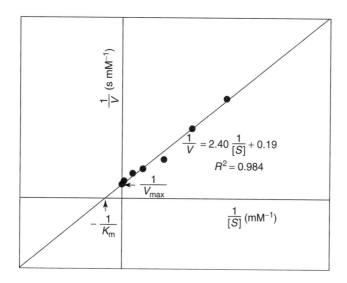

Figure 12.10. The Lineweaver–Burke plot of GPQG↓IWGQ and MMP-1.

$K_m = 2.40$ s $\times V_{max} = 2.40$ s $\times 5.26$ mM s$^{-1} = 12.63$ mM. As we know that $V_{max} = k_{cat}E_0$ and $E_0 = 1$ mM, we can calculate $k_{cat} = \frac{V_{max}}{E_0} = \frac{5.26 \text{ mM s}^{-1}}{1 \text{ mM}} = 5.26$ s^{-1}. Finally, we need to calculate the specificity constant, which, you will recall, is equal to $\frac{K_{cat}}{K_m}$. Therefore, for our system we calculate $\frac{K_{cat}}{K_m} = \frac{5.26 \text{ s}^{-1}}{12.63 \text{ mM}} = 0.416$ mM^{-1} s^{-1}.

When designing an enzyme-responsive drug delivery system, you would perform this type of experimental data collection and subsequent analysis for the sequence GPQG↓IWGQ and a variety of enzymes, so that you could compare the relative efficiencies of the peptide with each enzyme and determine the application your peptide sequence was best suited for.

12.6   KEY POINTS

- Stimuli-responsive polymers exhibit sharp changes in their physical properties upon exposure to specific stimuli.
- Stimuli that have been exploited for site-specific polymer-based drug delivery include temperature, pH, redox, and enzymatic activity.
- Numerous drug delivery devices have been adapted to include stimuli-responsive chemistries for drug delivery, including micelles, nanoparticles and nanogels, hydrogels, and soluble conjugates.
- A wide variety of drug classes have been incorporated and delivered using stimuli-responsive polymers, including nucleic acids, small, hydrophobic drugs, proteins, and peptides.

- Modifying the specific chemistry used in your stimuli-responsive drug delivery system often offers the ability to tune drug release behavior.

12.7 HOMEWORK QUESTIONS

1. Based on the observations of [27], explain how hydrophilicity and hydrophobicity of the three model drugs affect the phase transition temperature of poly(N-vinyl caprolactam) nanoparticles and drug loading and release.

2. Compile a list of NIPAAm copolymers from literature sources (include citations) and explain which one(s) are most suitable for drug delivery applications.

3. You have successfully synthesized a UCST polymer with phase transition temperature of 39 °C. Assuming a hydrogen bond strength (e.g., between water and the polymer in the solvated state) of 23.3 kJ mol^{-1} [150], 0.75 hydrogen bonds per monomer repeat in the polymer, and hydrophobic bonds (e.g., after collapse of the polymer) contribute solely to the ΔS term (where there are 0.33 bonds/monomer repeat unit of the polymer), what is ΔS after collapse/desolvation of the polymer? Assuming ΔG is -987 kJ mol^{-1}, how many repeat units exist within the polymer? Describe a way to exploit the UCST polymer for drug delivery. What drug characteristics must you consider to ensure effective delivery?

4. PharmaSys, Inc. is developing a new drug delivery system based on the work summarized in the References 61, 62. As already discussed, these poly(methacrylic acid-g-ethylene glycol) (P(MAA-g-EG)) hydrogels are collapsed in the stomach with mesh sizes of 70 Å but expand in the neutral-to-basic pH of the intestine, to a mesh size of ~210 Å. Specifically, PharmaSys is interested in developing these materials into nanometer-sized hydrogels ($d = 100$ nm) to deliver drugs to treat irritable bowel syndrome (IBS). IBS affects the ileum, which is the last part of the small intestine. The company is interested in using either Interferon ($r_s = 21$ Å), Rituximab ($r_s = 50$ Å), or ibuprofen ($r_s = 3.5$ Å) to reduce the inflammation associated with the IBS.

   a. On the basis of the pH-responsive behavior of the nanogels and the requirements of delivery to the small intestine, which drug would be most advantageous to develop? Recall the Stokes-Einstein equation and relationship between mesh size and hydrodynamic radius of hydrogels to make your recommendation.

   b. The typical residence times of the stomach and small intestine are 1 and 4 h, respectively. On the basis of this and the information above, how much of each drug will be released in the stomach and intestines? Does this information change your recommendations in a?

   c. On the basis of your results in part b, how might we improve the delivery system for intestine-specific delivery? Support your hypothesis mathematically.

5. You are designing a redox-responsive micelle system for delivery of an extracellularly- acting chemotherapeutic agent. Upon exposure to an oxidative environment, the micelle disintegrates and releases the encapsulated drug. Through meticulous experimentation, you have determined the rate of micelle disintegration as a function of the oxidative state (Fig. 12.11).

   You are hoping to use your delivery system to enhance localization of your chemotherapeutic drug to the tumor environment. However, you know that many elderly patients have arthritis, an inflammatory disease that is also characterized by an oxidative state. The oxidative state in the tissue is dependent largely on the extracellular presence of reactive oxygen species (such as hydrogen peroxide (H_2O_2)), reactive nitrogen species (such as nitric oxide (NO_3^-)), and Calcium (Ca^{2+}).

Agent	Concentration in tumor tissue	Concentration in arthritic joint
H_2O_2	25 mM	5 mM
NO_3^-	50 mM	10 mM
Ca^{2+}	3 μM	5 μM

Oxidative/Reductive agent	Standard reductive potential (V)
$H_2O_2(aq) + 2H^+(aq) + 2e^- \rightarrow 2H_2O(l)$	1.78
$NO_3^-(aq) + 4H^+(aq) + 3e^- \rightarrow NO(g) + 2H_2O(l)$	0.96
$Ca^{2+}(aq) + 2e^- \rightarrow Ca(s)$	-2.76

   a. What is the overall redox environment in each tissue?

   b. What will be the rate of micelle disintegration in each tissue?

   Assuming that the net volume of the tumor environment is approximately twice the overall size of the arthritic joints, but the residence time is the same, determine:

   c. What percentage of delivered micelles will disintegrate in the target tissue?

   d. Whether this is an appropriately designed delivery system, or does it need to be redesigned to reduce off-target effects? What would you change about the system to increase its specificity?

6. You have recently designed a novel, enzymatically-responsive drug delivery system. In your preliminary studies, you linked a model peptide drug to your carrier material (a long polymer chain intended to increase circulation time and targeted delivery to leaky vasculature) via the enzymatically degradable peptide sequence VPLS↓LYSG. Testing with this sequence generated the following enzyme kinetic data:

Enzyme	K_1, M^{-1} s^{-1}	K_{-1}, s^{-1}	K_{cat}, s^{-1}
MMP-2	65,000	2,000	36,500
MMP-9	45,000	50	24,000
MT1-MMP	7,500	2,500	6,000

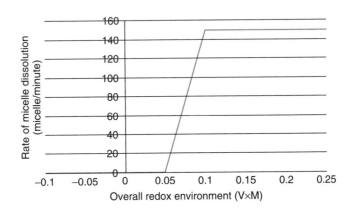

Figure 12.11. Rate of micelle dissolution as a function of local redox environment.

Using this data, determine:

a. The Michaelis constant for each enzyme.

b. The specificity constant for each enzyme.

You then performed research into the relative presence of these three enzymes in the body, both in healthy and diseased tissues. Using a tracking molecule, you determined that, after injection, some of the delivery system remains in the blood until being cleared by the kidneys. However, most of the delivery system quickly enters the tissue, mostly via the leaky vasculature into ischemic or tumor tissue (depending on the patient), where it remains for some time before being cleared from the body.

Tissue information					
		Blood	Healthy tissue	Ischemic tissue	Tumor
Amount of	MMP-2	0.25	1.25	20	55
Enzyme,	MMP-9	0.1	0.75	7.5	60
nM	MT1-MMP	0	1	15	3
Residence time, min		720	240	200	300
pH of tissue		7.4	7.2	6.0	6.5
Distribution of carrier system, %	Ischemic patient	20	5	75	–
	Cancer patient	20	5	–	75
Net volume of tissue, L	Ischemic patient	5	15	0.15	–
	Cancer patient	5	15	–	0.25

Using this information, and assuming you inject 10 moles of the carrier/drug material, determine:

a. V_{max} for each enzyme/tissue combination.
b. The amount of model drug that will be released in each tissue.
c. The therapeutic application you feel this delivery system is best suited for.

REFERENCES

1. Dirk S. Thermo- and pH-responsive polymers in drug delivery. Advanced Drug Delivery Reviews 2006;58(15):1655–1670.

2. Schild HG. Poly(N-isopropylacrylamide): experiment, Theory, and application. Progress in Polymer Science 1992;17:163–249.

3. Makhaeva EE, Tenhu H, Khokhlov AR. Conformational changes of poly(vinylcaprolactam) macromolecules and their complexes with ionic surfactants in aqueous solution. Macromolecules 1998;31(18):6112–6118.

4. Aoki T et al. Temperature-responsive interpenetrating polymer networks constructed with poly(acrylic acid) and poly(N,N-dimethylacrylamide). Macromolecules 1994;27(4): 947–952.

5. Principi T et al. Solution properties of hydrophobically modified copolymers of N-isopropylacrylamide and N-glycine acrylamide: a study by microcalorimetry and fluorescence spectroscopy. Macromolecules 2000;33(8):2958–2966.

6. Kuckling D et al. Temperature and pH dependent solubility of novel poly(N-isopropylacrylamide)-copolymers. Macromolecular Chemistry and Physics 2000;201(2):273–280.

7. Meewes M et al. Coil-globule transition of poly(N-isopropylacrylamide): a study of surfactant effects by light scattering. Macromolecules 1991;24(21):5811–5816.

8. da Silva G, Amelia MPS, et al. Thermo-responsiveness of poly(-diethylacrylamide) polymers at the air–water interface: The effect of a hydrophobic block. Journal of Colloid and Interface Science 2008;327(1):129–137.

9. Panayiotou M et al. Synthesis and characterisation of thermo-responsive poly(N,N'-diethylacrylamide) microgels. Reactive and Functional Polymers 2007;67(9):807–819.

10. Confortini O, Du Prez FE. Functionalized thermo-responsive poly(vinyl ether) by living cationic random copolymerization of methyl vinyl ether and 2-chloroethyl vinyl ether. Macromolecular Chemistry and Physics 2007;208(17):1871–1882.

11. Van Durme K et al. End-group modified poly(methyl vinyl ether): characterization and LCST demixing behavior in water. Journal of Polymer Science Part B: Polymer Physics 2006;44(2):461–469.

12. Verdonck B et al. Association behavior of thermo-responsive block copolymers based on poly(vinyl ethers). Polymer 2005;46(23):9899–9907.

13. Verdonck B, Goethals EJ, Du Prez FE. Block copolymers of methyl vinyl ether and isobutyl vinyl ether with thermo-adjustable amphiphilic properties. Macromolecular Chemistry and Physics 2003;204(17):2090–2098.

14. Sun S, Wu P. Infrared spectroscopic insight into hydration behavior of poly(N-vinylcaprolactam) in water. The Journal of Physical Chemistry B 2011;115(40): 11609–11618.

15. Maeda Y, Nakamura T, Ikeda I. Hydration and phase behavior of poly(N-vinylcaprolactam) and poly(N-vinylpyrrolidone) in water. Macromolecules 2001;35(1): 217–222.

16. Meeussen F et al. Phase behaviour of poly(N-vinyl caprolactam) in water. Polymer 2000;41(24):8597–8602.

17. Lozinsky VI et al. Synthesis of N-vinylcaprolactam polymers in water-containing media. Polymer 2000;41(17):6507–6518.

18. Bloksma MM et al. Poly(2-cyclopropyl-2-oxazoline): from rate acceleration by cyclopropyl to thermoresponsive properties. Macromolecules 2011;44(11):4057–4064.

19. Diehl C, Schlaad H. Thermo-responsive polyoxazolines with widely tuneable LCST. Macromolecular Bioscience 2009;9(2):157–161.

20. Park J-S, Kataoka K. Comprehensive and accurate control of thermosensitivity of poly(2-alkyl-2-oxazoline)s via well-defined gradient or random copolymerization. Macromolecules 2007;40(10):3599–3609.

21. Park J-S et al. Versatile synthesis of end-functionalized thermosensitive poly(2-isopropyl-2-oxazolines). Macromolecules 2004;37(18):6786–6792.

22. Dreher MR et al. Evaluation of an elastin-like polypeptide-doxorubicin conjugate for cancer therapy. J Control Release 2003;91(1–2):31–43.

23. Tsutsui H et al. Synthesis and temperature-responsive properties of novel semi-interpenetrating polymer networks consisting of a poly(acrylamide) polymer network and linear poly(acrylic acid) chains. Macromolecules 2006;39(6):2291–2297.

24. Li Y et al. Novel thermo-sensitive core-shell nanoparticles for targeted paclitaxel delivery. Nanotechnology 2009;20(6):065104.

25. Chen Y et al. Synthesis of hydroxypropylcellulose-poly(acrylic acid) particles with semi-interpenetrating polymer network structure. Biomacromolecules 2008;9(10):2609–2614.

26. Kono K et al. Highly temperature-sensitive liposomes based on a thermosensitive block copolymer for tumor-specific chemotherapy. Biomaterials 2010;31(27):7096–7105.

27. Vihola H et al. Binding and release of drugs into and from thermosensitive poly(N-vinyl caprolactam) nanoparticles. European Journal of Pharmaceutical Sciences 2002;16(1–2): 69–74.

28. Prabaharan M et al. Thermosensitive micelles based on folate-conjugated poly(N-vinylcaprolactam)-block-poly(ethylene glycol) for tumor-targeted drug delivery. Macromolecular Bioscience 2009;9(8):744–753.

29. Luxenhofer R et al. Doubly amphiphilic poly(2-oxazoline)s as high-capacity delivery systems for hydrophobic drugs. Biomaterials 2010;31(18):4972–4979.

30. Wang QF et al. Preparation and characterization of a positive thermoresponsive hydrogel for drug loading and release. Journal of Applied Polymer Science 2009;111(3):1417–1425.

31. Imaz A, Forcada J. N-vinylcaprolactam-based microgels for biomedical applications. Journal of Polymer Science Part A: Polymer Chemistry 2010;48(5):1173–1181.

32. Elizondo E et al. High loading of gentamicin in bioadhesive PVM/MA nanostructured microparticles using compressed carbon-dioxide. Pharmaceutical Research 2011;28(2): 309–321.

33. Kono K et al. Multi-functional liposomes having temperature-triggered release and magnetic resonance imaging for tumor-specific chemotherapy. Biomaterials 2011;32(5): 1387–1395.

34. Kono K et al. Temperature sensitization of liposomes by use of thermosensitive block copolymers synthesized by living cationic polymerization: effect of copolymer chain length. Bioconjugate Chemistry 2005;16(6):1367–1374.

35. Kiremitçi AS et al. Novel chlorhexidine releasing system developed from thermosensitive vinyl ether-based hydrogels. Journal of Biomedical Materials Research Part B: Applied Biomaterials 2007;83B(2):609–614.

36. Hruby M et al. Polyoxazoline thermoresponsive micelles as radionuclide delivery systems. Macromolecular Bioscience 2010;10(8):916–924.

37. Coughlan DC, Corrigan OI. Drug-polymer interactions and their effect on thermoresponsive poly(N-isopropylacrylamide) drug delivery systems. International Journal of Pharmaceutics 2006;313(1–2):163–174.

38. Coughlan DC, Quilty FP, Corrigan OI. Effect of drug physicochemical properties on swelling/deswelling kinetics and pulsatile drug release from thermoresponsive poly(N-isopropylacrylamide) hydrogels. Journal of Controlled Release 2004;98(1):97–114.

39. Rippke F, Schreiner V, Schwanitz HJ. The acidic milieu of the horny layer: new findings on the physiology and pathophysiology of skin pH. Am J Clin Dermatol 2002;3(4):261–272.

40. Fallingborg J. Intraluminal pH of the human gastrointestinal tract. Dan Med Bull 1999;46(3):183–196.

41. Owen DH, Katz DF. A vaginal fluid simulant. Contraception 1999;59(2):91–95.

42. Gupta KM et al. Temperature and pH sensitive hydrogels: an approach smart semen-triggered vaginal microbicidal vehicles. J Pharm Sci 2007;96(3):670–681.

43. Allsop P et al. Continuous intramuscular pH measurement during the recovery from brief, maximal exercise in man. Eur J Appl Physiol Occup Physiol 1990;59(6):465–470.

44. Dunning J et al. Coronary bypass grafting using crossclamp fibrillation does not result in reliable reperfusion of the myocardium when the crossclamp is intermittently released: a prospective cohort study. J Cardiothorac Surg 2006;1:45.

45. Khabbaz KR, Zankoul F, Warner KG. Intraoperative metabolic monitoring of the heart: II. Online measurement of myocardial tissue pH. Ann Thorac Surg 2001;72(6):S2227–S2233 discussion S2233–S2234, S2267–S2270.

46. Kumbhani DJ et al. Determinants of regional myocardial acidosis during cardiac surgery. Surgery 2004;136(2):190–198.

47. Newman RJ. Metabolic effects of tourniquet ischaemia studied by nuclear magnetic resonance spectroscopy. J Bone Joint Surg Br 1984;66(3):434–440.

48. Rehncrona S. Brain acidosis. Ann Emerg Med 1985;14(8):770–776.

49. Schneider LA et al. Influence of pH on wound-healing: a new perspective for wound-therapy? Arch Dermatol Res 2007;298(9):413–420.

50. Schmaljohann D. Thermo- and pH-responsive polymers in drug delivery. Advanced Drug Delivery Reviews 2006;58(15):1655–1670.

51. Qiu Y, Park K. Environment-sensitive hydrogels for drug delivery. Advanced Drug Delivery Reviews 2001;53(3):321–339.

52. Nicolazzi C et al. Anionic polyethyleneglycol lipids added to cationic lipoplexes increase their plasmatic circulation time. J Control Release 2003;88(3):429–443.

53. Garbern JC, Hoffman AS, Stayton PS. Injectable pH- and temperature-responsive poly(N-isopropylacrylamide-co-propylacrylic acid) copolymers for delivery of angiogenic growth factors. Biomacromolecules 2010;11(7):1833–1839.

54. Benoit DSW et al. pH-responsive polymeric siRNA carriers sensitize multidrug resistant ovarian cancer cells to doxorubicin via knockdown of polo-like kinase 1. Mol Pharm 2010;7(2):442–455.

55. Ray S, Maiti S, Sa B. Polyethyleneimine-treated xanthan beads for prolonged release of diltiazem: in vitro and in vivo evaluation. Arch Pharm Res 2010;33(4):575–583.

56. Zhang M et al. Biocleavable polycationic micelles as highly efficient gene delivery vectors. Nanoscale Res Lett 2010;5(11):1804–1811.

57. Brahim S, Narinesingh D, Guiseppi-Elie A. Release characteristics of novel pH-sensitive p(HEMA-DMAEMA) hydrogels containing 3-(trimethoxy-silyl) propyl methacrylate. Biomacromolecules 2003;4(5):1224–1231.

58. Murthy N et al. Design and synthesis of pH-responsive polymeric carriers that target uptake and enhance the intracellular delivery of oligonucleotides. J Control Release 2003;89(3):365–374.

59. Wong JB et al. Acid cleavable PEG-lipids for applications in a ternary gene delivery vector. Mol Biosyst 2008;4(6):532–541.

60. Borden KA et al. Interactions of synthetic polymers with cell membranes and model membrane systems. 13. On the mechanism of polyelectrolyte-induced structural reorganization in thin molecular films. Macromolecules 1987;20(2):454–456.

61. Nakamura K et al. Oral insulin delivery using P(MAA-g-EG) hydrogels: effects of network morphology on insulin delivery characteristics. J Control Release 2004;95(3):589–599.

62. Tuesca A et al. Complexation hydrogels for oral insulin delivery: effects of polymer dosing on in vivo efficacy. J Pharm Sci 2008;97(7):2607–2618.

63. Flanary S, Hoffman AS, Stayton PS. Antigen delivery with poly(propylacrylic acid) conjugation enhances MHC-1 presentation and T-cell activation. Bioconjugate Chemistry 2009;20(2):241–248.

64. Convertine AJ et al. Development of a novel endosomolytic diblock copolymer for siRNA delivery. J Control Release 2009;133(3):221–229.

65. Duvall CL et al. Intracellular delivery of a proapoptotic peptide via conjugation to a RAFT synthesized endosomolytic polymer. Molecular Pharmaceutics 2010;7(2):468–476.

66. Ha NTH, Fujimori K. Theoretical study of the copolymerization of styrene and maleic anhydride prepared in carbon tetrachloride and in N, N-dimethylformamide. Acta Polymerica 1998;49(8):404–410.

67. Mu Y et al. Bioconjugation of laminin peptide YIGSR with poly(styrene co-maleic acid) increases its antimetastatic effect on lung metastasis of B16-BL6 melanoma cells. Biochemical and Biophysical Research Communications 1999;255(1):75–79.

68. Maeda H. SMANCS and polymer-conjugated macromolecular drugs: advantages in cancer chemotherapy. Advanced Drug Delivery Reviews 2001;46(1–3):169–185.

69. Maeda H, Sawa T, Konno T. Mechanism of tumor-targeted delivery of macromolecular drugs, including the EPR effect in solid tumor and clinical overview of the prototype polymeric drug SMANCS. Journal of Controlled Release 2001;74(1–3):47–61.

70. Maeda H et al. Conjugation of poly(styrene-co-maleic acid) derivatives to the antitumor protein neocarzinostatin - pronounced improvements in pharmacological properties. Journal of Medicinal Chemistry 1985;28(4):455–461.

71. Henry SM et al. pH-responsive poly(styrene-alt-maleic anhydride) alkylamide copolymers for intracellular drug delivery. Biomacromolecules 2006;7(8):2407–2414.

72. Wu XL et al. Tumor-targeting peptide conjugated pH-responsive micelles as a potential drug carrier for cancer therapy. Bioconjug Chem 2010;21(2):208–213.

73. Criscione JM et al. Self-assembly of pH-responsive fluorinated dendrimer-based particulates for drug delivery and noninvasive imaging. Biomaterials 2009;30(23–24): 3946–3955.

74. You J-O, Auguste DT. Feedback-regulated paclitaxel delivery based on poly(N,N-dimethylaminoethyl methacrylate-co-2-hydroxyethyl methacrylate) nanoparticles. Biomaterials 2008;29(12):1950–1957.

75. Kavetskii RE, Osinskii SP, Bubnovskaya LN. Activation of glycolysis in tumor tissue by inorganic phosphate at low pH values. Bulletin of Experimental Biology and Medicine 1979;87(3):277–278.

76. Boussif O, Zanta MA, Behr JP. Optimized galenics improve in vitro gene transfer with cationic molecules up to 1000-fold. Gene Therapy 1996;3(12):1074–1080.

77. Bandyopadhyay P et al. Nucleotide exchange in genomic DNA of rat hepatocytes using RNA/DNA oligonucleotides. Targeted delivery of liposomes and polyethyleneimine to the asialoglycoprotein receptor. J Biol Chem 1999;274(15):10163–10172.

78. Breunig M et al. Mechanistic insights into linear polyethylenimine-mediated gene transfer. Biochimica Et Biophysica Acta-General Subjects 2007;1770(2):196–205.

79. Kichler A et al. Polyethylenimine-mediated gene delivery: a mechanistic study. Journal of Gene Medicine 2001;3(2):135–144.

80. Oh YK et al. Polyethylenimine-mediated cellular uptake, nucleus trafficking and expression of cytokine plasmid DNA. Gene Therapy 2002;9(23):1627–1632.

81. Durocher Y, Perret S, Kamen A. High-level and high-throughput recombinant protein production by transient transfection of suspension-growing human 293-EBNA1 cells. Nucleic Acids Res 2002;30(2).

82. Geisse S, Fux C. Recombinant protein production by transient gene transfer into mammalian cells. In: Guide to Protein Purification. 2nd ed. Vol. 466. 2009. p 223–238.

83. Iwai M et al. Polyethylenimine-mediated suicide gene transfer induces a therapeutic effect for hepatocellular carcinoma in vivo by using an Epstein-Barr virus-based plasmid vector. Biochem Biophys Res Commun 2002;291(1):48–54.

84. Kim J, Chen CP, Rice KG. The proteasome metabolizes peptide-mediated nonviral gene delivery systems. Gene Therapy 2005;12(21):1581–1590.

85. Pham PL, Kamen A, Durocher Y. Large-scale Transfection of mammalian cells for the fast production of recombinant protein. Molecular Biotechnology 2006;34(2):225–237.

86. Creusat G et al. Proton sponge trick for pH-sensitive disassembly of polyethylenimine-based siRNA delivery systems. Bioconjug Chem 2010;21(5):994–1002.

87. Segura T, Hubbell JA. Synthesis and in vitro characterization of an ABC triblock copolymer for siRNA delivery. Bioconjug Chem 2007;18(3):736–745.

88. Aigner A et al. Delivery of unmodified bioactive ribozymes by an RNA-stabilizing polyethylenimine (LMW-PEI) efficiently down-regulates gene expression. Gene Ther 2002;9(24):1700–1707.

89. Merdan T et al. Pegylated polyethylenimine-Fab' antibody fragment conjugates for targeted gene delivery to human ovarian carcinoma cells. Bioconjugate Chemistry 2003;14(5):989–996.

90. Kwon EJ, Bergen JM, Pun SH. Application of an HIV gp41-derived peptide for enhanced intracellular trafficking of synthetic gene and siRNA delivery vehicles. Bioconjug Chem 2008;19(4):920–927.

91. Standley SM et al. Acid-degradable particles for protein-based vaccines: enhanced survival rate for tumor-challenged mice using ovalbumin model. Bioconjugate Chemistry 2004;15:1281–1288.

92. Kwon EJ, Liong S, Pun SH. A truncated HGP peptide sequence that retains endosomolytic activity and improves gene delivery efficiencies. Mol Pharm 2010;7(4):1260–1265.

93. Leamon CP, Low PS. Folate-mediated targeting: from diagnostics to drug and gene delivery. Drug Discovery Today 2001;6(1):44–51.

94. Leamon CP, Weigl D, Hendren RW. Folate copolymer-mediated transfection of cultured cells. Bioconjug Chem 1999;10(6):947–957.

95. Saito G, Swanson JA, Lee KD. Drug delivery strategy utilizing conjugation via reversible disulfide linkages: role and site of cellular reducing activities. Advanced Drug Delivery Reviews 2003;55(2):199–215.

96. Haensler J, Szoka FC Jr. Polyamidoamine cascade polymers mediate efficient transfection of cells in culture. Bioconjug Chem 1993;4(5):372–379.

97. Harada Y et al. Highly efficient suicide gene expression in hepatocellular carcinoma cells by Epstein-Barr virus-based plasmid vectors combined with polyamidoamine dendrimer. Cancer Gene Therapy 2000;7(1):27–36.

98. Maruyama-Tabata H et al. Effective suicide gene therapy in vivo by EBV-based plasmid vector coupled with polyamidoamine dendrimer. Gene Ther 2000;7(1):53–60.

99. Rudolph C et al. In vivo gene delivery to the lung using polyethylenimine and fractured polyamidoamine dendrimers. Journal of Gene Medicine 2000;2(4):269–278.

100. Tanaka S et al. Targeted killing of carcinoembryonic antigen (CEA)-producing cholangiocarcinoma cells by polyamidoamine dendrimer-mediated transfer of an Epstein-Barr virus (EBV)-based plasmid vector carrying the CEA promoter. Cancer Gene Ther 2000;7(9):1241–1250.

101. Kale AA, Torchilin VP. Design, synthesis, and characterization of pH-sensitive PEG-PE conjugates for stimuli-sensitive pharmaceutical nanocarriers: the effect of substitutes at the hydrazone linkage on the ph stability of PEG-PE conjugates. Bioconjug Chem 2007;18(2):363–370.

102. St. Pierre T, Chiellini E. Biodegradability of synthetic polymers used for medical and pharmaceutical applications: part 1—principles of hydrolysis mechanisms. Journal of Bioactive and Compatible Polymers 1986;1(4).

103. Middleton JC, Tipton AJ. Synthetic biodegradable polymers as orthopedic devices. Biomaterials 2000;21(23):2335–2346.

104. Gillies ER, Goodwin AP, Frechet JM. Acetals as pH-sensitive linkages for drug delivery. Bioconjug Chem 2004;15(6):1254–1263.

105. Shen Y et al. Prodrugs forming high drug loading multifunctional nanocapsules for intracellular cancer drug delivery. J Am Chem Soc 2010;132(12):4259–4265.

106. Bruyere H, Westwell AD, Jones AT. Tuning the pH sensitivities of orthoester based compounds for drug delivery applications by simple chemical modification. Bioorganic & Medicinal Chemistry Letters 2010;20(7):2200–2203.

107. Sethuraman VA, Na K, Bae YH. pH-responsive sulfonamide/pei system for tumor specific gene delivery: an in vitro study. Biomacromolecules 2005;7(1):64–70.

108. Brown TL, LeMay HE, Bursten BE, editors. Chemistry, The Central Science. 7 ed. Upper Saddle River, NJ: Prentice-Hall; 1997.

109. Schafer FQ, Buettner GR. Redox environment of the cell as viewed through the redox state of the glutathione disulfide/glutathione couple. Free Radical Biology and Medicine 2001;30(11):1191–1212.

110. Go Y-M, Jones DP. Redox compartmentalization in eukaryotic cells. Biochimica et Biophysica Acta (BBA) - General Subjects 2008;1780(11):1273–1290.

111. Wu G et al. Glutathione Metabolism and its Implications for Health. The Journal of Nutrition 2004;134(3):489–492.

112. Napoli A et al. Glucose-oxidase based self-destructing polymeric vesicles. Langmuir 2004;20(9):3487–3491.

113. Napoli A et al. Oxidation-responsive polymeric vesicles. Nature Materials 2004;3(3): 183–189.

114. Napoli A et al. New synthetic methodologies for amphiphilic multiblock copolymers of ethylene glycol and propylene sulfide. Macromolecules 2001;34(26):8913–8917.

115. Velluto D et al. PEG-b-PPS-b-PEI micelles and PEG-b-PPS/PEG-b-PPS-b-PEI mixed micelles as non-viral vectors for plasmid DNA: tumor immunotoxicity in B16F10 melanoma. Biomaterials 2011;32(36):9839–9847.

116. Velluto D, Demurtas D, Hubbell JA. PEG-b-PPS diblock copolymer aggregates for hydrophobic drug solubilization and release: cyclosporin A as an example. Mol Pharm 2008;5(4):632–642.

117. Kakizawa Y et al. Electrochemical control of vesicle formation with a double-tailed cationic surfactant bearing ferrocenyl moieties. Langmuir 2001;17(26):8044–8048.

118. Song N et al. Preparation and in vitro properties of redox-responsive polymeric nanoparticles for paclitaxel delivery. Colloids and Surfaces B: Biointerfaces 2011;87(2):454–463.

119. Heredia KL et al. Reversible siRNA-polymer conjugates by RAFT polymerization. Chemical Communications 2008;28:3245–3247.

120. Foster S et al. Intracellular delivery of a protein antigen with an endosomal-releasing polymer enhances CD8 T-Cell production and prophylactic vaccine efficacy. Bioconjugate Chemistry 2010;21(12):2205–2212.

121. Kommareddy S, Amiji M. Poly(ethylene glycol)-modified thiolated gelatin nanoparticles for glutathione-responsive intracellular DNA delivery. Nanomedicine-Nanotechnology Biology and Medicine 2007;3(1):32–42.

122. Liu J et al. Redox-responsive polyphosphate nanosized assemblies: A smart drug delivery platform for cancer therapy. Biomacromolecules 2011;12(6):2407–2415.

123. Napoli A et al. Oxidation-responsive polymeric vesicles. Nat Mater 2004;3(3):183–189.

124. Napoli A et al. New synthetic methodologies for amphiphilic multiblock copolymers of ethylene glycol and propylene sulfide. Macromolecules 2001;34(26):8913–8917.

125. Velluto D, Demurtas D, Hubbell JA. PEG-b-PPS diblock copolymer aggregates for hydrophobic drug solubilization and release: cyclosporin A as an example. Molecular Pharmaceutics 2008;5(4):632–642.

126. Kondo T, Kanai T, Uosaki K. Control of the charge-transfer rate at a gold electrode modified with a self-assembled monolayer containing ferrocene and azobenzene by electro- and photochemical structural conversion of cis and trans forms of the azobenzene moiety. Langmuir 2001;17(20):6317–6324.

127. Power-Billard KN, Spontak RJ, Manners I. Redox-active organometallic vesicles: aqueous self-assembly of a diblock copolymer with a hydrophilic polyferrocenylsilane polyelectrolyte block. Angewandte Chemie International Edition 2004;43(10):1260–1264.

128. Duvall CL et al. Intracellular delivery of a proapoptotic peptide via conjugation to a RAFT synthesized endosomolytic polymer. Molecular Pharmaceutics 2009;7(2):468–476.

129. Alberts B, Wilson JH, Hunt T. Molecular Biology of the Cell. 5th ed. New York: Garland Sciencexxxiii, 1601; 2008. p 90.

130. Lehninger AL, Nelson DL, Cox MM. Lehninger Principles of Biochemistry. 3rd ed. New York: Worth Publishers; 2000.

131. Hamosh M, Scow RO. Lingual lipase and its role in the digestion of dietary lipid. The Journal of Clinical Investigation 1973;52(1):88–95.

132. Fox SI. Human physiology. 6th ed. Boston: WCB/McGraw-Hillxx; 1999. p 731.

133. Whitcomb DC, Lowe ME. Human pancreatic digestive enzymes. Digestive Diseases and Sciences 2007;52(1):1–17.

134. Chourasia MK, Jain SK. Pharmaceutical approaches to colon targeted drug delivery systems. Journal of Pharmacy and Pharmaceutical Sciences 2003;6(1):33–66.

135. Inaoka T et al. Molecular-cloning of human Cdna for cathepsin-K - novel cysteine proteinase predominantly expressed in bone. Biochemical and Biophysical Research Communications 1995;206(1):89–96.

136. Yegneswaran B, Pitchumoni CS. When should serum amylase and lipase levels be repeated in a patient with acute pancreatitis? Cleveland Clinic Journal of Medicine 2010;77(4):230–231.

137. Polette M et al. MT-MMP expression and localisation in human lung and breast cancers. Virchows Archiv-an International Journal of Pathology 1996;428(1):29–35.

138. Perillie PE, Finch SC. Alkaline phosphatase activity of exudative leukocytes in acute leukemia. Blood 1961;18:572–580.

139. Madlener M, Parks WC, Werner S. Matrix metalloproteinases (MMPs) and their physiological inhibitors (TIMPs) are differentially expressed during excisional skin wound repair. Experimental Cell Research 1998;242(1):201–210.

140. Muhs BE et al. Temporal expression and activation of matrix metalloproteinases-2,-9, and membrane type 1 - Matrix metalloproteinase following acute hindlimb ischemia. Journal of Surgical Research 2003;111(1):8–15.

141. Sintov A, Levy RJ. Polymeric drug delivery of enzymatically degradable pendant agents: peptidyl-linked procainamide model system studies. International Journal of Pharmaceutics 1997;146(1):55–62.

142. Aimetti AA, Tibbitt MW, Anseth KS. Human neutrophil elastase responsive delivery from poly(ethylene glycol) hydrogels. Biomacromolecules 2009;10(6):1484–1489.

143. Sakiyama-Elbert SE, Panitch A, Hubbell JA. Development of growth factor fusion proteins for cell-triggered drug delivery. Faseb Journal 2001;15(7):1300–1302.

144. Hovgaard L, Brondsted H. Dextran hydrogels for colon-specific drug-delivery. Journal of Controlled Release 1995;36(1–2):159–166.

145. Park C et al. Enzyme responsive nanocontainers with cyclodextrin gatekeepers and synergistic effects in release of guests. Journal of the American Chemical Society 2009;131(46):16614–16615.

146. Pechar M et al. Poly(ethylene glycol) multiblock copolymer as a carrier of anti-cancer drug doxorubicin. Bioconjugate Chemistry 2000;11(2):131–139.

147. Baker GL et al. Functionalization of Polyglycolides by "Click" Chemistry. USA: Board of Trustees of Michigan State University; 2009. p 26.

148. Fairbanks BD et al. A Versatile Synthetic Extracellular Matrix Mimic via Thiol-Norbornene Photopolymerization. Advanced Materials 2009;21(48):5005.

149. Hubbell JA, Patterson J. Enhanced proteolytic degradation of molecularly engineered PEG hydrogels in response to MMP-1 and MMP-2. Biomaterials 2010;31(30):7836–7845.

150. Suresh SJ, Naik VM. Hydrogen bond thermodynamic properties of water from dielectric constant data. Journal of Chemical Physics 2000;113(21):9727–9732.

151. Idziak I et al. Thermosensitivity of aqueous solutions of poly(N,N-diethylacrylamide). Macromolecules 1999;32(4):1260–1263.

152. Mikheeva LM et al. Microcalorimetric study of thermal cooperative transitions in poly(N-vinylcaprolactam) hydrogels. Macromolecules 1997;30(9):2693–2699.

153. Shibayama M, Norisuye T, Nomura S. Cross-link density dependence of spatial inhomogeneities and dynamic fluctuations of poly(N-isopropylacrylamide) gels. Macromolecules 1996;29(27):8746–8750.

154. Van Durme K et al. Influence of poly(ethylene oxide) grafts on kinetics of LCST behavior in aqueous poly(N-vinylcaprolactam) solutions and networks studied by modulated temperature DSC. Macromolecules 2004;37(3):1054–1061.

13

AFFINITY-BASED DRUG DELIVERY

Andrew S. Fu and Horst A. von Recum

Department of Biomedical Engineering, Case Western Reserve University,
Cleveland, OH, USA

13.1 INTRODUCTION

Much like how affinity in an interpersonal sense describes a spontaneous or natural liking for someone, affinity in a chemical sense characterizes the natural tendency for two molecules to bind or associate. In general, such an affinity can be based on a variety of interactions: ionic interactions, hydrophobic interactions, hydrogen binding, and van der Waals forces. Affinity-based drug delivery systems (DDSs) utilize these molecular interactions to control the loading and release of drugs.

Unlike some of the more "traditional" DDSs, such as diffusion-, swelling-, erosion-, or stimuli-based DDSs, affinity-based DDSs offer some unique possibilities to tailor the rate of drug release through mechanisms that are less dependent of the properties of the polymer matrix (e.g., geometry, pore size, degradation rate, sensitivity to changes in pH, temperature, and glucose concentration). As a result, one of the advantages of affinity-based DDSs is that they have the potential to deliver multiple drugs at different rates, assuming that each of the drugs has a different affinity to the delivery device. A potential application could be the regeneration of blood

Engineering Polymer Systems for Improved Drug Delivery, First Edition.
Edited by Rebecca A. Bader and David A. Putnam.
© 2014 John Wiley & Sons, Inc. Published 2014 by John Wiley & Sons, Inc.

vessels, where the delivery of growth factors such as vascular endothelial growth factor and platelet-derived growth factor at different rates has proven to be critical [1]. Another unique advantage is the potential to reload or refill an affinity-based DDS, which may act as a drug reservoir after the initial dose had been delivered. Commercially available reloadable DDSs typically consist of an injectable depot, and reloading requires device access and needle injection into the depot. Affinity-based reloading differs by allowing the drug to be injected near the vicinity of the DDS, where selective and specific reloading of the drug occurs at a molecular level. The ability to reload a DDS is particularly advantageous for treating diseases such as diabetes, ocular disease, and recurrent malignant gliomas, where repetitive, long-term administrations of insulin, retinoids, and chemotherapy agents, respectively, are invaluable.

One of the most important parameters in an affinity-based DDS is the association constant between the drug and the DDS. The chapter will start with a discussion of the basics of association constants and some of the methods used to determine them. Next, various affinity-based DDSs and their applications will be discussed. The goal of this section is not to present an exhaustive review of all affinity-based DDSs, but to highlight a few that are representative. For a more in-depth review of many affinity-based DDSs, the reader may refer to a recent article by Wang and von Recum [2]. Finally, basic mathematical modeling of affinity-based DDSs will be discussed.

13.2 ASSOCIATION CONSTANT

Release from an affinity-based DDS is governed by the association constant between the drug and the DDS. A high association constant suggests a high affinity between the drug and the DDS, which implies prolonged release of the drug. The goal of an effective drug delivery platform is to maintain local drug concentration within a therapeutic window for extended periods. In some cases, a rapid initial release, followed by more sustained release, may be needed for the drug to rapidly reach an effective therapeutic concentration, while in other cases the "burst effect" could lead to potential toxic effects. Nevertheless, the common goal is to exert control over release rate and duration, which can be achieved through varying the association constant between the drug and the DDS.

13.2.1 Host–Guest Binding Model

Most affinity-based DDSs can be mathematically described through a host–guest binding model:

$$H + G \underset{k_2}{\overset{k_1}{\rightleftharpoons}} H \cdot G \tag{13.1}$$

A drug acts as the guest (G), while an affinity moiety of the DDS acts as the host (H). k_1 and k_2 represent the on-rate and the off-rate constants, respectively. The rate at which the concentration of the receptor–ligand complex changes is

$$\frac{d[H \cdot G]}{dt} = k_1[H][G] - k_2[H \cdot G] \tag{13.2}$$

At chemical equilibrium, association constant (K_a) can be determined by the following:

$$k_1[H][G] = k_2[H \cdot G] \Rightarrow K_a = \frac{k_1}{k_2} = \frac{[H \cdot G]}{[H][G]} \tag{13.3}$$

Assuming that the total concentration of guest is the sum of the free and bound guest concentration, that is

$$[G]_t = [G] + [H \cdot G] \tag{13.4}$$

Eq. 13.3 can further be simplified as

$$K_a = \frac{k_1}{k_2} = \frac{[H \cdot G]}{[H]([G]_t - [H \cdot G])} \tag{13.5}$$

In a typical study, the total concentration of guest is a fixed quantity. As a result, K_a becomes of a function of two variables, $[H]$ and $[H \cdot G]$.

Another related concept is the dissociation constant (K_d), which is simply the inverse of K_a. Both K_a and K_d quantify the relative importance of the on-rate and off-rate constants. Although K_a and K_d can be used generally to describe the affinity between the drug and the DDS, it is important to distinguish the different roles played by on-rate and off-rate constants under different circumstances. For instance, the on-rate constant should dictate drug loading and reloading processes, while the off-rate constant plays a more important role in sustaining drug release.

13.2.2 Methods to Determine Association Constant

13.2.2.1 Absorbance Spectrometry. Optical spectrometry is one of the most commonly used methods to determine K_a. When a drug and its host form a complex in a solution, a shift may occur in the absorption spectrum. The addition of different concentrations of host molecules to a constant concentration of the drug solution will result in different degrees of complexation at equilibrium. A relationship can be established between the absorbance reading of the solution and the concentration of the host molecule, given by

$$\frac{1}{A - A_0} = \frac{1}{K_a(b \Delta \varepsilon [G_0])} \cdot \frac{1}{[H]} + \frac{1}{b \Delta \varepsilon [G_0]} \tag{13.6}$$

A is the absorbance at any given concentration of the host molecule, and A_0 is the absorbance in the absence of host molecule. $[G_0]$ represents the concentration of the drug molecule, which is held constant. b and $\Delta \varepsilon$ represent the transmission distance

TABLE 13.1. Absorbance (A) Readings for Different Concentrations of FM at a Constant Concentration of Drug A

[FM] (mM)	A
0	0.0121
24.6	0.0631
41.8	0.0919
59.1	0.1203
76.6	0.1466
96.1	0.1791

What is the association constant between FM and compound A?

and the change in molar absorptivity associated with Beer's Law, respectively. For our interest, b and $\Delta\varepsilon$ values are not needed to determine the association constant K_a. The quantity $b\Delta\varepsilon[G_0]$ can be viewed as a constant. When $1/(A - A_0)$ is plotted against $1/[H]$, K_a = y-intercept/slope. Eq. 13.1 is more commonly known as the Benesi–Hildebrand equation [3]. Although beyond the scope of this chapter, the derivations of the Benesi–Hildebrand equation can be found in *Binding Constants: The Measurement of Molecular Complex Stability* by Connors [4].

13.3 WORKED EXAMPLE

You are designing an affinity-based DDS to deliver a drug called compound A. This particular DDS is a molecular imprinting polymer (MIP) consisting of a functional monomer (FM) that is known to associate with drug A. You add different concentrations of FM to a constant concentration of drug A. After chemical equilibrium is reached, absorbance readings are obtained at a wavelength of 350 nm (Table 13.1).

Solution

Using the absorbance data, a double reciprocal plot of $1/A - A_0$ versus $1/[FM]$ can be obtained (Fig. 13.1).

Least-squares linear regression gives an estimate for the slope and the y-intercept. As a result, K_a can be determined by

$$K_a = \frac{y - \text{intercept}}{\text{slope}} = \frac{1.57}{447.04} = 3.52 \times 10^{-3} \text{mM}^{-1}$$

One of the limitations of using the Benesi–Hildebrand equation and the double reciprocal plot to estimate K_a is the unequal weighting of data points. As is evident in the previous example, the slope is more sensitive to errors associated with larger

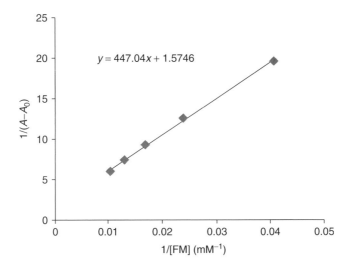

Figure 13.1. Determination of K_a from Eq. 13.6.

y values. A more accurate estimation for K_a can be obtained by using nonlinear regression analysis based on a modified Eq. 13.6, that is,

$$A = \frac{K_a[H]B}{1 + K_a[H]} + A_0; \quad (B = b\Delta\varepsilon[G_0]) \quad (13.7)$$

Using the curve-fitting tool in MATLAB, K_a was estimated to be $2.20 \times 10^{-3}\,\mathrm{mM}^{-1}$ (Fig. 13.2).

13.3.1 Fluorescence Spectrometry

When a drug is fluorescent, it is useful to use fluorescence spectrometry to determine its K_a with the host molecule. After the fluorescent drug molecule forms a full or partial inclusion complex with the host molecule, the fluorescent signal is often enhanced [5]. This is generally due to the isolation of the drug molecules from their aqueous environment, which diminishes intermolecular quenching. Experiments can be designed to add an increasing amount of host molecules to a constant amount of drug and to establish a relationship between the fluorescence intensity and the concentration of the host molecule:

$$\frac{1}{F - F_0} = \frac{1}{K_a(F_\infty - F_0)[H]} + \frac{1}{F_\infty - F_0} \quad (13.8)$$

This variation of the Benesi–Hildebrand equation can be derived from a modified Stern–Volmer equation [6]. F and F_0 are the fluorescence intensities in the presence and absence of $[H]$, respectively. F_∞ is the fluorescence intensity when $[H]$

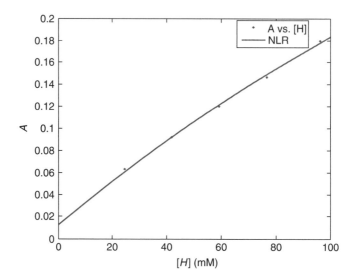

Figure 13.2. Determination of K_a from Eq. 13.7.

is extremely high. For our interest, F_∞ is not needed to determine K_a. Using a similar approach as in the previous section, after plotting $1/(F - F_0)$ versus $1/[H]$, $K_a = $ y-intercept/slope.

13.3.2 Surface Plasmon Resonance

Surface plasmon resonance (SPR) spectroscopy is a technique used in a variety of biosensors in order to analyze molecular interactions in real time. In a typical experiment, the host molecule is immobilized on a carboxymethylated-dextran sensor chip, over which an aqueous solution carrying the drug molecule passes through a flow cell. As the drug binds to the immobilized host at the sensor surface, it causes an increase in the refractive index, which is then converted to an SPR response signal (R). In essence, all concentration terms can be expressed in terms of R. Assume the concentration of the free drug is held constant in the flow cell; then the binding can be described by

$$\frac{dR}{dt} = k_1[G](R_{max} - R) - k_2 R \tag{13.9}$$

where dR/dt represents the rate of change of the SPR response signal, R_{max} and R are the maximum and measured response signal, and $[G]$ is the injection concentration of the drug. At equilibrium, Eq. 13.8 can be rewritten as

$$\frac{R_{eq}}{[G]} = -K_a R_{eq} + K_a R_{max} \tag{13.10}$$

Hence, the association constant K_a can be determined from a plot of $R_{eq}/[G]$ versus R_{eq}.

SPR analysis provides a great alternative for studying K_a, especially when the drug is not suitable for absorbance or fluorescence spectrometry. However, because SPR measurements depend on the mass of the material binding to the sensor surface, very small analytes may give very small responses.

13.3.3 Docking Simulations

As an alternative to experimentally determining K_a, molecular simulations can be used to predict affinity interactions between a drug and a DDS. Molecular modeling represents drug and host molecules numerically and simulates their interaction in a three-dimensional (3-D) environment through a process called *docking*. During docking, a drug molecule will be presented to a host molecule in different orientations, possible through intermolecular motion. The goal of the simulation is to minimize the free energy of the system by finding the "best fit" between the drug and the host molecule. After the binding orientation is established, a scoring function can be applied to estimate the strength of the association between the drug and the host molecule.

A wide variety of scoring functions have been developed based on intermolecular forces, bond angles, and number and types of bonds. Some scoring functions are trained based on databases, such as the Cambridge Structural Database. Attempts have also been made to use hybrid or consensus scoring functions during docking simulations, although the efficacy of this approach is debated [7, 8].

One of the common scoring functions is based on a generic force field, which is the sum of the van der Waals and electrostatic forces between the drug and the host molecule. An application using generic force field to minimize the energy of binding can be found at the Cyclodextrin Knowledge Base (interactions.cyclodextrin.net/web), a Web-based simulation software for predicting the interaction between cyclodextrin (CD) and different molecules.

Let us assume a researcher wants to choose a CD-based polymer for delivering an anticancer drug doxorubicin. The three potential candidates are α-, β-, and γ-CD, which consist of six, seven, and eight D-glucopyranose units, respectively, in a ring formation. More D-glucopyranose units result in a larger cavity for binding. The researcher uses the docking simulation software and generates the results shown in Table 13.2 and Fig. 13.3.

TABLE 13.2. Free Energy of Binding and K_a Obtained from Molecular Simulation of Doxorubicin Complexation with CD

	Free Energy of Binding (kcal)	K_a (M^{-1})
Dox and α-CD	−3.40	39
Dox and β-CD	−4.04	347
Dox and γ-CD	−5.98	550

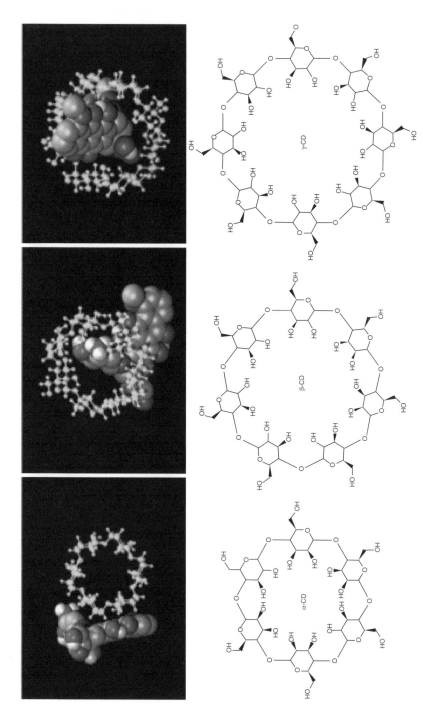

Figure 13.3. Molecular modeling results between doxorubicin and α-, β-, and γ-CD (top) and molecular structure of α-, β-, and γ-CD (bottom).

The docking simulations suggest that the size of the opening of the glucose rings plays an important role in the association with doxorubicin. On one hand, the simulation failed to predict a complexation between doxorubicin and α-CD, which has the smallest opening among the three CD molecules. On the other hand, γ- and β-CDs were predicted to form partial complexations with doxorubicin. The estimated association constant and free energy of binding values suggest that doxorubicin has the strongest affinity toward γ-CD and that the complexation is most favorable. Overall, the estimated association constants coincide with experimental values [9]. Through this series of docking simulations, the researcher gains valuable information regarding the affinity between doxorubicin and various types of CDs, which may help in the design of drug release and drug loading experiments.

Molecular modeling is a cost- and time-efficient tool for estimating the affinity between a drug and the host molecule. However, estimates from docking simulations are subject to a variety of errors. The scoring functions cannot taken into account all molecular interactions that affect affinity, nor can a computer algorithm test all possible orientations in which a drug can be presented to a host molecule in an aqueous environment. In particular, once a least energy fit is determined, it is not always certain this is the best fit. Modeling is also heavily limited by software and computation power. In most situations, it is critical to conduct the necessary benchtop experiments to determine K_a, and the K_a obtained from docking simulations should be used as a reference to aid in the design of experiments.

13.4 AFFINITY-BASED DRUG DELIVERY SYSTEMS

13.4.1 Cyclodextrin-Based Polymers

As described previously, CD is a cyclic oligosaccharide consisting of α-(1,4)-linked-D-glucopyranose units. The 3-D structure of CD resembles that of a toroid, with primary hydroxyl groups extending from the smaller opening and secondary hydroxyl groups extending from the larger opening. This arrangement gives CD a hydrophilic outer surface and a relatively more hydrophobic interior. In aqueous solutions, CDs can act as host molecule to form inclusion complexes with guest molecules, often hydrophobic in nature (Fig. 13.4). The driving forces for such complexation include the release of high energy water molecules from the cavity, formation of charge-transfer complexes, hydrogen bonding, and van der Waals forces [10, 11].

Because no covalent bonds are established when a drug forms an inclusion complex with CD, the drug can reversibly dissociate from the complex. The propensity for dissociation may be viewed as a probability function governed by the affinity between the drug and CD. At any given time, a higher affinity or larger association constant suggests a lower probability for the drug to dissociate from the complex. Comprehensive studies have been done to determine the K_a between CD and many hydrophobic molecules [12, 13].

Owing to its ability to modify the physicochemical properties of drugs, CD, in its monomer form, is widely used in pharmaceutical industries to increase the solubility,

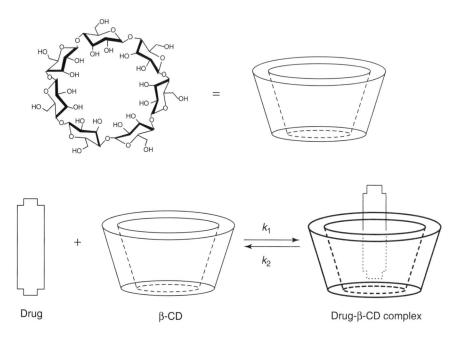

Figure 13.4. Formation of inclusion complex between drug and β-CD.

bioavailability, and stability of poorly soluble drugs [14]. However, effective drug delivery is not limited to increasing the drug's bioavailability; it is equally important to be able to control the rate of drug release to meet specific therapeutic needs. CD, in its polymer form, can be cross-linked to form insoluble DDSs for the controlled delivery of a variety of therapeutic agents. For example, von Recum and coworkers published a series of work on controlled delivery of antibiotics using CD-based hydrogels [15–18]. CD-based hydrogel synthesis conditions and various types and concentration of cross-linkers, such as lysine triisocyanate and hexamethylene diisocyanate, are optimized for the delivery of rifampin (RM), novobiocin (NB), and vancomycin (VM) [18]. A dextran hydrogel was used as a non-affinity control because of its similarity in chemical structure (a polysaccharide) and macromer molecular weight (MW). *In vitro* release of RM, NB, and VM from CD-based hydrogels were slower and more linear than the release from dextran hydrogels. In a zone-of-inhibition study, RM- and NB-loaded hydrogels were able to persistently kill *Staphylococcus aureus* at least 30–90 days (depending on the drug), whereas the release from dextran hydrogels failed to clear a zone after 20 days, even in the best release condition. Antibiotic-loaded CD coatings were also applied to metal screws and polymer meshes [17] to prevent prosthetic device infections. In an *in vivo* animal model, VM-loaded CD-coated meshes were able to prevent infection of *S. aureus* for at least 4 weeks [16].

    CD-based delivery systems can be modified to achieve different release rates. For instance, Rodriguez-Tenreiro and coworkers used ethyleneglycol diglycidylether to cross-link various types of CDs, such as β-CD, methyl-β-CD, hydroxypropyl-β-CD, and sulfobutyl-β-CD, for the controlled delivery of estradiol [19]. The difference in CD types resulted in differences in the affinity between estradiol and the cross-linked gels. Estradiol loading was found to be positively correlated with K_a, while the release rate was negatively correlated with K_a. Different release rates can also be obtained by modifying the drug rather than the device. Thatiparti et al. modified RM to contain either one or two PEG-adamantane (Ad) arms [15]. Ad is known to have a high affinity for CD. Mutiplexing interactions between RM-PEG-adamantane and CD in a CD-based hydrogel allowed for additional binding domains, which led to prolonged release of RM. In the same work, coumermycin, a dimeric form of the antibiotic NB, was found to have a much higher impact on release than could be explained by diffusivity change alone, suggesting the possibility of interactions with two CD domains per drug.

13.4.2 Molecular Imprinting

Molecular imprinting is similar to a lock–key model: a polymer matrix, acting as a lock, is created to have affinity toward a molecule of interest, acting as a key. The binding of the molecule to the resulting polymer matrix, known as a *molecular imprinting polymer*, is highly specific because the key is used as a template molecule to make the lock. FMs with affinity to the template molecule is cross-linked and self-assembled to form a polymer. The template is then removed from the polymer, leaving the polymer with cavities or specific binding sites for the template molecule (Fig. 13.5). Since the size, geometry, and functional groups associated with the binding cavity can all be modified, an MIP can be customized for the controlled deliver of a variety of therapeutic agents.

13.4.2.1 Covalent Versus Noncovalent Imprinting. One of the important criteria for designing an effective MIP is the choice of imprinting mode. There are two predominant ways to establish interactions between the FM and the template molecule: covalent bonding and noncovalent bonding. In general, covalent imprinting, although offering great specificity, is not very desirable for drug delivery because of the difficulty to design an MIP in which covalent bond formation and cleavage are

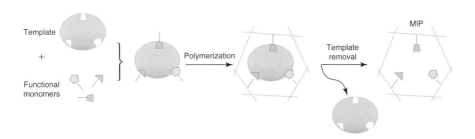

Figure 13.5. Schematic of molecular imprinting.

readily reversible under mild conditions. Noncovalent imprinting, relying on weak intermolecular forces such as hydrogen bonding, hydrophobic interactions, and metal coordination, is a much more popular choice for drug delivery due to the availability of a wide variety of monomers that can interact with any given template.

Noncovalent imprinting can occur in both an organic solvent and water. Because water may interfere with the weak intermolecular interactions between the monomer and the template, MIPs prepared in organic solvents offer stronger recognition. However, since most DDSs function in an aqueous environment, it is preferable that the imprinting takes place in water. Research has suggested that effective MIPs can be prepared in water by either incorporating a large number of a single type of interaction [20, 21] or a concoction of different types of interactions [22].

Oral and Peppas used a cross-linked and multiarm PEG star polymer network for an MIP designed to recognize D-glucose [20]. They hypothesized that the use of a monomer with a large number of functional sites increases the probability of intermolecular interactions and the subsequent specificity of recognizing D-glucose. They showed that the PEG star polymer network was effective at distinguishing D-glucose from other sugars. Interestingly, between the two types of star polymers, the 31-arm version showed better capacity in D-glucose uptake than the 75-arm version, suggesting that more arms or more functional sites do not necessarily mean more uptake. Instead, it is likely that there is an optimal number for functional sites given a specific application. Oral and Peppas, in another work, also suggest that, with a large number of interaction sites, noncovalent imprinting in water with poly(hydroxyethyl methacrylate) polymers can have selectivity despite nonspecific binding [21].

Another approach to improve recognition of noncovalent imprinting prepared in an aqueous environment is to simultaneously incorporate more than one type of intermolecular interactions [22]. For example, Piletsky et al. combined 2-acryloylamido-2,2'-dimethylpropane sulfonic acid, an electrostatic interacting monomer, with bisacryloyl β-CD, a hydrophobic interacting monomer in an MIP prepared in water. Two enantiomers of phenylalanine were used as template molecules: D-and L-phenylalanine. In both cases, the MIPs showed selectivity in recognizing their respective enantiomers. Through testing with a series of imprinted and nonimprinted reference polymers, the authors concluded that recognition is dependent on both hydrophobic and electrostatic interactions.

13.4.2.2 *Metal-Complexed MIP.*

Although imprinting using metal coordination is technically a type of noncovalent imprinting, it is unique enough to deserve its own section. One of the biggest advantages of implementing metal coordination in imprinting is that metal ions are highly versatile in associating with many biological molecules [23]. For example, Cu^{+2} and Fe^{+2} are commonly utilized to target the imidazole groups of histidine residues in proteins. Likewise, Ni^{+2} and Zn^{+2} are known to interact with phosphoryl groups. Further, the paramagnetic nature of metal ions, such as Cu^{+2}, can be exploited for characterizing the interactions using electron spin resonance spectroscopy [24].

In one of the earliest examples of using metal coordination in MIP, Dhal and Arnold demonstrated that, by using a copper-containing monomer and various bis(imidazole) substrates as templates during polymerization, the resulting MIPs can recognize bis(imidazole) substrates that differ slightly in the placement of the imidazole ligand [25]. The strength, specificity, and directionality of the metal coordination interactions are believed to be more comparable to those of covalent interactions than the weaker hydrogen bonding or electrostatic interactions. Meanwhile, the release and binding kinetics of metal-complexed MIPs are favorable for biological molecules, and the polymerization process can occur in aqueous solution.

Another unique characteristic of metal-complexed MIP is that the metal ions can be exchanged after templating to modify the affinity between the MIP and the template molecule. For a chromatographic separation application, Plunkett and Arnold were able to separate highly similar bis(imidazole)-containing substrate by replacing the Cu^{+2} in a copper-complexed MIP with Zn^{+2} [26]. By the exchange of metal ions, theoretically, different affinities and thus different rates of release can be achieved with a single MIP when delivering an array of drugs or biological molecules that are similar in structure.

13.4.3 Heparin-Based Delivery Systems

Heparin is a type of sulfated glycosaminoglycan with known affinity toward heparin-binding growth factors such as the basic fibroblast growth factor (bFGF). More specifically, the sulfated groups on heparin can bind with binding domains of the growth factors based on electrostatic interactions [27, 28]. As a result, the incorporation of heparin into a DDS can modulate the release of these growth factors. In addition, heparin can improve the bioactivity of the growth factors by temporarily stabilizing them or protecting them from degradation [28–33].

One of the earliest heparin-based delivery systems was developed by Edelman et al. [29]. Heparin–sepharose-bound bFGF were encapsulated in calcium alginate microspheres. The binding between heparin and bFGF contributed to preserving the bioactivity of bFGF. Heparinase, a temperature-sensitive enzyme that cleaves the heparin bond, was used to facilitate and control the release of bFGF. Similar strategies were implemented for delivering bFGF with heparinized collagen matrices [30]. Wissink et al. immobilized heparin to collagen using 1-ethyl-3-(3-dimethylaminopropyl) carbodiimide and N-hydroxysuccinimide for cross-linking. Immobilization of increasing amounts of heparin led to the binding of increasing amounts of bFGF to the collagen matrix and improved human umbilical vein endothelial cell seeding.

The Sakiyama–Elbert group has worked extensively with heparin and heparin-like affinity systems [31–34]. In one study, a bi-domain peptide that binds to both fibrin and heparin was covalently cross-linked to a fibrin matrix [32]. The peptide serves to immobilize heparin, which in turn binds to and stabilizes bFGF. The delivery system, mimicking the extracellular matrix, and its ability to provide slow passive release of growth factor were tested in a neuronal cell culture assay to confirm the bioactivity of bFGF. A similar system using a bi-domain peptide was developed to deliver the beta-nerve growth factor (β-NGF) and other members of the neurotrophin family, such as brain-derived neurotrophic factor (BDNF) and neurotrophin-3 (NT-3)

[33]. The affinity between these neurotrophins and heparin, although much weaker than that between bFGF and heparin, were shown to slow down the diffusion-based release from a fibrin matrix. The prolonged release of neurotrophins is especially relevant in the field of nerve regeneration where the healing process can take weeks to months.

The release rate of the previously described heparin-based system is dependent on the affinity between the bi-domain peptide and heparin. Modulating the release rate remains a challenge. With the help of combinatorial phage display libraries, Maxwell et al. identified and tested a group of short peptide sequences with varying affinities for heparin [31]. The theory was that the previously mentioned bi-domain peptide could be exchanged with one of the identified sequences. Mathematical modeling and experimental work suggested that the incorporation of peptides with varying affinity for heparin was able to modulate the release rate of heparin-bound neural growth factor and its biological activity in a neurite extension model.

Heparin-like affinity systems were also developed to modulate the release rate. If a peptide sequence can be synthesized to resemble the growth factor binding domain of heparin, then an affinity system would only need two components: the peptide sequence and the polymer matrix. Willerth et al. screened a phage display library consisting of 12 amino acid random peptide sequences against β-NGF-conjugated chromatography resin to identify peptide sequences of varying affinity for NGF [34]. Selected peptides were incorporated into fibrin matrices for the delivery of NGF. Variability in the affinity between different peptides and NGF resulted in variability in release rates. NGF release from fibrin matrix alone was faster than release from peptide-incorporated fibrin matrices.

A different approach to create a heparin-like affinity system was developed by Freeman et al. using an alginate hydrogel [35]. Uronic acids in non-sulfated alginate were sulfated to resemble the sulfated groups on heparin, and hydrogels of alginate/alginate-sulfate were fabricated. Through SPR analysis, K_as between 10 heparin-binding proteins and alignate-sulfate were found to be comparable or one order of magnitude higher than those obtained between the proteins and heparin. In an *in vivo* study, the delivery of bFGF from an alginate/alginate-sulfate scaffold induced twice the number of blood vessel formations compared to a control. A similar alginate/alginate-sulfate system was developed to deliver hepatocyte growth factor to improve tissue blood perfusion and to induce mature blood vessel network formation in a hindlimb ischemia model [36].

Fucoidans, sulfate-containing polysaccharides extracted from brown algae, are also known to bind to heparin-binding growth factors such as FGF-1 and FGF-2[37]. Nakamura et al. developed a chitosan/fucoidan complex hydrogel for immobilizing and delivering FGF-2 [38]. The interaction between FGF-2 and fucoidan enhanced the growth factor's bioactivity and protected it from inactivation by heat and proteolysis. Overall, heparin-like systems, mostly containing sulfated polysaccharides, can be viewed as simplified versions of the traditional heparin systems because controlled release can be achieved without using heparin and a heparin-binding bi-domain peptide.

13.4.4   Other Affinity-Based Delivery Systems

Albumin is another attractive candidate to use in affinity-based delivery systems because of its natural affinity for various drugs and peptides, as well as its biocompatibility. Oss-Ronen and Seliktar conjugated serum albumin to poly(ethylene glycol) to synthesize a mono-PEGylated albumin hydrogel [39]. The release kinetics of these hydrogels was examined using the drug naproxen and two types of recombinant insulin, Actrapid and modified Levemir. Despite having affinity for albumin, naproxen exhibited the fastest release rate because of its low MW. Modified Levemir, which has affinity for albumin, showed significantly slower release than Actrapid, which is similar in MW but has no affinity for albumin. To further improve these hydrogels for use as 3-D cell culture scaffolds, PEGylated fibrinogen was incorporated, along with mono-PEGylated albumin, to form a composite hydrogel system. The addition of PEGylated fibrinogen was meant to compensate for the lack of known cell adhesion sites on the albumin backbone [40].

Novel affinity-based delivery systems have also been developed for non-heparin-binding growth factors. For example, Soontornworajit et al. used an aptamer-functionalized hydrogel for the delivery of PDGF-B [41]. Based on a model aptamer which had known affinity for PDGF-B, a series of anti-PDGF aptamers are generated either by randomizing the nonessential nucleotide tail or by mutating the essential nucleotides. The study showed that the aptamer affinity was significantly affected by mutations of the essential nucleotides, whereas variations in the nonessential nucleotides had a smaller effect. Different release rates were achieved by adjusting the affinity of the aptamers. Another related study suggested that the oligonucleotide tails of the aptamers are important in inducing intermolecular hybridization and initiating aptamer–protein dissociation [42]. Attachment of oligonucleotide tails and increasing hybridizing length were found to have a synergistic effect on the affinity between the aptamer and the protein.

Metal ions can be incorporated into not only MIPs but also polymer matrices for affinity-based drug delivery. Lin and Metters developed an affinity-based hydrogel based on PEG-diacrylate and a metal-ion-chelating ligand glycidyl methacrylate-iminodiacetic acid (GMIDA) to retard the release of a model protein hexa-histidine-tagged fluorescence protein (hisGFP) [43]. GMIDA is known to have higher affinity towards copper ions than nickel ions. The study showed that tunable and sustained release could be accomplished by increasing the GMIDA: hisGFP ratio or interchanging nickel ions with copper ions. In another study, Shen et al. modified the surface of submicrometer particles with MgO for the controlled delivery of ibuprofen. The alkalinity of MgO created affinity with acidic ibuprofen molecules and slowed the release rate. In addition, the release rate of ibuprofen could be adjusted by varying the content of MgO [44]. In addition to copper, nickel, and magnesium, calcium ions can also be included into polymer matrices to modulate drug release. Margiotta et al. added calcium in a silica xerogel for the delivery of an antitumor agent containing bisphosphonate [45]. The affinity between calcium and bisphosphonate was found to be important in modulating the release rate and stabilizing the formulation.

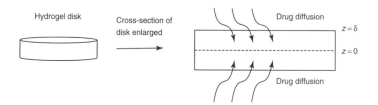

Figure 13.6. Geometry of a β-CD-based hydrogel.

13.5   MATHEMATICAL MODELING OF AFFINITY-BASED SYSTEMS

Mathematical modeling plays an important role in the design of biomaterials for tissue engineering and drug delivery by identifying key release mechanisms and parameters. Simulated release profiles can help predict the effect of various design parameters and minimize the number of experimental studies. This section, which was originally described by Fu et al. [46] and reprinted with permission from Springer, will focus on an in-depth examination of a β-CD-based hydrogel system and how to mathematically describe its *in vitro* drug release.

Consider the geometry in Fig. 13.6. The β-CD hydrogel has a thin disk geometry. Diffusion of the drug will occur via the top and bottom surfaces in the z direction. Diffusion in the radial direction can be assumed to be negligible because the top and bottom surface areas are much larger than the surrounding surface area. Before the *in vitro* drug release experiment in aqueous solution, we load the hydrogel with drug until chemical equilibrium has been established.

13.5.1   Mass Transport Dynamics

The system diagram (Fig. 13.7) shows the transport processes in the hydrogel, where the sum of the local concentrations of free and bound β-CD are constant everywhere because they are immobile, $C_T = C_C + C_{\text{LoC}}$.

Therefore, the net rate of binding is

$$R_b = k_1 C_L C_C - k_2 C_{\text{LoC}} = k_1 C_L (C_T - C_{\text{LoC}}) - k_2 C_{\text{LoC}} \qquad (13.11)$$

The concentration of free ligand in the hydrogel changes by diffusion and reaction:

$$\frac{\partial C_L}{\partial t} = D \frac{\partial^2 C_L}{\partial z^2} - R_b \quad (0 < z < \delta) \qquad (13.12)$$

The concentration of bound ligand in the hydrogel changes according to

$$\frac{\partial C_{\text{LoC}}}{\partial t} = R_b$$

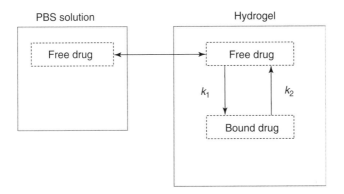

Figure 13.7. System diagram of *in vitro* drug release in a phosphate buffer solution (PBS).

At the center, symmetry applies:

$$z = 0: \quad \frac{\partial C_L}{\partial z} = 0$$

At the boundary of the hydrogel and solution, $z = \delta : C_L = 0$.
The initial conditions for release from the hydrogel are

$$t = 0: \quad C_L = C_L^{\text{eq}}; \quad C_{\text{LoC}} = C_{\text{LoC}}^{\text{eq}}$$

where C_L^{eq} and $C_{\text{LoC}}^{\text{eq}}$ are known concentration of free and bound drug when loading reaches equilibrium.

The rate of release (RR) is

$$\frac{\mathrm{d}M_R}{\mathrm{d}t} = RR = -AD \left.\frac{\partial C_L}{\partial z}\right|_{z=\delta}$$

$$M_R = 0, t = 0 \tag{13.13}$$

13.5.2 Dimensionless Model

In the previous section, we established the governing equations for the mass transport dynamics of the affinity-based system. To reduce the complexity of the current model, we will employ dimensional analysis to reduce the number of parameters. The model can be simplified when expressed with the following dimensionless variables:

$$\tau = k_2 t; \quad C_L^* = \frac{C_L}{C_0}; \quad C_{\text{LoC}}^* = \frac{C_{\text{LoC}}}{C_0}; \quad z^* = \frac{z}{\delta}; \quad R_b^* = \frac{R_b}{C_0 k_2}$$

where $C_0 = C_L^{\text{eq}} + C_{L \cdot C}^{\text{eq}}$ and is a known constant.

The dimensionless rate of binding is

$$R_b^* = \frac{R_b}{C_0 k_2} = \left[\frac{k_1 C_0}{k_2}\right] C_L^* \left(\left[\frac{C_T}{C_0}\right] - C_{\text{LoC}}^*\right) - C_{\text{LoC}}^* \qquad (13.14)$$

The dimensionless concentration of free drug in the hydrogel changes according to

$$(C_0 k_2)\frac{\partial C_L^*}{\partial \tau} = \left(\frac{D C_0}{\delta^2}\right)\frac{\partial^2 C_L^*}{\partial z^{*2}} - C_0 k_2 R_b^* \Rightarrow \frac{\partial C_L^*}{\partial \tau} = \left[\frac{D}{k_2 \delta^2}\right]\frac{\partial^2 C_L^*}{\partial z^{*2}} - R_b^* \qquad (13.15)$$

The dimensionless concentration of bound drug in the hydrogel changes according to

$$\frac{\partial C_{\text{LoC}}^*}{\partial \tau} = R_b^* \qquad (13.16)$$

The dimensionless boundary condition at the hydrogel center is

$$z^* = 0: \quad \frac{\partial C_L^*}{\partial z^*} = 0$$

For the release phase, the dimensionless initial conditions are

$$\tau = 0: \quad C_L^* = \frac{C_L^{\text{eq}}}{C_0}; \quad C_{\text{LoC}}^* = \frac{C_{\text{LoC}}^{\text{eq}}}{C_0}$$

and at the boundary of the hydrogel, the solution is $z^* = 1: \; C_L^* = 0$

The dimensionless rate of release of drug from the hydrogel into the surroundings is

$$\frac{dM_R^*}{d\tau} = RR^* = -\frac{1}{2}\left[\frac{D}{k_2 \delta^2}\right]\frac{\partial C_L^*}{\partial z^*}\bigg|_{z^* = 1}$$

$$M_R^* = 0, \quad \tau = 0 \qquad (13.17)$$

The dimensionless parameter groups associated with the binding and transport processes are

$$P_1 = \left[\frac{k_1 C_0}{k_2}\right]; \quad P_2 = \left[\frac{D}{k_2 \delta^2}\right]; \quad P_3 = \left[\frac{C_T}{C_0}\right]$$

After dimensional analysis, we can conclude that our model outputs of interest, namely free and bound drug concentration and release rate, are dependent on three dimensionless parameters. P_1 and P_2 contain the parameters k_1, k_2, and D, which are often unknown and cumbersome to determine experimentally. P_3 should be a known constant because both C_T and C_0 are known constants.

P_1 and P_2 are coefficients of the diffusion and affinity term of the governing equations. Another important result from dimensional analysis is that now we can compare the relative importance of diffusion and affinity terms. The governing equations can be further simplified by eliminating the diffusion or affinity terms based on whether $P_1/P_2 \gg 1$ or $P_1/P_2 \ll 1$.

13.5.3 Methods of Lines

The dimensionless model can be solved numerically using the method of lines, in which the spatial derivatives are discretized. We can discretize the derivatives with respect to z^*, starting with

$$\Delta = \frac{1}{N}, \quad z_i^* = 1\Delta \quad (i = 0, 1, 2 \ldots N) \tag{13.18}$$

Discretized first derivatives are either forward or backward differences; discretized second derivatives are central differences. The discretized governing equations are

$$\frac{dC_{L,i}^*}{d\tau} = P_2 \frac{C_{L,i+1}^* - 2C_{L,i}^* + C_{L,i-1}^*}{\Delta^2} - R_{b,i}^* \quad (i = 1, 2 \ldots N - 1) \tag{13.19}$$

$$\frac{dC_{\text{LoC},i}^*}{d\tau} = R_{b,i}^* \quad (i = 1, 2 \ldots N - 1) \tag{13.20}$$

where $R_{b,i}^* = P_1 C_{L,i}^* (P_3 - C_{\text{LoC},i}^*) - C_{\text{LoC},i}^*$

$$\frac{dM_R^*}{d\tau} = RR^* = -\frac{1}{2} P_2 \frac{C_{L,N}^* - C_{L,N-1}^*}{\Delta} \tag{13.21}$$

The discretized initial conditions are

$$\tau = 0: \quad C_L^* = \frac{C_L^{\text{eq}}}{C_0}; \quad C_{\text{LoC}}^* = \frac{C_{\text{LoC}}^{\text{eq}}}{C_0}; \quad M_R^* = 0;$$

The discretized boundary conditions are

$$i = 0: \quad \frac{\partial C_{L,0}^*}{\partial z^*} = 0 \Rightarrow C_{L,1}^* = C_{L,0}^*$$

$$i = N: \quad C_{L,N}^* = 0$$

These are incorporated into the equations for $i = 1$ and $i = N - 1$, respectively:

$$i = 1: \quad \frac{dC_{L,1}^*}{d\tau} = P_2 \frac{C_{L,2}^* - C_{L,1}^*}{\Delta^2} - R_{b,1}^* \tag{13.22}$$

$$i = N - 1: \quad \frac{dC_{L,N-1}^*}{d\tau} = P_2 \frac{-2C_{L,N-1}^* + C_{L,N-2}^*}{\Delta^2} - R_{b,N-1}^* \tag{13.23}$$

The resulting system of differential-difference equations can be solved numerically using "ode15s" in MATLAB.

13.6   CHALLENGES AND FUTURE DIRECTIONS

Since the word "drug" in drug delivery encompasses not only drugs but also other therapeutic agents such as growth factors, proteins, and nucleic acids, it is perhaps impossible to design a deliver-it-all affinity-based system. It is important to recognize that different affinity-based systems have their own limitations. One of the limitations of heparin and heparin-like affinity systems is that the delivery is limited to mostly heparin-binding growth factors. Likewise, CD-based polymer systems specialize in the delivery of small hydrophobic molecules or drugs modified with small hydrophobic groups. An ideal platform would be customizable for the delivery of a variety of therapeutic agents. Special attention should be drawn to the application of these affinity-based DDSs. Because most of these systems are intended for *in vivo* use, it is important to aim for mild synthesis conditions by using less toxic solvents and polymers. It is also desirable to create stimulus-responsive affinity-based systems; ideally, the stimulus should be able to modulate the release rate of the DDS.

It is interesting to note how many affinity-based systems have their roots in other applications. For instance, CD was originally used in pharmaceutical industries for improving drug solubility, while MIPs were initially popular for chromatographic separation and chemical sensors. Inspiration has also been drawn from natural binding phenomenon, such as the affinity between metal ions and many biological molecules (which was also first exploited commercially in chromatography). As our basic understanding of biological systems continues to improve, we should be confident that new binding phenomena will be discovered and exploited, leading to new affinity-based delivery systems.

13.7   KEY POINTS

- Affinity-based DDSs utilize molecular interactions to control the loading and release of drugs.
- The affinity in an affinity-based DDS is governed by the K_a between the drug and the DDS.
- A variety of analytical methods as well as molecular modeling can be used to estimate K_a.
- CD-based polymer systems can be used to delivery small hydrophobic molecules.
- MIPs can be customized in terms of the size, geometry, and functional groups associated with the binding cavity for controlled delivery of a variety of therapeutic agents.
- Heparin and heparin-like affinity systems specialize in the controlled delivery a variety of heparin-binding growth factors.

13.8 HOMEWORK PROBLEMS

1. Before trying to deliver a fluorescently tagged growth factor using a heparin-based polymer, a student wants to use fluorescence spectrometry to determine the association constant between the growth factor and heparin. The following fluorescence spectrometry data is given:

[Heparin] (mM)	F
20	1163
17	961
10	608
6.25	375
4	256
0	52

   (A) Estimate K_a using the Benesi–Hildebrand equation.
   (B) Modify the Benesi–Hildebrand equation and use nonlinear regression analysis to achieve a more accurate estimate of K_a.

2. Based on the example given with the CD-based hydrogel in a thin disk geometry and assuming similar release conditions, consider an alternative system that has a spherical geometry:

   (A) Derive the governing equations to describe the rate of drug release along with initial and boundary conditions.
   (B) Represent the equations as well as initial and boundary conditions in dimensionless form.
   (C) Apply method of lines and establish a system of ordinary differential equations that can be used to solve for the concentration of drug with respect to time.

REFERENCES

1. Richardson TP et al. Polymeric system for dual growth factor delivery. Nat Biotechnol 2001;19(11):1029–1034.
2. Wang NX, von Recum HA. Affinity-based drug delivery. Macromol Biosci 2011;11(3):321–332.
3. Benesi H, Hildebrand J. A spectrophotometric investigation of the interaction of iodine with aromatic hydrocarbons. J Am Chem Soc 1949;71(8):2703–2707.
4. Connors K. Binding Constants: The Measurement of Molecular Complex Stability. New York: John Wiley & Sons, Inc.; 1987.

5. Connors KA. The stability of cyclodextrin complexes in solution. Chem Rev 1997;97(5): 1325–1357.

6. Patonay G et al. A systematic study of pyrene inclusion complexes with alpha-cyclodextrins, beta-cyclodextrins, and gamma-cyclodextrins. J Phys Chem 1986;90(9):1963–1966.

7. Englebienne P, Moitessier N. Docking ligands into flexible and solvated macromolecules. 4. Are popular scoring functions accurate for this class of proteins? J Chem Inf Model 2009;49(6):1568–1580.

8. Oda A et al. Comparison of consensus scoring strategies for evaluating computational models of protein-ligand complexes. J Chem Inf Model 2006;46(1):380–391.

9. Husain N et al. Complexation of doxorubicin with β- and γ-cyclodextrins. Appl Spectrosc 1992;46(4):652–658.

10. Liu L, Guo QX. The driving forces in the inclusion complexation of cyclodextrins. J Inclusion Phenom Macrocyclic Chem 2002;42(1–2):1–14.

11. Ross PD, Rekharsky MV. Thermodynamics of hydrogen bond and hydrophobic interactions in cyclodextrin complexes. Biophys J 1996;71(4):2144–2154.

12. Rekharsky MV, Inoue Y. Complexation thermodynamics of cyclodextrins. Chem Rev 1998;98(5):1875–1917.

13. Connors KA. Population characteristics of cyclodextrin complex stabilities in aqueous-solution. J Pharm Sci 1995;84(7):843–848.

14. Loftsson T, Duchene D. Cyclodextrins and their pharmaceutical applications. Int J Pharm 2007;329(1–2):1–11.

15. Thatiparti TR et al. Multiplexing interactions to control antibiotic release from cyclodextrin hydrogels. Macromol Biosci 2011;11(11):1544–1552.

16. Harth KC et al. Antibiotic-releasing mesh coating to reduce prosthetic sepsis: an In vivo study. J Surg Res 2010;163(2):337–343.

17. Thatiparti TR, Shoffstall AJ, von Recum HA. Cyclodextrin-based device coatings for affinity-based release of antibiotics. Biomaterials 2010;31(8):2335–2347.

18. Thatiparti TR, von Recum HA. Cyclodextrin complexation for affinity-based antibiotic delivery. Macromol Biosci 2010;10(1):82–90.

19. Rodriguez-Tenreiro C et al. Estradiol sustained release from high affinity cyclodextrin hydrogels. Eur J Pharm Biopharm 2007;66(1):55–62.

20. Oral E, Peppas NA. Responsive and recognitive hydrogels using star polymers. J Biomed Mater Res A 2004;68(3):439–447.

21. Oral E, Peppas NA. Hydrophilic molecularly imprinted poly(hydroxyethyl-methacrylate) polymers. J Biomed Mater Res A 2006;78A(1):205–210.

22. Piletsky SA, Andersson HS, Nicholls IA. Combined hydrophobic and electrostatic interaction-based recognition in molecularly imprinted polymers. Macromolecules 1999;32(3):633–636.

23. Dhal PK. Metal-ion coordination in designing molecularly imprinted polymeric receptors. In: Sellergren B, editor. Molecularly Imprinted Polymers: Man-Made Mimics of Antibodies and Their Application in Analytical Chemistry. Amsterdam: Elsevier Science B.V; 2001.

24. Dhal PK, Arnold FH. Template-mediated synthesis of metal-complexing polymers for molecular recognition. J Am Chem Soc 1991;113(19):7417–7418.

25. Dhal PK, Arnold FH. Metal-coordination interactions in the template-mediated synthesis of substrate-selective polymers - recognition of Bis(imidazole) substrates by copper(Ii) iminodiacetate containing polymers. Macromolecules 1992;25(25):7051–7059.

26. Plunkett SD, Arnold FH. Molecularly imprinted polymers on silica - selective supports for high-performance ligand-exchange chromatography. J Chromatogr, A 1995;708(1):19–29.

27. Mulloy B. The specificity of interactions between proteins and sulfated polysaccharides. An Acad Bras Cienc 2005;77(4):651–664.

28. Mach H et al. Nature of the interaction of heparin with acidic fibroblast growth-factor. Biochemistry 1993;32(20):5480–5489.

29. Edelman ER et al. Controlled and modulated release of basic fibroblast growth-factor. Biomaterials 1991;12(7):619–626.

30. Wissink MJB et al. Improved endothelialization of vascular grafts by local release of growth factor from heparinized collagen matrices. J Control Release 2000;64(1–3):103–114.

31. Maxwell DJ et al. Development of rationally designed affinity-based drug delivery systems. Acta Biomater 2005;1(1):101–113.

32. Sakiyama-Elbert SE, Hubbell JA. Development of fibrin derivatives for controlled release of heparin-binding growth factors. J Control Release 2000;65(3):389–402.

33. Sakiyama-Elbert SE, Hubbell JA. Controlled release of nerve growth factor from a heparin-containing fibrin-based cell ingrowth matrix. J Control Release 2000;69(1):149–158.

34. Willerth SM et al. Rationally designed peptides for controlled release of nerve growth factor from fibrin matrices. J Biomed Mater Res A 2007;80A(1):13–23.

35. Freeman I, Kedem A, Cohen S. The effect of sulfation of alginate hydrogels on the specific binding and controlled release of heparin-binding proteins. Biomaterials 2008; 29(22):3260–3268.

36. Ruvinov E, Leor J, Cohen S. The effects of controlled HGF delivery from an affinity-binding alginate biomaterial on angiogenesis and blood perfusion in a hindlimb ischemia model. Biomaterials 2010;31(16):4573–4582.

37. Belford DA, Hendry IA, Parish CR. Investigation of the ability of several naturally-occurring and synthetic polyanions to bind to and potentiate the biological-activity of acidic fibroblast growth-factor. J Cell Physiol 1993;157(1):184–189.

38. Nakamura S et al. Effect of controlled release of fibroblast growth factor-2 from chitosan/fucoidan micro complex-hydrogel on in vitro and in vivo vascularization. J Biomed Mater Res A 2008;85A(3):619–627.

39. Oss-Ronen L, Seliktar D. Polymer-conjugated albumin and fibrinogen composite hydrogels as cell scaffolds designed for affinity-based drug delivery. Acta Biomater 2011;7(1):163–170.

40. Gonen-Wadmany M, Oss-Ronen L, Seliktar D. Protein-polymer conjugates for forming photopolymerizable biomimetic hydrogels for tissue engineering. Biomaterials 2007;28(26):3876–3886.

41. Soontornworajit B et al. Aptamer-functionalized in situ injectable hydrogel for controlled protein release. Biomacromolecules 2010;11(10):2724–2730.

42. Soontornworajit B et al. Affinity hydrogels for controlled protein release using nucleic acid aptamers and complementary oligonucleotides. Biomaterials 2011;32(28):6839–6849.

43. Lin CC, Metters AT. Metal-chelating affinity hydrogels for sustained protein release. J Biomed Mater Res A 2007;83A(4):954–964.

44. Shen SC et al. Submicron particles of SBA-15 modified with MgO as carriers for controlled drug delivery. Chem Pharm Bull 2007;55(7):985–991.

45. Margiotta N et al. Bisphosphonate complexation and calcium doping in silica xerogels as a combined strategy for local and controlled release of active platinum antitumor compounds. Dalton Trans 2007;29:3131–3139.

46. Fu AS et al. Experimental studies and modeling of drug release from a tunable affinity-based drug delivery platform. Ann Biomed Eng 2011;39(9):2466–2475.

INDEX

Engineering Polymer Systems for Improved Drug Delivery, First Edition.
Edited by Rebecca A. Bader and David A. Putnam.
© 2014 John Wiley & Sons, Inc. Published 2014 by John Wiley & Sons, Inc.